Mosby's
EMT-B Certification Preparation and Review

Mosby's EMT-B Certification Preparation and Review

Third Edition

Daniel Mack, NREMT-P

President
Alternative Medical Education Concepts, Inc.
Cincinnati, Ohio

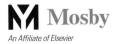 Mosby
An Affiliate of Elsevier

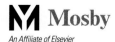

Executive Editor: Claire Merrick
Developmental Editor: Lisa Brightwell
Project Manager: Deborah L. Vogel
Project Specialist: Ann E. Rogers
Book Design Manager: Judi Lang
Cover Design: Michael Warrell

THIRD EDITION

Mosby, Inc.
An Affiliate of Elsevier
11830 Westline Industrial Drive
St. Louis, Missouri 63146

Printed in United States of America.

Library of Congress Cataloging in Publication Data
Mack, Daniel.
    Mosby's EMT-B certification preparation and review/Daniel Mack.—3rd ed.
        p. cm.
    Previous ed. published under title: JEMS EMT-B certification preparation and review. 2nd ed. 1996.
    ISBN 0-323-01434-8
    1. Emergency medicine—Examinations, questions, etc. 2. Emergency medical technicians—Examinations, questions, ect. I. Title: EMT-B certification preparation and review. II. Mack, Daniel, JEMS EMT-B certification preparation and review.

RC86.9 .M34 2002
616.02'5'076—dc21   2001030875

04 05 06 07 08 SG/KPT 9 8 7 6 5 4

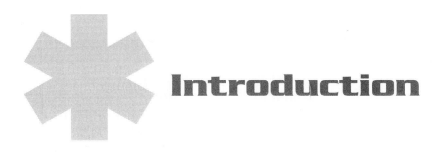

Introduction

USING THIS REVIEW MANUAL

The questions in this manual appear primarily in a multiple-choice format. This type of question tests not only knowledge of the correct answer but also the ability to understand why an answer is incorrect. Other formats, such as matching and fill-in-the-blank, are also used in this manual. These types of questions accomplish two things. First, they allow the reviewer to perform different question-analysis functions. In the field, the EMT must analyze information in a variety of ways; the answer isn't there to choose from a list. Second, the use of different question types breaks the monotony of single-format questions. Keep in mind, however, that the National Registry test and certain other state tests contain only multiple-choice questions.

This review manual is not meant to take the place of a textbook or EMT instructor. Nor is it intended to simulate an actual test. There are key differences between a review manual and a test—each serves a different purpose. Due to the limited amount of space on an EMT test, there are relatively few questions in comparison to the amount of information presented in the EMT course. The test cannot be all-encompassing. Many tests are computer generated; that is, questions are chosen randomly from a large bank of test questions. There is no way for the student to know exactly what will be covered. On the other hand, a review manual presents the opportunity for all or most of the critical items presented in the EMT curriculum to be covered. This allows the EMT to review specific areas of the material or, if questions are chosen randomly, a variety of information.

 Enrichment Questions

This manual includes enrichment questions that cover information that may or may not have been presented in your EMT class. **These are at the end of each chapter or section and follow the heading that is clearly identified by a "star of life" icon.** Your examination may not contain questions covering this information, but knowing this information may prove helpful when taking the exam and when working in the field. It can provide you with a better understanding of why patients with medical problems present in a particular way, or why certain types of care are most effective. This can increase your confidence and your abilities as an EMT.

■ GETTING THE MOST FROM PRACTICE QUESTIONS

Questions on specific subjects are grouped together, allowing the EMT or student to focus on specific problem areas. This will also help the reader identify areas in which additional study is needed. As you read each question, see if you can answer it without looking at the answer choices. If you answer correctly, read the rationale for the answer anyway. There may be additional helpful information included in the answer rationale.

If you answer a question incorrectly, look for a pattern. Try to determine why the answer was incorrect.

- *Is there a particular subject area you are having difficulty with, or is the missed question isolated?* If you are having difficulty with an entire subject area or a portion thereof, place emphasis on studying this section of your EMT text.

- *Did you not know or did you forget the information being tested?* If you were unfamiliar with the subject content, spend extra time reviewing this material. If your time is limited, do not waste valuable study time reviewing information you already know. Concentrate on the parts of the EMT text that cover the topics you feel the least familiar with. Look for key points and definitions. Try to remember concepts, not rote answers.

- *Did you misunderstand the content or concept when reading the EMT text or covering the material in class?* Or did you draw a wrong conclusion when studying the topic? Talk with your instructor or a knowledgeable EMT. Try to explain the subject using your own words and ask what part of your explanation is incorrect. Ask for help in adjusting any misunderstanding. And don't be afraid to consult other EMT texts to compare the information presented. Each EMT text has its strong points. You may find a different textbook presents clearer, easier-to-understand information on a particular subject.

- *Did you actually know the correct answer but simply misread the question or answer choices?* You may need to take more time to carefully read the question and answer choices. Recognizing that you have difficulty reading and comprehending test questions may be as important as identifying specific areas in which additional study of the EMT materials is needed.

- *Did you read too much into the question?* The only information you are expected to consider is the information presented in the stem. Do not try to determine what happened before or might happen after the fictional "event" referred to in the question.

- *Were you overconfident?* A positive attitude is good, but overconfidence can cause even the most competent EMT to fail.

HELPFUL TIPS FOR SURVIVING EMT TESTS

Very few people enjoy taking tests. Test taking can be even more stressful for EMT students taking an initial certification test, or for certified EMTs taking a recertification test.

Most of us got into this field because of a desire to be an EMT. It was or is a personal goal we wanted to meet. For many EMTs and EMT students, some time has elapsed since high school or college. When you were in school, the daily expectation of tests or quizzes kept you in a "test taking" frame of mind. It has likely been quite some time since you had to take such a critical test. And to make matters worse, you find yourself faced with a test that will decide the course of your EMS career path.

But remember, you've come this far and you *can* pass the test. Although you may never enjoy test taking, it can be less stressful if you follow some simple, helpful hints. The more relaxed you are, the more clearly you will think. Those who write the test do not want you to fail, but they do want you to be challenged. Keeping a level head and using your sense of reasoning and problem solving will allow you to meet that challenge.

■ BEFORE THE TEST

- **Schedule time for both personal and group study.** Each has its advantages. When you study alone, you have a chance to go over material you are unsure of. When you study in a group, you can learn from your partners and help others.

- **Get plenty of rest.** It's hard to think clearly if you're tired.

- **Dress comfortably.** Wear layered clothing so you can add or remove clothing if the testing room is too hot or too cold.

- **Avoid overeating** or eating foods that may be hard to digest, such as spicy or greasy foods. Instead, eat low-fat or complex-carbohydrate foods, such as nuts, pasta, or yogurt. If your test is in the morning, eat breakfast if this is what you normally do.

- **Avoid too much caffeine,** which can affect attention and concentration. Do not drink alcohol before the test (there will be plenty of time for this after the test). And while you should not self-medicate, there are a number of medications your doctor can prescribe if you suffer from severe test anxiety that hampers your performance.

- **Don't cram.** Although you may feel that cramming for the test the night before will help, in general this is not the case. Cramming tends to clutter the mind and confuse the test taker.

- **Give yourself enough time** to reach the test location and try to arrive early. Running late for a test will only increase your anxiety level. Also, by arriving early, you will have an opportunity to choose your seat wisely. Although this may not seem important, a seat in an area that is too hot, too cold, too noisy, or uncomfortable for any other reason can cause additional anxiety.

- **Try to relax.** If you have some favorite relaxation techniques, use them before starting the test. Relaxation and stress-reduction exercises can also be practiced during the test, provided they do not distract the other students. A simple exercise is to sit up straight and close your eyes. Take five deep breaths, counting each one and exhaling completely each time. As you count each breath, focus on relaxing all the muscles in your body.

- **Have confidence in your ability to pass the test.** Maintain a positive "I-can-pass-this-test" attitude. Put forth your best effort, and imagine how good you'll feel when you receive word that you have passed.

- **Evaluate your past test-taking experiences.** If you have had a history of not doing well on written examinations, there is a possibility you may suffer from a reading or learning disability. Professionals at the counseling center at your local training facility, community college, or university can help you determine if this is the case. If you do have a diagnosed learning disability, they can provide you with strategies to help compensate for it. Also, in some cases, certifying agencies will allow reasonable accommodations such as longer testing times if you have a documented learning disability.

■ TIPS FOR TAKING MULTIPLE-CHOICE TESTS

- **Carefully read all the directions** before starting the test to be sure you understand what you are supposed to do. If you don't understand test instructions, ask the test proctor for clarification.

- **Read the entire question before attempting to answer it.** Important background information is often contained in the sentences leading up to the actual question. You don't want to lose any points because you have misread a question.

- **Answer the question by yourself.** After reading the entire question, try to answer it without looking at the choices. Then look at the choices to see if your answer is the same as, or close to, one of the choices.

- **Read *all* of the choices.** Even if the first choice seems to be the correct answer, read the other choices so you do not overlook a better choice.

- **Read carefully.** Give all the words in the question and the answer choices equal attention. A missed or misread word can mean the difference between a correct answer and an incorrect answer.

- **Remember the fundamentals.** In most cases, confirming scene safety, ensuring an open airway, and correcting life-threatening problems take precedence. Look for answers that deal with these aspects of patient management.

- **Skip questions you don't know.** If you are unsure of an answer, leave the corresponding number on the answer sheet blank and proceed to the next question. Be careful not to get answer numbers out of sequence. Don't forget to go back to unanswered questions after completing the exam.

- **Don't take a question personally.** Don't get upset over a question or answer choice you don't like. This will only increase your anxiety and tension.

- **Keep on track.** Be sure the number on the answer sheet corresponds to the number of the question. Check periodically to ensure the question number and answer number correspond.

- **Trust your intuition.** It is usually best to trust your first answer choice. Only change an answer if you feel you must.

- **Check all the options.** If time permits or if you are having difficulty deciding on an answer, read the question using each of the answer choices given. Reading the question and each answer choice together in their entirety allows you to focus on choices that make sense both logically and grammatically.

- **Don't look for patterns.** The answers to multiple-choice questions do not follow a pattern, so don't try to find one. Trying to find a pattern will only add to any confusion you may already feel.

- **Don't count on "tricks."** Be cautious of using test-taking "tricks" such as "when in doubt mark C" or "there will never be more than three of the same letter in a row." People who design high-stakes examinations know about these "tricks" and design tests to reduce their effectiveness.

- **Narrow down your choices.** If you do not immediately recognize the correct answer, eliminate any choice that you are sure is incorrect, so you have fewer answers to choose from. If you can narrow the number of choices to two plausible answers, you have greatly increased your chances of getting the answer right.

- **Look for absolutes,** such as "never," "always," or "every." These types of words may indicate that the choice is wrong.

- **Look for key words** in the question such as "immediately," "initially," "first," or "most." These may help you identify which answer choice is the best.

- **Carefully read any question using the words "not" or "except."** These types of questions are used to determine whether you can tell what should not be done or if you know an exception. Many tests try to avoid such questions, but some still use them.

- **Be wary of any distractors** that contain words or information you have never seen, even if they seem to be plausible choices.

- **Follow the text.** Base your answers on what you learned from the text, not an experience other practicing EMTs may have had with their patients.

- **Use all your resources.** If you are allowed to use a sheet of paper to solve problems, take advantage of it.

- **Know which scoring system is used.** Generally, it is best to answer every question. However, some tests are scored using a system that does not penalize for unanswered questions but does penalize incorrect responses to discourage guessing. On this type of test it is better to leave questions blank if you are not very sure of the correct answer. Be sure you understand the system that will be used to grade the examination you are taking.

■ Managing Your Time

- **Know how much time is allotted** for the test and how many questions you must answer. For instance, the National Registry test allows 2 hours and 30 minutes to complete 150 questions (which averages out to 1 minute per question). In most cases, you will be given more time than you are likely to need. Relax and do not be overly time conscious early on.

- **Use all the allotted time.** Your knowledge is what is being tested—not your ability to finish early.

- **Answer the easiest questions first.** Save the harder questions for last. Doing so will allow you to spend more time on the harder questions.

- **Answer all questions** if that is of benefit to you (check the scoring method). Make sure you go back to all the questions you have left blank. If unanswered questions count against you, take a guess if you still don't know the answer.

- **Review your answers** if you have time left at the end of the examination. Sometimes the content of a later question or answer may remind you of information that could affect a previous answer.

- **Check your answer sheet.** Be sure each choice marked on the answer sheet corresponds to the choice you want. Even if you know the answer to a question, errors in marking can cause the choice to be scored as incorrect. Also check to be sure you did not leave any questions unanswered (if appropriate).

A word of caution applies when using this or any review manual. Do not view this book as a review manual to pass the National Registry test or any other particular test. If you are taking the National Registry test, some questions may be presented differently. Do not become overly confident simply because you have completed a review manual. Passing tests does not make you a good EMT. Instead, if you try to be the most knowledgeable and best EMT you can be, passing the test will be an added bonus. We wish you the best in your endeavors to become, or remain, the best EMT you can be.

NOTE TO THE READER: The Author and publisher have made every attempt to ensure that the patient care procedures presented in this text are accurate and represent accepted practices in the United States. They are not provided as standards of care. It is the reader's responsibility to follow patient care protocols established by medical direction physicians and to remain current in the delivery of emergency care.

ACKNOWLEDGMENTS

No book such as this could be completed without the hard work of dedicated reviewers. After looking at questions for hours on end, it is only with the input of these unsung heroes that a manual can be of any quality. A special word of thanks goes to:

Neil Coker, BS, EMT-P—Your insight into ways to refine questions and distractors, as well as your knowledge of EMS education, was invaluable. It seemed that when I wasn't exactly sure how to put something into words, you knew just how to say it simply and clearly.

Eric Powell, MS, NREMT-P—Thanks for your many encouraging comments and your attention to detail. It's great to have someone with your level of experience and who is still so active in the field as part of the review team.

A. Keith Wesley, MD, FACEP—Your willingness to assist with such a "basic" manual reinforced my belief that we truly are all in this together, regardless of what level of care we provide. Your clarifications regarding the nuances of emergency care issues lent a special touch to the vision of this book. I hope we can work together again in the future.

■ TO THE STAFF AT HARCOURT HEALTH SCIENCES:

To Claire Merrick—I value our relationship and the support you have given me over the years with various projects. You have helped me to fulfill a lifelong dream.

To Lisa Brightwell—I know it's been a learning experience, but you've been a joy to work with. I hope I haven't made it too complicated.

To Derril Trakalo—Thanks for helping to make these projects successful. It's only through good marketing that we can get useful books into the hands of those who need them. (By the way, if there are any books or videos that you don't want to ship back…)

Contents

Mosby's
EMT-B Certification Preparation and Review

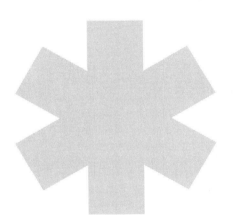

1

The Human Body

D.O.T. Curriculum Objectives Covered in This Chapter:

Lesson 1-4

CHAPTER 1 REVIEW QUESTIONS

■ THE SKELETAL SYSTEM

1. The functions of the skeletal system include:
   a. protecting vital organs
   b. providing form
   c. providing for body movement
   d. all of the above

2. The main function of the bone marrow is:
   a. regulation of body temperature
   b. production of insulin
   c. production of red blood cells
   d. regulation of body metabolism

3. Using the list below, label Figure 1-1.
   mandible
   maxilla
   nasal bone
   orbit
   zygomatic bone

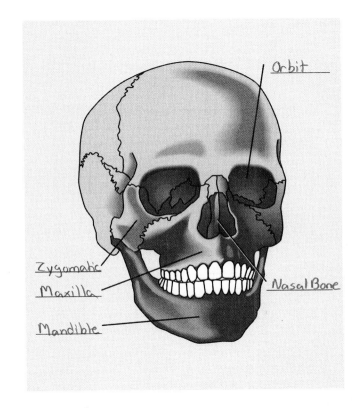

Figure 1-1

4. The largest bone of the pelvis is the:
   a. ischium
   b. ilium
   c. pubis
   d. acetabulum

5. The rib cage is composed of:
   a. 12 pairs of ribs, all attached to the sternum
   b. 10 pairs of ribs, eight attached to the sternum and two floating
   c. 10 pairs of ribs, all attached to the sternum
   d. 12 pairs of ribs, 10 attached to the sternum and two floating

6. The lower, moveable section of the jaw is the:
   a. maxilla
   b. mastoid
   c. mandible
   d. malleolus

7. The upper segment of the sternum is the:
   a. acetabulum
   b. angle of Louis
   c. manubrium
   d. xiphoid

8. The small, finger-like projection of cartilage at the inferior end of the sternum is the:
   a. mastoid process
   b. xiphoid process
   c. styloid process
   d. lenticular process

9. The heel bone is also known as the:
   a. calcaneus
   b. metacarpal
   c. carpal
   d. tarsal

10. The greater trochanter is part of the:
    a. radius
    b. lumbar spine
    c. tibia
    d. femur

11. The kneecap is also called the:
    a. parietal
    b. peristalsis
    c. perineum
    d. patella

12. Using the given list of sections of the spine, label Figure 1-2.
    cervical
    coccyx
    lumbar
    thoracic
    sacrum

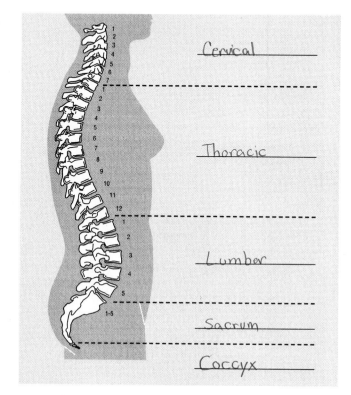

Cervical

Thoracic

Lumbar

Sacrum

Coccyx

Figure 1-2

13. The collar bone is the:
    a. scapula
    b. clavicle
    c. acromion process
    d. ilium

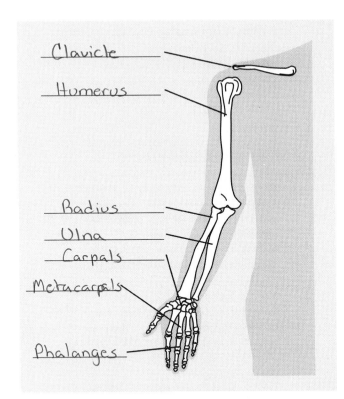

Clavicle

Humerus

Radius

Ulna

Carpals

Metacarpals

Phalanges

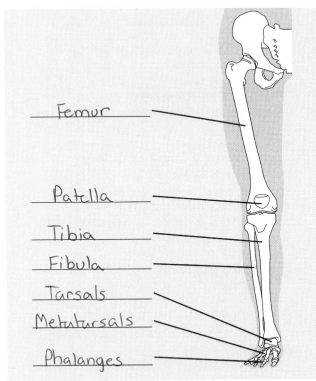

Femur

Patella

Tibia

Fibula

Tarsals

Metatarsals

Phalanges

Figure 1-3
Upper extremities (top).
Lower extremities (bottom).

14. Using the list of bones below, label the upper and lower extremities on Figure 1-3. (NOTE: Some answers may be used more than once.)

carpals	**patella**
clavicle	**phalanges**
femur	**radius**
fibula	**tarsals**
humerus	**tibia**
metacarpals	**ulna**
metatarsals	

15. Three bones lying directly underneath the skin that can be palpated throughout their entire length are the:
    a. femur, tibia, and fibula
    b. humerus, radius, and ulna
    c. tibia, clavicle, and ulna
    d. femur, clavicle, and humerus

16. An example of a ball-and-socket joint would be the:
    a. elbow
    b. finger
    c. ankle
    d. hip

17. The knee joint is an example of a:
    a. hinge joint
    b. ball-and-socket joint
    c. floating joint
    d. false joint

18. Using the list below, label the major bones of the pelvis on Figure 1-4.
    ilium
    ischium
    pubis
    sacrum

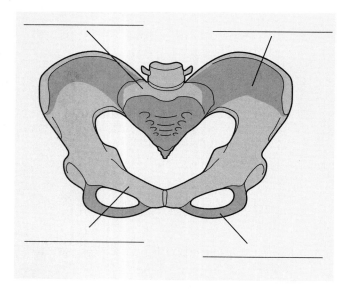

Figure 1-4

19. The type of muscle found in the gastrointestinal tract is:
    a. skeletal
    b. cardiac
    c. smooth
    d. striated

20. The type of muscle that allows you to move an arm or a leg is:
    a. skeletal
    b. smooth
    c. cardiac
    d. involuntary

21. The ability of cardiac muscle to contract on its own is known as:
    a. self-regulation
    b. focality
    c. autopacing
    d. automaticity

✱ **ENRICHMENT QUESTIONS**

22. Concerning the function of muscles, the true statement is:
    a. muscles don't pull; they only push
    b. muscles don't push; they only pull
    c. muscles both push and pull
    d. muscles neither push nor pull

23. The diaphragm differs from most skeletal muscles in that it:
    a. primarily acts as an involuntary muscle
    b. is not striated
    c. is formed from smooth muscle
    d. is formed from cardiac muscle

24. An example of striated muscle would be:
    a. skeletal muscle
    b. smooth muscle
    c. gastrointestinal tract muscle
    d. urinary tract muscle

25. The function of tendons is to:
    a. connect bone to bone
    b. cover bone ends at joints
    c. connect muscle to bone
    d. connect muscles to muscles

26. The function of ligaments is to:
    a. connect muscle to bone
    b. connect bone to bone
    c. connect muscles to muscles
    d. lubricate joints

27. The fibrous membrane that covers the muscle tissue is known as the:
    a. meninges
    b. pleura
    c. fascia
    d. dura mater

28. Circular muscles that contract to constrict the opening of a tube or duct are:
    a. somatic muscles
    b. cardiac muscles
    c. sigmoid muscles
    d. sphincter muscles

■ THE SKIN

29. Two main functions of the skin are:
    a. blood cell production and waste disposal
    b. temperature regulation and fluid absorption
    c. protection and temperature regulation
    d. waste disposal and fluid absorption

30. The outermost layer of the skin is known as the:
    a. epidermis
    b. superdermis
    c. subcutaneous tissue
    d. hyperdermis

31. The sweat glands and hair follicles are contained in the:
    a. dermis
    b. subcutaneous tissue
    c. pleura
    d. epidermis

32. Directly beneath the dermis lies the:
    a. bone
    b. subcutaneous layer
    c. meninges
    d. subfascia layer

✳ ENRICHMENT QUESTION

33. Sebaceous glands secrete:
    a. acids
    b. sweat
    c. saliva
    d. oils

■ THE NERVOUS SYSTEM

34. The two anatomical divisions of the nervous system are the:
    a. central nervous system and peripheral nervous system
    b. automatic nervous system and somatic nervous system
    c. central nervous system and automatic nervous system
    d. peripheral nervous system and systemic nervous system

35. The central nervous system consists of the:
    a. brain and spinal cord
    b. nervous and integumentary systems
    c. automatic nervous system and spinal cord
    d. brain and cranial nerves

36. The two main types of nerves that enter and leave the spinal cord are:
    a. neuron and proton
    b. peripheral and motor
    c. lateral and medial
    d. sensory and motor

✳ ENRICHMENT QUESTION

37. Higher functions, such as thought, decision making, and communication, are the responsibility of the:
    a. autonomic nervous system
    b. somatic nervous system
    c. central nervous system
    d. cranial nervous system

For questions 38 through 40, refer to Figure 1-5.

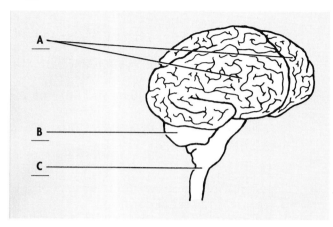

Figure 1-5

38. Structure *A* is the:
   a. cerebellum
   b. medulla
   c. cerebrum
   d. brainstem

39. Structure *B* is the:
   a. cerebrum
   b. cerebellum
   c. medulla
   d. frontal lobe

40. Structure *C* is the:
   a. brainstem
   b. cerebellum
   c. cerebrum
   d. temporal lobe

41. Involuntary functions, such as breathing, heart rate, and digestion, are controlled by the:
   a. cerebrum
   b. brainstem
   c. cerebellum
   d. occipital lobe

42. Higher functions, such as voluntary activities, thought, memory, and sensory reception are controlled by the:
   a. cerebellum
   b. autonomic nervous system
   c. cerebrum
   d. cranial nerves

43. The three layers of special tissue that cover the brain and spinal cord are the:
   a. meninges
   b. dura mater
   c. meniscus
   d. pleura

44. The autonomic nervous system controls:
   a. digestion
   b. heart rate
   c. sweating
   d. all of the above

45. Stimulation of the sympathetic nervous system:
   a. inhibits sweating
   b. increases heart rate
   c. constricts the pupils
   d dilates blood vessels

■ THE RESPIRATORY SYSTEM

46. The leaf-shaped structure that prevents food or liquids from entering the trachea is the:
   a. uvula
   b. epigastrium
   c. pharynx
   d. epiglottis

47. Tidal volume refers to the:
   a. volume of blood passing through the lungs each minute
   b. amount of oxygen in a breath
   c. volume of air per breath
   d. volume of air moved in a minute

48. The two gases normally exchanged during breathing are:
    a. oxygen and carbon monoxide
    b. nitrogen and oxygen
    c. carbon dioxide and nitrogen
    d. oxygen and carbon dioxide

49. The structure commonly referred to as the "Adam's apple" is the:
    a. cricothyroid membrane
    b. thyroid cartilage
    c. sixth tracheal ring
    d. carina

50. The major muscle associated with breathing mechanics is the:
    a. trapezius
    b. sternomastoid
    c. pectoral
    d. diaphragm

51. The exchange of gases within the lungs takes place in the:
    a. bronchi
    b. pleural space
    c. alveoli
    d. trachea

52. When blood enters the capillaries in the lungs, it is:
    a. high in oxygen and low in carbon dioxide
    b. low in oxygen and high in carbon dioxide
    c. low in oxygen and low in carbon dioxide
    d. high in oxygen and high in carbon dioxide

53. When blood enters the capillaries at the body tissue level, it is:
    a. low in oxygen and low in carbon dioxide
    b. high in oxygen and high in carbon dioxide
    c. low in oxygen and high in carbon dioxide
    d. high in oxygen and low in carbon dioxide

54. The primary stimulus for breathing in normal healthy humans is the:
    a. oxygen level in arterial blood
    b. carbon monoxide level in arterial blood
    c. carbon dioxide level in arterial blood
    d. oxygen level in venous blood

■ THE CIRCULATORY SYSTEM

55. The chambers of the heart that receive blood from the veins are the:
    a. atria
    b. ventricles
    c. aorta
    d. vallecula

56. The chambers of the heart that pump blood into the arteries are the:
    a. atria
    b. ventricles
    c. varices
    d. auricles

57. The heart muscle receives oxygen and nourishment via the:
    a. coronary arteries
    b. ventricles
    c. pulmonary arteries
    d. subclavian arteries

58. The major artery originating directly from the heart is the:
    a. carotid
    b. innominate
    c. aorta
    d. subclavian

59. Blood is pumped to the body by the:
    a. left atrium
    b. left ventricle
    c. right atrium
    d. right ventricle

60. Blood is pumped to the lungs by the:
    a. left atrium
    b. left ventricle
    c. right atrium
    d. right ventricle

61. The functions of the blood include:
    a. carrying oxygen and removing waste products
    b. combating infections
    c. clotting capabilities
    d. all of the above

62. The purpose of valves within the circulatory system is to:
    a. shunt blood from one area to another
    b. prevent blood from flowing backward
    c. regulate the blood pressure
    d. sense the volume of blood in the body

63. The lower extremities receive blood from the:
    a. femoral arteries
    b. brachial arteries
    c. radial arteries
    d. carotid arteries

64. The blood vessels that transport blood away from the heart are:
    a. veins
    b. capillaries
    c. arteries
    d. venules

65. In the foot, a pulse can be felt at the:
    a. dorsalis pedis artery
    b. inferior vena cava
    c. aorta
    d. innominate artery

66. The blood vessels that transport blood toward the heart are:
    a. arteries
    b. veins
    c. capillaries
    d. venules

67. The blood vessels that connect veins and arteries are:
    a. arterioles
    b. ventricles
    c. capillaries
    d. venules

68. White blood cells are responsible for:
    a. carrying oxygen
    b. carrying carbon dioxide
    c. removing wastes
    d. defending against infection

69. The liquid component of blood is known as:
    a. whole blood
    b. plasma
    c. lymph
    d. interstitial fluid

70. Red blood cells are responsible for:
    a. carrying oxygen
    b. maintaining blood acidity
    c. carrying carbon monoxide
    d. filtering blood impurities

71. The small cellular fragments in the blood essential to the formation of blood clots are:
    a. lymphocytes
    b. leukocytes
    c. electrolytes
    d. platelets

72. Using the following list of components of the circulatory system, label Figure 1-6.
    aorta
    inferior vena cava
    left atrium
    left ventricle
    pulmonary artery
    pulmonary veins
    right atrium
    right ventricle
    superior vena cava

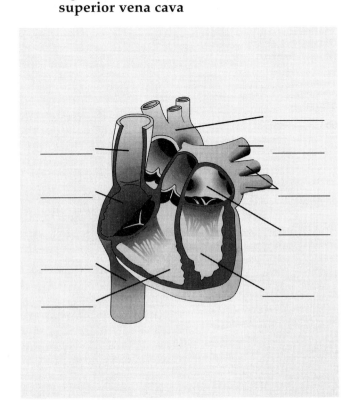

Figure 1-6

73. The muscular wall that separates the right and left sides of the heart is the:
    a. pericardium
    b. sacrum
    c. septum
    d. diaphragm

74. The amount of blood in an average-size adult is:
    a. 5 pints
    b. 5 liters
    c. 5 units
    d. 5 gallons

75. The average amount of blood in a 1-year-old child is:
    a. 8 pints
    b. 3 liters
    c. 800 cc
    d. 3 to 5 units

■ GENERAL ANATOMY AND PHYSIOLOGY

76. The endocrine system is responsible for producing:
    a. hormones
    b. red blood cells
    c. sugar and glucose
    d. white blood cells

77. The spine is located on the body's:
    a. ventral side
    b. cephalic side
    c. anterior side
    d. dorsal side

78. In anatomical terms, the umbilicus is on the:
    a. anterior abdomen
    b. caudal abdomen
    c. posterior abdomen
    d. lateral abdomen

79. A body structure that is above another is:
    a. lateral
    b. superior
    c. distal
    d. inferior

80. The hand is on the:
    a. lateral end of the arm
    b. proximal end of the arm
    c. distal end of the arm
    b. medial end of the arm

81. When describing something that appears or is present on both sides of the body, EMTs should use the term:
    a. hemilateral
    b. bilateral
    c. trilateral
    d. bigeminy

82. Using the list below, label the three imaginary dividing lines in Figure 1-7.
    midaxillary line
    midclavicular line
    midline

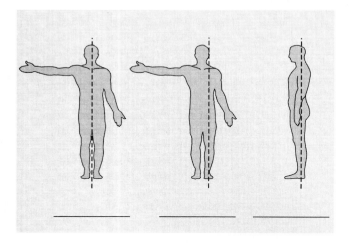

Figure 1-7

83. An unconscious patient is found lying face down. This patient would be described as being found in the:
    a. supine position
    b. lateral recumbent position
    c. shock position
    d. prone position

84. The directional term that is used to describe something that is away from the midline, or toward the side, is:
    a. medial
    b. proximal
    c. lateral
    d. distal

85. The one third of the femur that is closest to the hip would be described as the:
    a. lateral one third of the femur
    b. proximal one third of the femur
    c. distal one third of the femur
    d. medial one third of the femur

86. Your patient has a gunshot wound on his back about 4" below the level of his diaphragm. This entry site would best be described as being on the:
    a. anterior abdomen
    b. lateral abdomen
    c. inferior abdomen
    d. posterior abdomen

87. Match the list of directional terms below to their definitions.

anterior	medial
distal	posterior
inferior	proximal
lateral	superior

    _____ toward the trunk

    _____ away from the trunk

    _____ toward the back

    _____ toward the front

    _____ toward the midline

    _____ away from the midline

    _____ toward the top of the body

    _____ toward the bottom of the body

88. Before transporting a female patient to the hospital, medical direction instructs you to place her in the Trendelenburg position. To accomplish this, you would position your patient:
    a. lying on her right side in a horizontal position with her knees bent
    b. lying face down with the foot of the cot raised
    c. lying on her back with her feet elevated approximately 8 to 12 inches at her hips and with her body flat
    d. lying on her back with the foot of the cot raised higher than the head while maintaining a straight incline to the head of the cot

89. Your patient is responsive only to painful stimuli. Since there is no reason to suspect a spinal injury, you place him in the recovery position. This position is also referred to as the:
    a. supine position
    b. lateral recumbent position
    c. prone position
    d. Fowler's position

90. To place a patient in the recovery position, you would:
    a. elevate the foot end of the cot and position the patient lying face down
    b. elevate the foot end of the cot and position the patient lying face up
    c. position the patient lying on his left or right side
    d. position the patient lying on his back and elevate his head about 6 inches

91. A patient who is immobilized on a backboard is generally placed in the:
    a. prone position
    b. supine position
    c. lateral recumbent position
    d. shock position

92. A 68-year-old female patient is complaining of mild chest discomfort with minimal shortness of breath. She appears to be most comfortable in the Fowler's position. The Fowler's position is best described as:
    a. lying on one's side with the head of the cot slightly elevated
    b. lying on one's side with the head of the cot slightly lowered
    c. sitting straight upright or leaning slightly forward
    d. lying on one's back with the upper body elevated at a 45- to 60-degree angle

 ENRICHMENT QUESTIONS

93. Using the following list of body cavities, label Figure 1-8.
    abdominal
    cranial
    pelvic
    spinal
    thoracic

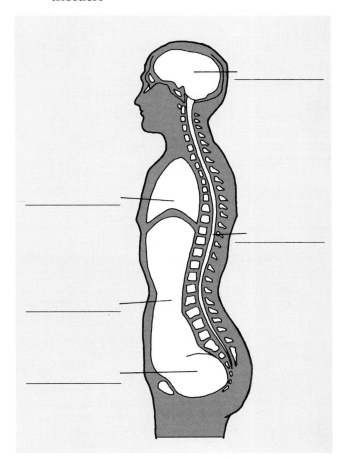

Figure 1-8

94. The pelvic cavity contains the:
    a. colon
    b. kidneys
    c. appendix
    d. bladder

95. Referring to Figure 1-9, label the following organs with the abdominal quadrants in which they are primarily located.
(NOTE: some organs may be in more than one quadrant.)

_____ appendix

_____ gallbladder

_____ large intestine

_____ left kidney

_____ liver

_____ pancreas

_____ right kidney

_____ small intestine

_____ spleen

_____ stomach

96. The immune system includes the:
a. liver, spleen, and lymph glands
b. heart, lungs, and blood vessels
c. stomach, small intestines, and large intestines
d. kidneys, pancreas, and gallbladder

97. A major function of the pancreas is the production of:
a. bile
b. insulin
c. adrenalin
d. epinephrine

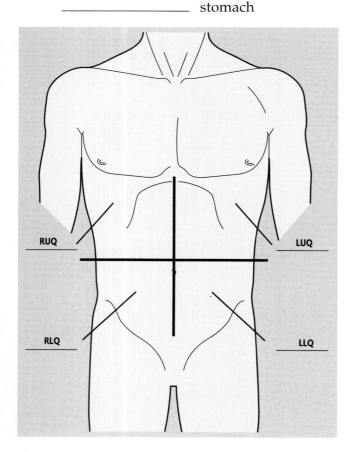

Figure 1-9

Chapter 1

main function of Bone marrow
largest bone in pelvis
upper segment of sternum
greater trochanter
sebaceous glands secrete?
circulatory system

1) d ✓	36) d	68) d
2) c ✓	37) c	69) b
3)	38) c	70) b
4) a	39) b	71) d
5) d ✓	40) a	73) a
6) c ✓	41) c	74) b
7) b	42) c	75) c
8) b	43) a	76) b
9) a	44) d	77) a
10) b	45) b	78) a
11) d	46) d	79) b
13) b	47) d	80) c
15) c	48) d	81) b
16) d	49) a	83) d
17) a	50) d	84) c
19) d	51) c	85) b
20) a	52) a	86) d
21) d	53) c	88) c
22) c	54) a	89) b
23) a	55) a	90) c
24) c	56) a	91) b
25) c	57) b	92) c
26) b	58) c	95) d
27) d	59) a	96) d
28) a	60) b	97) b
29) c	61) d	
30) a	62) b	
31) a	63) a	
32) d	64) b	
33) d	65) a	
34) a	66) d	
35) c	67) c	

ANSWERS TO CHAPTER 1 REVIEW QUESTIONS

■ THE SKELETAL SYSTEM

1. **d.** All of the above. The skeletal system protects vital organs, provides form for the body, and provides for body movement. It also produces blood cells.

2. **c.** Bone marrow produces red blood cells.

3. Using the list below, label Figure 1-1.
   mandible
   maxilla
   nasal bone
   orbit
   zygomatic bone

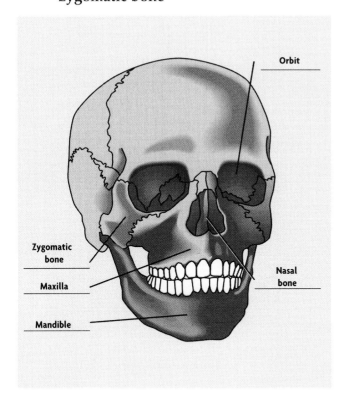

Figure 1-1

4. **b.** The ilium is the largest bone of the pelvis. The ischium and pubis are the other two bones of the pelvis. The acetabulum is the rounded cavity of the pelvis into which the femoral head fits.

5. **d.** The human body contains 12 pairs of ribs. Ten pairs attach to the sternum. The lower two pairs do not, and are therefore "floating."

6. **c.** The mandible is the lower, moveable section of the jaw. The maxilla is the upper jaw. The malleolus is either of the rounded projections on each side of the ankle joint. The mastoid is the prominent bony mass at the base of the skull.

7. **c.** The manubrium is the upper segment of the sternum. The main, middle segment of the sternum is the body. The angle of Louis is a bony prominence at the level of the second rib, which marks the junction of the manubrium and body of the sternum. The acetabulum is the rounded cavity of the pelvis into which the femoral head fits.

8. **b.** The xiphoid process is the cartilaginous projection at the lower end of the sternum. The styloid process and mastoid process are both part of the skull. The lenticular process is part of the incus bone of the middle ear.

9. **a.** The calcaneus is the heel bone. The carpals and metacarpals are bones of the hand and wrist. The tarsals are bones of the ankle.

10. **d.** The greater trochanter is the proximal part of the femur.

11. **d.** The patella is the kneecap. Parietal pertains to the wall of a cavity. Peristalsis is the wavelike movement by which tubular organs propel their contents, and the perineum is the area of skin between the vagina or scrotum and the anus.

12. Using the given list of sections of the spine, label Figure 1-2.
    cervical
    coccyx
    lumbar
    thoracic
    sacrum

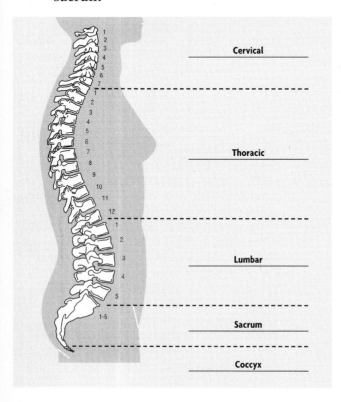

Cervical

Thoracic

Lumbar

Sacrum

Coccyx

Figure 1-2

13. **b.** The clavicle is the collar bone. The scapula is the shoulder blade. The acromion process is the highest point of the shoulder, and the costal cartilage connects the ribs to the sternum. The ilium is one of the three bones that are fused together to form each pelvic bone.

14. Using the list of bones below, label the upper and lower extremities on Figure 1-3.

carpals	patella
clavicle	phalanges
femur	radius
fibula	tarsals
humerus	tibia
metacarpals	ulna
metatarsals	

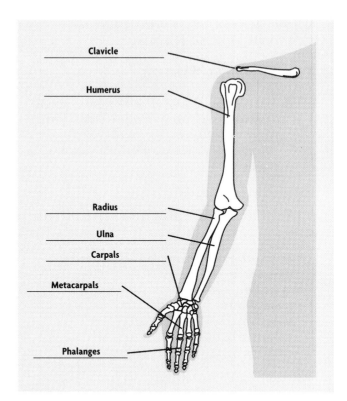

Clavicle

Humerus

Radius

Ulna

Carpals

Metacarpals

Phalanges

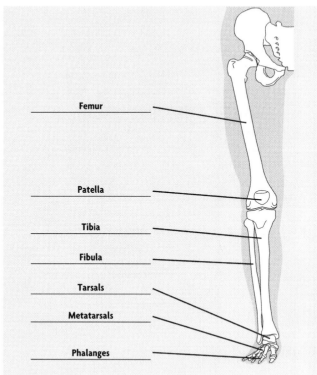

Femur

Patella

Tibia

Fibula

Tarsals

Metatarsals

Phalanges

Figure 1-3
Upper extremities (top).
Lower extremities (bottom).

15. **c.** The tibia, clavicle, and ulna lie directly underneath the skin and can be palpated along their entire lengths.

16. **d.** The hip is an example of a ball-and-socket joint, as is the shoulder.

17. **a.** The knee and elbow are hinge joints. A false joint is one that forms subsequent to a fracture.

18. Using the list below, label the major bones of the pelvis on Figure 1-4.
ilium
ischium
pubis
sacrum

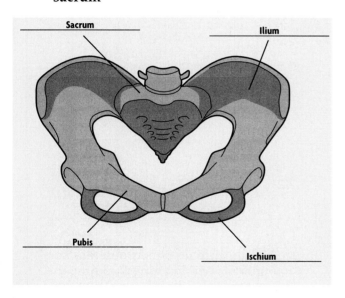

Figure 1-4

19. **c.** The gastrointestinal tract is made up of smooth muscle. Smooth muscles are also referred to as involuntary muscles.

20. **a.** Skeletal muscles allow us to move. They are also classified as voluntary muscles.

21. **d.** Automaticity refers to cardiac muscle's ability to contract on its own.

✳ ENRICHMENT QUESTIONS

22. **b.** Muscles do *not* push; they *only* pull.

23. **a.** The diaphragm acts primarily as an involuntary muscle even though it is formed of striated skeletal muscle.

24. **a.** Skeletal muscles are striated muscles. Skeletal muscles are also classified as voluntary muscles. The gastrointestinal tract and urinary tract muscles are smooth muscles. Smooth muscles are also referred to as involuntary muscles.

25. **c.** Tendons connect muscle to bone.

26. **b.** Ligaments connect bone to bone. They also help form and strengthen joints.

27. **c.** The fascia is the fibrous membrane that encases muscle tissue. The meninges cover the brain and spinal cord. Dura mater is one of the meninges, and the pleura is tissue in the chest cavity that surrounds the lungs and lines the cavity walls.

28. **d.** Sphincter muscles are circular muscles that, when contracted, close natural body openings. Examples of sphincter muscles would be the anus and the valves between the various sections of the GI tract.

■ THE SKIN

29. **c.** The skin provides temperature regulation and protection to underlying structures. Because it is rich in nerve endings, it also allows information to be transmitted from the environment to the brain. The skin also senses heat, cold, touch, pressure, and pain.

30. **a.** The epidermis is the outermost layer of skin. The dermis is the second layer of the skin. *Epi* means "upon"; therefore *epidermis* means upon the dermis.

31. **a.** The dermis contains sweat glands and hair follicles.

32. **b.** The subcutaneous layer is a layer of fatty tissue that lies under the dermis.

✳ ENRICHMENT QUESTION

33. **d.** Oils are secreted by sebaceous glands.

■ THE NERVOUS SYSTEM

34. **a.** The two anatomical divisions of the nervous system are the central nervous system and peripheral nervous system.

35. **a.** The brain and spinal cord make up the central nervous system.

36. **d.** Sensory and motor nerves are the two main types of nerves that enter and leave the spinal cord.

✳ ENRICHMENT QUESTION

37. **c.** The central nervous system is responsible for higher mental functions, including thought, decision making, and communication. In addition, it plays an important role in regulating body functions.

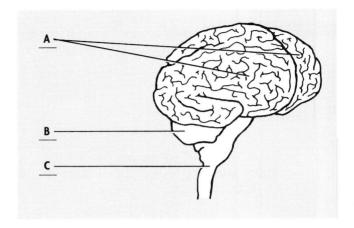

Figure 1-5

38. **c.** Structure *A* is the cerebrum.

39. **b.** Structure *B* is the cerebellum.

40. **a.** Structure *C* is the brainstem.

41. **b.** The brainstem controls involuntary functions.

42. **c.** The cerebrum is responsible for voluntary functions, thought, memory, and sensory reception.

43. **a.** The meninges cover the brain and spinal cord. The dura mater is the outer of the three layers of the meninges. The arachnoid and pia mater are the other two. The word "PAD" can be used to remember the order of the three layers. Starting from the brain and working out, the layers are: *P*ia mater, *A*rachnoid, *D*ura mater. A meniscus is a fibrocartilage that serves as a cushion between two bones meeting in a joint, and the pleura is the membrane that covers the lungs and lines the thoracic cavity.

44. **d.** The autonomic nervous system controls the body's involuntary activities, such as digestion, heart rate, and sweating.

45. b. Stimulation of the sympathetic nervous system increases heart rate. It also constricts blood vessels, causes bronchodilation, and stimulates sweating. Stimulation of the parasympathetic nervous system slows heart rate and dilates blood vessels, along with other effects.

■ THE RESPIRATORY SYSTEM

46. d. The epiglottis prevents food or liquids from entering the trachea. The uvula is the structure that hangs down from the soft palate above the back of the tongue. The cardiac sphincter closes the esophageal opening of the stomach. Epigastrium refers to the area of the abdomen between the umbilicus and the xiphoid process.

47. c. Tidal volume refers to the volume of air per breath. It is a measure of how deeply the patient is breathing.

48. d. Oxygen and carbon dioxide are normally exchanged during breathing.

49. b. The thyroid cartilage is commonly referred to as the Adam's apple. It is part of the larynx.

50. d. The diaphragm is the major muscle involved in breathing. It also separates the thoracic cavity from the abdominal cavity. Intercostal muscles are also involved in breathing.

51. c. The exchange of gases during breathing takes place in the alveoli. The alveoli, resembling small grape clusters, are the "work stations" of the lungs.

52. b. Blood entering the capillaries in the lungs is low in oxygen and high in carbon dioxide.

53. d. Since blood reaching the body tissues has come from the lungs, it is high in oxygen and low in carbon dioxide.

54. c. In healthy humans, the most sensitive and rapid-responding system for breathing stimulus monitors the carbon dioxide level in arterial blood. A secondary stimulus is a low level of oxygen in arterial blood.

■ THE CIRCULATORY SYSTEM

55. a. The atria receive blood. They are the upper chambers of the heart. Atria is plural; the singular form is atrium. The vallecula is the depression between the epiglottis and the root of the tongue.

56. b. The ventricles pump the blood. They are the lower chambers of the heart. Varices are dilated, twisted blood vessels. The atria are sometimes referred to as the auricles.

57. a. The coronary arteries supply the heart muscle with blood. Pulmonary arteries carry blood to the lungs.

58. c. The aorta is the major artery in the body and comes directly off the heart. It is also the largest artery. The carotid, subclavian, and innominate (or brachiocephalic) arteries branch off the arch of the aorta.

59. b. The left ventricle pumps blood to the body. The left atrium receives blood from the lungs.

60. d. Blood is pumped to the lungs by the right ventricle. The right atrium receives blood from the body.

61. **d.** All of the above. Blood carries oxygen, removes waste products including carbon dioxide, carries antibodies that combat infections, and carries clotting factors.

62. **b.** Valves prevent blood from flowing backward. Valves are found in the venous system and the heart.

63. **a.** The lower extremities receive blood from the femoral arteries.

64. **c.** The blood vessels that transport blood away from the heart are arteries.

65. **a.** In the foot, a pulse can be felt at the dorsalis pedis artery. The inferior vena cava is the major vein that supplies the heart with blood from the lower body and the innominate artery branches off the aorta.

66. **b.** The blood vessels that transport blood toward the heart are veins. Venules connect veins to capillaries.

67. **c.** The blood vessels that connect veins and arteries are capillaries. Arterioles connect arteries to capillaries, and the ventricles are chambers of the heart.

68. **d.** White blood cells defend against infection. They are also known as leukocytes (*leuko* meaning white and *cyte* meaning cell).

69. **b.** Plasma is the liquid component of blood. It carries the blood cells and nutrients. Lymph is a fluid composed of a number of substances; it is returned to general circulation via the lymphatic system. Interstitial fluid is fluid that occupies the space outside the blood vessels.

70. **a.** Red blood cells carry oxygen. They are also known as erythrocytes (*erythro* meaning red and *cyte* meaning cell). Hemoglobin is a protein component of red blood cells that allows them to carry oxygen. Red blood cells give blood its color.

71. **d.** Platelets are small, cellular fragments in the blood that are essential to clot formation. T-lymphocytes play a part in immune response.

72. Using the following list of components of the circulatory system, label Figure 1-6:
    aorta
    inferior vena cava
    left atrium
    left ventricle
    pulmonary artery
    pulmonary veins
    right atrium
    right ventricle
    superior vena cava

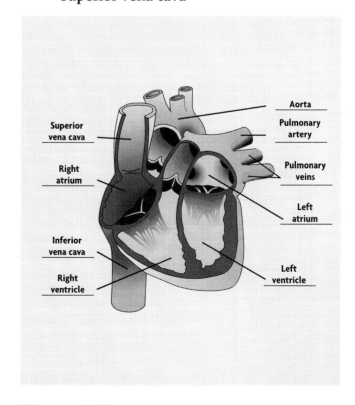

Figure 1-6

73. **c.** The right and left sides of the heart are separated by a muscular wall known as the septum. The pericardium is the fibrous sac that surrounds the heart. The sacrum is one of three bones that make up the pelvic ring, and the diaphragm is the muscle that separates the thoracic cavity from the abdominal cavity.

74. **b.** An average-size adult has 5 liters (approximately 10 pints) of blood. Blood volume may be less in females and smaller males. Generally, about $\frac{1}{12}$ to $\frac{1}{15}$ (or 7%) of body weight is blood. A unit of blood equals 500 cc (half a liter).

75. **c.** The average amount of blood in a 1-year-old child is approximately 800 cc.

▪ GENERAL ANATOMY AND PHYSIOLOGY

76. **a.** The endocrine system is responsible for producing chemicals called hormones.

77. **d.** The spine is located on the dorsal side. Ventral refers to the belly side, cephalic is toward the head, and anterior is toward the front.

78. **a.** Anatomically, the umbilicus is on the anterior abdomen. Caudal is toward the tail, posterior means following or located behind, and lateral refers to away from the midline.

79. **b.** A body structure that is above another is said to be superior. Inferior refers to a structure below another.

80. **c.** The hand is on the distal end of the arm, that is, near the end of an extremity or farther from the midline. Proximal refers to the end of an extremity closer to the midline. Medial refers to close to the midline, and lateral is farther from the midline.

81. **b.** The term *bilateral* is used to describe the right and left relative to each other.

82. Using the list below, label the three imaginary dividing lines in Figure 1-7.
midaxillary line
midclavicular line
midline

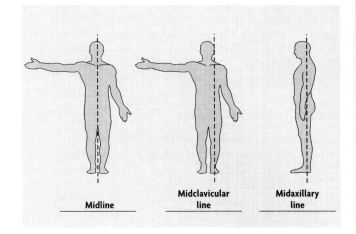

Figure 1-7

83. **d.** A patient who is lying face down is said to be in the prone position.

84. **c.** The term lateral refers to something that is away from the midline or middle, or toward the side.

85. **b.** The portion of the femur closest to the hip would be the proximal portion, that is, the portion closer to the torso or trunk of the body.

86. **d.** Posterior refers to the back. Therefore, this wound would best be described as being on the posterior abdomen.

87. Match the list of directional terms below to their definitions.

_____ proximal _____	toward the trunk
_____ distal _____	away from the trunk
_____ posterior _____	toward the back
_____ anterior _____	toward the front
_____ medial _____	toward the midline
_____ lateral _____	away from the midline
_____ superior _____	toward the top of the body
_____ inferior _____	toward the bottom of the body

88. **d.** To place a patient in the Trendelenburg position, position the patient lying on her back with the foot of the cot raised higher than the head while maintaining a straight incline to the head of the cot. This is not just a matter of elevating the legs at the hips; the entire body is on an incline.

89. **b.** The recovery position is also referred to as the lateral recumbent position.

90. **c.** To place a patient in the recovery position, you would position the patient lying on his left or right side. In most cases during transport in an ambulance, the patient is positioned on his left side so that he is facing the EMT providing care.

91. **b.** A patient who is lying on his back, such as on a backboard, is in the supine position.

92. **d.** A patient placed in the Fowler's position can be described as lying on her back with her upper body elevated at a 45- to 60-degree angle.

■ **ENRICHMENT QUESTIONS**

93. Using the following list of body cavities, label Figure 1-8.
 abdominal
 cranial
 pelvic
 spinal
 thoracic

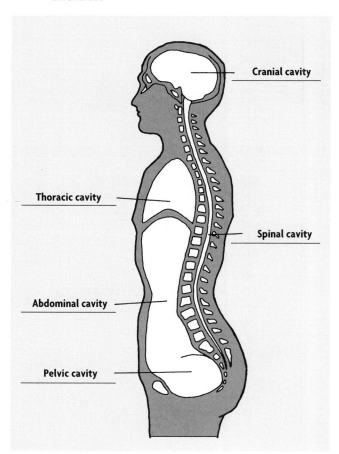

Cranial cavity

Thoracic cavity

Spinal cavity

Abdominal cavity

Pelvic cavity

Figure 1-8

94. **d.** The bladder is in the pelvic cavity. Also in the pelvic cavity are the rectum and internal female reproductive organs.

95. Referring to Figure 1-9, label the following organs with the abdominal quadrants in which they are primarily located.
(NOTE: some organs may be in more than one quadrant.)

RLQ	appendix
RUQ	gallbladder
RUQ, LUQ, RLQ, LLQ	large intestine
LUQ	left kidney
RUQ	liver
RUQ, LUQ	pancreas
RUQ	right kidney
RLQ, LLQ	small intestine
LUQ	spleen
LUQ	stomach

96. **a.** The liver, spleen, lymph glands, and white blood cells are all part of the immune system.

97. **b.** The islets of Langerhans in the pancreas produce the hormone insulin. Some of the primary functions of insulin are to increase glucose metabolism by cells and to increase glucose transport into cells.

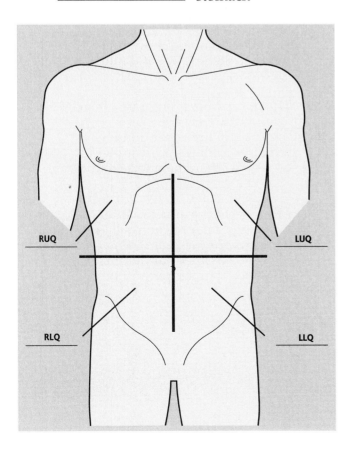

Figure 1-9

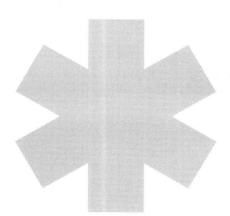

2

Vital Signs and Patient History

CHAPTER 2 REVIEW QUESTIONS

1. The chief complaint is a:
   a. list of what is currently wrong with the patient
   b. brief, short description of why EMS was called
   c. history of the present illness
   d. description of the patient's medical history

2. When assessing a child, the most important aspect is the:
   a. patient's blood pressure
   b. patient's pulse rate
   c. parent's general reactions
   d. EMT's general impression of the patient

3. Baseline vital signs consist of assessing:
   a. pulse, breathing, blood pressure, skin, and pupils
   b. breathing, pulse, medical history, and age
   c. age, sex, blood pressure, and pulse
   d. pulse, breathing, skin, and race

4. When determining a patient's breathing rate:
   a. instruct the patient to breathe in a normal, relaxed manner
   b. place the patient in a sitting position
   c. do not let the patient know you are counting breathing rate
   d. ask the patient about his/her chief complaint and medical history

5. The normal adult breathing rate is:
   a. 5 to 10 times per minute
   b. 8 to 16 times per minute
   c. 12 to 20 times per minute
   d. 16 to 28 times per minute

6. The normal breathing rate for a child is:
   a. 10 to 20 times per minute
   b. 15 to 30 times per minute
   c. 25 to 40 times per minute
   d. slower than the normal adult rate

7. The normal breathing rate for an infant is:
   a. slower than the normal adult rate
   b. 10 to 25 times per minute
   c. 20 to 40 times per minute
   d. 25 to 50 times per minute

8. The adequacy of a patient's breathing can be assessed by checking the:
   a. respiratory rate, blood pressure, and lung sounds
   b. respiratory rate, depth of respirations, and skin color
   c. depth of respirations, pulse rate, and blood pressure
   d. skin color, capillary refill time, and pulse rate

9. The EMT should be concerned if an adult has a breathing rate of:
   a. <6 or >12
   b. <8 or >24
   c. <8 or >18
   d. <14 or >20

10. Breathing characterized by occasional, gasping breaths is known as:
    a. Kussmaul breathing
    b. agonal breathing
    c. grunting breathing
    d. sonorous breathing

11. The pulse may be defined as:
    a. the number of times the heart contracts each minute
    b. the pressure in an artery
    c. a wave of blood that courses through an artery as the heart contracts
    d. blood flowing through a vein

12. When checking a carotid pulse, the EMT should:
    a. check only one side at a time
    b. check both sides simultaneously
    c. only perform carotid pulse checks on patients over age 65
    d use the thumb of the hand closest to the head

13. The most common place to check a pulse in a conscious adult patient is the:
    a. brachial artery
    b. radial artery
    c. carotid artery
    d. femoral artery

14. The EMT should check a pulse for:
    a. rate and quality
    b. volume and strength
    c. flow and rate
    d. quality and volume

15. When describing a patient's pulse, the term "quality" refers to its:
    a. strength and regularity
    b. rhythm and rate
    c. rate and regularity
    d. strength and rate

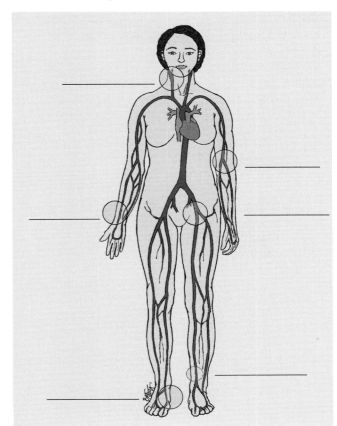

Figure 2-1

16. Using the key pulse points listed below, label Figure 2-1.
    brachial
    carotid
    dorsalis pedis
    femoral
    posterior tibial
    radial

17. To quickly assess a patient's skin temperature:
    a. touch the patient's skin with the back of the hand
    b. touch the patient's skin with the palm of the hand
    c. kiss the patient's forehead
    d. touch the patient's lips with the back of the hand

18. Capillary refill should be checked:
    a. on patients over 16 years old
    b. on all patients
    c. on any patient in shock
    d. on patients less than 6 years old

19. When checking capillary refill time, color should normally return within:
    a. ½ to 1 second
    b. 2 seconds
    c. 4 seconds
    d. 10 seconds

20. For the medical emergencies below, note which of the following you would expect the patient's skin color to be.
    cyanotic
    flushed
    jaundiced
    pale or pink

    _____ hypoglycemia

    _____ heat emergency with dry skin

    _____ liver dysfunction

    _____ normal skin

    _____ late stage carbon monoxide poisoning

    _____ insufficient circulation

    _____ inadequate oxygenation

    _____ hypoperfusion

21. The best place to check a patient for jaundice is:
    a. the white area of the eye
    b. the lowest areas of the body
    c. the gums
    d. the skin of the thigh

22. Skin color may be most easily assessed by checking any of the following areas *except* the:
    a. conjunctiva
    b. oral mucosa
    c. nail beds
    d. chest

23. The skin of a patient who is in hypoperfusion (shock) is most likely be:
    a. flushed, cool, and dry
    b. cyanotic, warm, and dry
    c. flushed, warm, and moist
    d. pale, cool, and moist

24. When checking pupils, the EMT should remember that:
    a. cataracts do not affect pupil response
    b. unequal pupils generally occur early in head injuries
    c. medications may affect pupillary response
    d. bright lights will not affect the pupil check

25. Blood pressure can be defined as:
    a. the pressure blood exerts against the walls of the arteries
    b. the volume of blood in an artery
    c. the pressure exerted by blood against the walls of the veins
    d. the difference between the arterial pressure and venous pressure

26. The blood pressure should be checked:
    a. only if the patient's pulse feels weak
    b. on every patient regardless of their age
    c. on patients older than 3 years of age
    d. only on patients who have sustained trauma

27. The first sound noted when taking a blood pressure by auscultation is the:
    a. diastolic pressur
    b. systolic pressure
    c. mean arterial pressure
    d. venous pressure

28. The diastolic pressure corresponds to:
    a. the pressure exerted against the walls of the arteries when the heart is pumping
    b. the difference between the resting pressure and pumping pressure
    c. the pressure exerted against the walls of the arteries when the left ventricle is at rest
    d. half the systolic pressure

29. Systolic blood pressure may indicate a serious problem if it is:
    a. >90 mm Hg
    b. >130 mm Hg
    c. <100 mm Hg
    d. <140 mm Hg

30. Obtaining a blood pressure by feeling a pulse rather than by listening with a stethoscope is known as:
    a. auscultating a blood pressure
    b. palpating a blood pressure
    c. pulsing a blood pressure
    d. tamponading a blood pressure

31. Vital signs of an unstable patient should be checked:
    a. every 5 minutes
    b. every 10 minutes
    c. every 15 minutes
    d. only if a medical intervention is performed

Questions 32 to 36 refer to the acronym S-A-M-P-L-E.

32. When the EMT takes a patient history, the letter *P* refers to:
    a. location of "pain"
    b. presence of "paralysis"
    c. events "preceding" the injury or illness
    d. "pertinent" past medical history

33. The letter *M* refers to:
    a. present "medications"
    b. ability to "move" all extremities
    c. time of the last "meal"
    d. name of the patient's "MD"

34. The letter *E* refers to:
    a. length of time from onset of problem until "EMS" was called
    b. "events" leading up to the injury or illness
    c. whether the situation should be classified as a true "emergency"
    d. whether there is a need for "extrication"

35. The letter *L* refers to:
    a. the patient's "life-style"
    b. things that "lead" up to the event
    c. the patient's "last" oral intake
    d. checking the patient's "lung" sounds

36. When routinely questioning a patient about allergies (the *A* in S-A-M-P-L-E), the EMT is most concerned with allergies to:
    a. medications
    b. food
    c. environmental factors
    d. all of the above

37. Something related to a patient's medical problem that the EMT sees, feels, or hears is a:
    a. symptom
    b. syndrome
    c. sign
    d. scenario

38. Mark each entry in the following list as a **sign**, a **symptom**, or **both**.

    _____ chest pain

    _____ cyanosis

    _____ apnea

    _____ difficulty breathing

    _____ nausea

    _____ sweating

    _____ cool skin

    _____ headache

    _____ dizziness

    _____ paleness

    _____ deformed extremity

    _____ vomiting

    _____ swelling

    _____ double vision

    _____ numbness

    _____ wheezing

✳ **Enrichment Questions**

39. When using a stethoscope, the earpieces should:
    a. face backward
    b. be placed in the most comfortable position
    c. face away from the patient
    d. face forward

40. The diaphragm of the stethoscope is best used for listening to:
    a. high-frequency sounds
    b. low-frequency sounds
    c. heart sounds
    d. gallops

41. The normal pulse rate for an adult is:
    a. 50 to 70 beats per minute
    b. 60 to 100 beats per minute
    c. 80 to 120 beats per minute
    d >110 beats per minute

42. The normal pulse rate for a child is:
    a. 60 to 80 beats per minute
    b. 80 to 100 beats per minute
    c. <80 beats per minute
    d. >120 beats per minute

43. The pulse rate for an infant is normally:
    a. 50 to 80 beats per minute
    b. 80 to 100 beats per minute
    c. 100 to 140 beats per minute
    d. 170 to 200 beats per minute

44. Normal pupils are:
    a. unequal and constrict when exposed to light
    b equal and constrict when exposed to light
    c. dilated and become unequal when exposed to light
    d. constricted and dilate when exposed to light

45. To obtain an accurate reading, the blood pressure cuff should:
    a. be the length of the forearm
    b. cover about ⅔ of the patient's upper arm
    c. be twice the diameter of the arm
    d. be placed even with the bend in the patient's elbow

46. An error in blood pressure measurement may be the result of:
    a. incorrect cuff size
    b. operator error
    c. loud background noise
    d. all of the above

47. If the EMT encounters difficulty hearing a blood pressure, the sounds may be augmented by:
    a. slowly inflating the cuff
    b. lowering the arm before inflating the cuff
    c. elevating the arm before inflating the cuff
    d. rapidly deflating the cuff

48. To obtain an accurate reading, a blood pressure cuff should be deflated at a rate of:
    a. 1 to 2 mm Hg per second
    b. 2 to 3 mm Hg per second
    c. 3 to 4 mm Hg per second
    d. 4 to 5 mm Hg per second

49. When charting vital signs on a run report, the most important thing to note is the:
    a. name of the EMT taking the vital signs
    b. arm used to take the pulse and blood pressure
    c. position the patient was in while vital signs were taken
    d. time the vital signs were taken

50. A second set of vital signs should always be checked before the patient reaches the hospital to:
    a. make the run report appear more complete
    b. confirm that the first set is correct
    c. compare with the initial set for changes
    d. provide the EMT with additional practice in taking vital signs

51. A pulse oximeter shows the:
    a. exchange of oxygen and carbon dioxide in the lungs
    b. patient's respiratory rate
    c. percentage of hemoglobin saturated with oxygen in the blood
    d. strength of a patient's pulse

52. A pulse oximeter will not provide accurate information if the patient's medical problems are related to:
    a. an asthma attack
    b. carbon monoxide poisoning
    c. congestive heart failure
    d. emphysema

■ Additional Points for Discussion ■

1. The medications taken by a patient can give the EMT a clue regarding what kind of medical problems a patient has. Because many patients are poor historians (especially the elderly), it is good for the EMT to be familiar with prescription medications commonly taken for certain medical problems. Review previous emergency calls to which you have responded. What medications are most commonly associated with the following problems?

   • Heart problems:

   • Breathing problems:

   • High blood pressure (hypertension):

   • Diabetes mellitus:

   • Seizure disorders:

   • Abdominal disorders:

   • Behavioral problems:

2. Using a drug reference book, research some of the medications you have listed and become familiar with their actions and side effects.

ANSWERS TO CHAPTER 2 REVIEW QUESTIONS

1. **b.** The chief complaint is a brief, short description of why EMS was called, such as "chest pain" or "difficulty breathing."

2. **d.** The EMT's general impression of a sick or injured child is more important than vital signs. Children can maintain what appear to be normal vital signs but their condition can suddenly deteriorate.

3. **a.** Baseline vital signs consist of checking pulse, breathing, blood pressure, skin, and pupils.

4. **c.** When determining the breathing rate, do not let the patient know you are counting breaths as this can affect the way the patient breathes. The patient does not need to be sitting up and should not talk during the assessment.

5. **c.** The normal adult breathing rate is 12 to 20 times a minute.

6. **b.** The normal breathing rate for a child is 15 to 30 times a minute.

7. **d.** Infants may breathe 25 to 50 times a minute. The rate is faster than the adult rate because of an infant's rapid metabolism.

8. **b.** The adequacy of a patient's breathing can be assessed by checking the respiratory rate, depth of respirations, and skin color.

9. **b.** If the breathing rate falls below eight breaths a minute in an adult, the EMT should be concerned. Rapid breathing rates may also provide cause for alarm. Sustained rates of 24 breaths a minute or greater may result in insufficient air volume. Sustained rates of greater than 28 breaths a minute are especially dangerous. Some people, such as athletes, may normally breathe slower. Always consider how the patient's problem and overall condition relate to the breathing rate and care for the patient accordingly.

10. **b.** Agonal breathing is characterized by occasional, gasping breaths, and most commonly occurs immediately before death. Kussmaul breathing is characterized by rapid, deep breathing.

11. **c.** The pulse may be defined as a wave of blood that courses through an artery as the heart contracts. It is not the number of times heart contracts each minute. There are times, such as when a patient has a rapid heart rate, that the heart may not completely refill. It does contract, but no pulse is felt as there is not enough blood in the ventricles to push out.

12. **a.** When checking a carotid pulse, check only one side at a time. Checking both sides simultaneously may obstruct blood flow to the brain. Rubbing the carotid artery may cause a drop in pulse rate, especially in the elderly. Never use the thumb to check any pulses; it has its own pulse.

13. **b.** EMTs most commonly check a radial pulse in any patient over 1 year of age. If the radial pulse cannot be felt, assess the carotid pulse. For children younger than 1 year, check the brachial pulse.

14. **a.** The pulse should be checked for rate and quality. Quality refers to volume (strong or weak) and regularity. If it is irregular, check for a regular irregularity (e.g., an extra beat every second or third beat) or irregular irregularity (e.g., no pattern to the irregularity).

15. **a.** The quality of a patient's pulse is determined by its strength and regularity.

16. Match the key pulse points listed below to their location in Figure 2-1.
    brachial
    carotid
    dorsalis pedis
    femoral
    posterior tibial
    radial

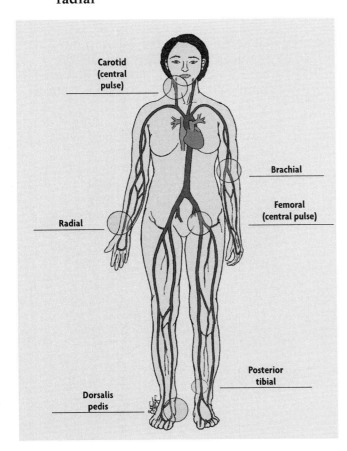

Figure 2-1

17. **a.** A patient's temperature can most easily be felt with the back of the EMT's hand. Exact temperature is not as important as noting the presence of a possible fever or possible hypothermia. Lip contact should be avoided to preclude possible infection transmission.

18. **d.** Capillary refill time should only be checked on patients younger than 6 years. Remember that if the patient's extremities are cold, capillary refill time will not be an accurate indicator.

19. **b.** When checking capillary refill, the color should return within 2 seconds.

20.
pale	hypoglycemia
flushed	heat emergency with dry skin
jaundiced	liver dysfunction
pink	normal skin
flushed	carbon monoxide poisoning
pale	insufficient circulation
cyanotic	inadequate oxygenation
pale	hypoperfusion

21. **a.** Jaundice manifests early in the white area of the eye. This area is easy to see, and no clothing must be removed to view it.

22. **d.** When checking for abnormal skin colors, examine the patients conjunctiva (eyes), oral mucosa (gums and lips), or nail beds. The chest is not a good area for assessing skin color.

23. **d.** The skin of a patient in hypoperfusion (shock) is most likely to be pale, cool, and moist.

24. **c.** Medications and cataracts may affect papillary response. Although unequal pupils may be seen in head injuries, they are usually a late sign. The EMT must also remember that many people have normally unequal pupils. Always check pupils in subdued light.

25. **a.** Blood pressure is the pressure blood exerts against the walls of the arteries.

26. **c.** Blood pressure should be checked on all patients older than 3 years.

27. **b.** The first sound noted when taking a blood pressure by auscultation is the systolic pressure. The point when the sounds fade or disappear during deflation of the cuff corresponds with the diastolic pressure.

28. **c.** The diastolic reading corresponds to the pressure exerted against the walls of the arteries when the left ventricle is at rest. The systolic reading is the pressure during ventricular contraction.

29. **c.** A systolic blood pressure less than 100 mm Hg may indicate a serious problem, especially if the patient has associated signs and symptoms of trauma or a medical problem.

30. **b.** Palpating a blood pressure. To do this, the EMT feels a pulse below the blood pressure cuff, then inflates the cuff. When the pulse is no longer felt, the cuff is inflated another 30 mm Hg. The pressure is then released. The first pulse felt as the cuff is deflated is the systolic pressure. Palpated blood pressures should be noted as the systolic pressure over "P" (e.g., 126/P).

31. **a.** Vital signs on an unstable patient should be checked every 5 minutes. If the patient is stable, the vital signs should be checked every 15 minutes.

32. **d.** The letter *P* refers to "pertinent" past medical history, such as previous illnesses or injuries.

33. **a.** The letter *M* refers to the patient's present "medications."

34. **b.** The letter *E* relates to the "events" that led up to or caused the injury or illness.

35. **c.** The letter *L* refers to the patient's "last" oral intake, whether solids or liquids.

36. **d.** All of the above. The allergies an EMT is concerned with are allergies to medications, food, or environmental factors, such as pollen or insect stings.

37. **c.** A sign is something the EMT sees, feels, or hears. A symptom is something the patient tells the EMT. A syndrome is a collection of symptoms. The *S* in S-A-M-P-L-E refers to "signs and symptoms."

38.

symptom	chest pain
sign	cyanosis
sign	apnea
both	difficulty breathing
symptom	nausea
sign	sweating
sign	cool skin
symptom	headache
symptom	dizziness
sign	paleness
sign	deformed extremity
sign	vomiting
sign	swelling
symptom	double vision
symptom	numbness
sign	wheezes

✳ **Enrichment Questions**

39. **d.** The earpieces of a stethoscope should face forward to match the natural direction of the EMT's ear canals.

40. **a.** The diaphragm of the stethoscope best amplifies high-frequency sounds, such as breath sounds. The bell is used to listen to low-frequency sounds, such as heart sounds. Gallops are types of heart sounds.

41. **b.** The normal adult pulse range is 60 to 100 beats per minute. Remember that the overall patient picture is more important than focusing on the patient's exact pulse rate.

42. **b.** The normal pulse range for a child is 80 to 100 beats per minute. In younger children, the pulse rate may normally be greater than 100.

43. **c.** The pulse rate of an infant is normally 100 to 140 beats per minute. The pulse rate of a newborn may be as high as 150 to 160.

44. **b.** Normal pupils are equal and constrict when exposed to light.

45. **b.** The blood pressure cuff should cover about ⅔ of the patient's upper arm. The width of the blood pressure cuff bladder should be at least 20% greater than the diameter of the patient's arm or 40% of the limb circumference. The bottom of the cuff should lie about an inch above the bend of the elbow.

46. **d.** All of the above. Incorrect cuff size, operator error, and loud background noise can all cause inaccurate blood pressure measurements.

47. **c.** Elevating the arm prior to inflating the cuff may reduce venous congestion, which makes it difficult to hear blood pressure sounds. The cuff should be rapidly, not slowly, inflated in 7 seconds or less. The cuff should then be deflated slowly.

48. **b.** A blood pressure cuff should be deflated at a rate of 2 to 3 mm Hg per second.

49. **d.** EMTs should always note the time vital signs were taken. The name of the EMT will appear elsewhere on the report. The arm used and patient position are not usually noted, but may be noted if the information is significant.

50. **c.** There should always be a minimum of two sets of vital signs recorded on every patient for the sake of comparison. A second set of vital signs should always be checked and compared for changes with the first set. The second set does not confirm the accuracy of the first set; it is an appropriate and important addition to a run report.

51. **c.** A pulse oximeter shows the percentage of saturated hemoglobin in the blood. Normally, hemoglobin is saturated with oxygen. However, hemoglobin may also be saturated with carbon monoxide, and a pulse oximeter cannot differentiate what the hemoglobin is bound with. Most pulse oximeters also show a pulse rate but not its strength. They also do not show a respiratory rate.

52. **b.** Pulse oximeters can provide useful information when managing patients with respiratory difficulty associated with problems such as asthma, emphysema, and congestive heart failure. They provide inaccurate information, however, when placed on a patient with carbon monoxide poisoning since the oximeter cannot differentiate carbon monoxide in the blood from oxygen in the blood.

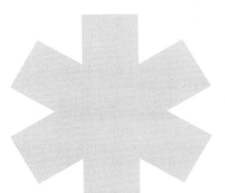

3

Airway Control and Oxygen Administration

D.O.T. Curriculum Objectives Covered in This Chapter:

Lesson 2-1
Lesson 8-1

CHAPTER 3 REVIEW QUESTIONS

1. When filled, an "E" tank will hold approximately:
   a. 350 L of oxygen
   b. 625 L of oxygen
   c. 2,000 L of oxygen
   d. 3,000 L of oxygen

2. When an oxygen tank is full, the normal pressure in the tank is approximately:
   a. 1,000 psi
   b. 1,400 psi
   c. 2,000 psi
   d. 2,800 psi

3. The date circled in Figure 3-1 is the date:
   a. the tank was manufactured
   b. for the next hydrostatic test
   c. the tank was placed in service
   d. of the last hydrostatic test

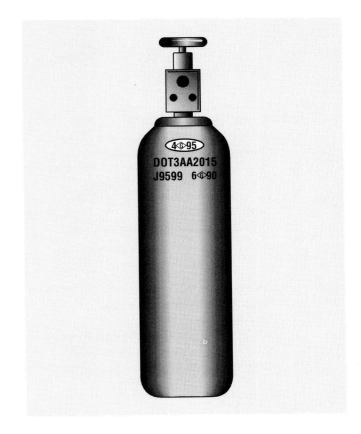

Figure 3-1

4. The safe working pressure of the tank in Figure 3-1 would be:
   a. 1,500 psi
   b. 1,750 psi
   c. 2,015 psi
   d. 3,000 psi

5. The tanks most commonly used in portable oxygen units are:
   a. "A" and "B" tanks
   b. "D" and "M" tanks
   c. "E" and "G" tanks
   d. "D" and "E" tanks

6. To "crack" the valve of an oxygen tank means to:
   a. quickly open and close the valve to blow out dust
   b. strike the valve stem sharply to loosen any dirt stuck in the valve opening
   c. damage the valve by dropping the tank
   d. seal the valve with tape after filling to prevent dust and dirt from entering it

7. When using supplemental oxygen with a pocket mask or bag-valve-mask device, the proper flow rate is:
   a. less than 3 L/min if the patient has a history of respiratory illness
   b. 6 L/min if the patient is only in respiratory arrest
   c. 12 L/min if the patient is a child
   d. 15 L/min in all cases

8. A nasal cannula will oxygenate patients:
   a. even if they breathe through their mouth
   b. only if they breathe through their nose
   c. as well as a nonrebreather mask
   d. even if a nasal obstruction is present

9. Oxygen may be administered to a laryngectomy patient by:
   a. inserting supply tubing into the stoma
   b. placing a cannula in the patient's nose
   c. placing a child- or infant-size mask over the patient's stoma
   d. placing a mask on the patient and instructing him to breathe only through his mouth

10. Patients in shock caused by trauma should be given oxygen:
    a. at high flow, unless they have a history of asthma
    b. at high flow via a nonrebreather reservoir mask
    c. using the device best tolerated by the patient
    d. only after removal from a wrecked vehicle due to the possibility of a fire occurring

11. The proper oxygen flow rate for a nonrebreather mask is:
    a. 3 L/min if there is a history of asthma
    b. 6 L/min if the patient will not tolerate high flow
    c. 9 L/min if the patient complains of dry mouth
    d. 15 L/min in all cases

12. The reservoir of a nonrebreather mask should:
    a. fully deflate with each patient ventilation to allow the EMT to assess depth of breaths
    b. be inflated prior to placing the mask on the patient
    c. be filled with the patient's expired air
    d. be removed if the patient insists that he or she is not getting enough air

13. A nasal cannula can be used if:
    a. the patient will not tolerate a nonrebreather mask
    b. the patient complains of a dry mouth
    c. a low oxygen tank pressure is discovered
    d. the patient is breathing primarily through the nose

14. There is no advantage to using nasal cannulas with oxygen flow rates greater than:
    a. 2 L/min
    b. 4 L/min
    c. 6 L/min
    d. 9 L/min

Questions 15 through 19 refer to Figures 3-2, 3-3, and 3-4.

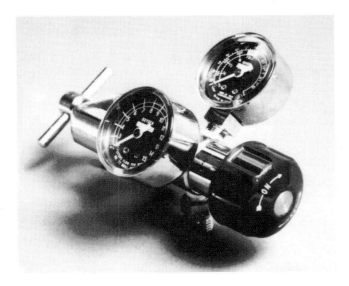

Figure 3-2

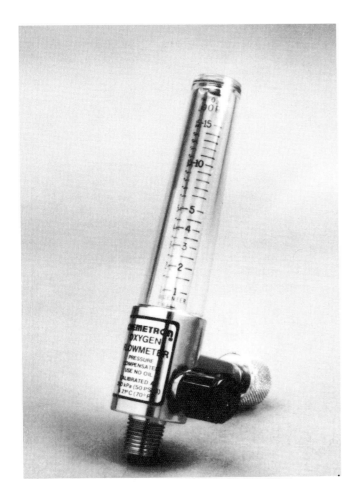

Figure 3-3

15. Figure 3-2 is an example of a:
    a. pressure-compensated flowmeter
    b. Bourdon gauge flowmeter
    c. ball valve flowmeter
    d. Thorpe-tube–type flowmeter

16. Figure 3-3 is an example of a:
    a. Bourdon gauge flowmeter
    b. ball valve flowmeter
    c. Venturi tube flowmeter
    d. pressure-compensated flowmeter

17. Figure 3-4 is an example of a:
    a. constant flow selector valve
    b. pressure-compensated flowmeter
    c. Thorpe-tube–type flowmeter
    d. Venturi tube flowmeter

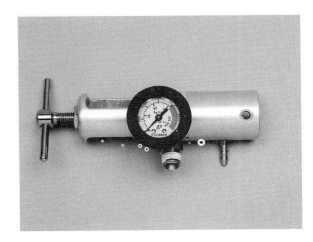

Figure 3-4

18. A disadvantage associated with the flowmeter in Figure 3-2 is that it:
    a. cannot be used with a "D" tank
    b. is difficult to calibrate
    c. does not compensate for backpressure
    d. cannot provide flow rates greater than 5 L/min

19. A potential problem with the flowmeter in Figure 3-3 is that it:
    a. is affected by gravity
    b. cannot be used with onboard ambulance oxygen systems
    c. is not accurate
    d. cannot be used to administer oxygen to infants or children

20. To administer oxygen to a conscious child who will not tolerate a mask, the EMT may need to:
    a. increase the flow rate to a cannula
    b. administer oxygen using a blow-by technique to increase the concentration of the surrounding air
    c. place an adult mask over the child's entire face
    d. place a child mask tightly over the child's face and restrain the patient's hands

21. The airway that is least likely to stimulate vomiting in a semiconscious patient with an intact gag reflex is the:
    a. oropharyngeal airway
    b. nasopharyngeal airway
    c. dual-lumen airway
    d. endotracheal airway

22. When a single rescuer is using a bag-valve-mask or flow-restricted, oxygen-powered ventilation device, the EMT should:
    a. only use an adjunctive airway in adult patients
    b. only use an adjunctive airway for infants or children
    c. always use an adjunctive airway if the patient tolerates it
    d. only use a nasopharyngeal airway

23. To determine the proper size of an oral airway to be inserted, measure from the:
    a. patient's Adam's apple to the corner of the mouth
    b. angle of the patient's jaw to the Adam's apple
    c. angle of the patient's jaw to the clavicle
    d. patient's earlobe to the corner of the mouth

24. To insert an oral airway in an adult, insert the airway:
    a. upside down, then rotate it 180 degrees
    b. by pushing the tip along the tongue
    c. until the flange lies immediately behind the teeth
    d. so the flange lies 1" beyond the lips

25. To determine the proper size of a nasopharyngeal airway to be inserted, measure from the:
    a. patient's upper lip to the Adam's apple
    b. tip of the patient's nose to the earlobe
    c. patient's nostril to the chin
    d. corner of the patient's mouth to the Adam's apple

26. When inserting a nasopharyngeal airway:
    a. force the airway if resistance is met
    b. attempt to insert the airway in the left nostril first
    c. do not try the other nostril if resistance is felt when inserting the airway in the first nostril
    d. lubricate the airway with a water-based jelly first

27. If a patient is not breathing, the EMT should:
    a. immediately begin ventilating with an appropriate ventilation device
    b. wait until oxygen is available to begin ventilations
    c. delay ventilations until an adjunctive airway is available
    d. never ventilate an adult patient at a rate greater than 12 times per minute

28. The EMT should assist with ventilation of an adult patient if the breathing rate falls below:
    a. 8 breaths per minute
    b. 12 breaths per minute
    c. 14 breaths per minute
    d. 16 breaths per minute

29. A bag-valve-mask should be connected to oxygen:
    a. only if the patient is cyanotic
    b. only when ventilating infants or children
    c. only if the patient has no history of breathing problems
    d. whenever it is available

30. The advantage of using a flow-restricted, oxygen-powered ventilation device versus a bag-valve-mask is that:
    a. an oral or nasal airway is not needed
    b. it does not need a mask
    c. it is easier for one rescuer to use
    d. it requires no training to use

31. A flow-restricted, oxygen-powered ventilation device should not be used on:
    a. infants and small children
    b. any trauma patient
    c. patients who are breathing
    d. patients without a gag reflex

32. A flow-restricted, oxygen-powered ventilation device:
    a. can be used if the oxygen tank becomes empty
    b. provides only 60% oxygen
    c. provides flow rates of 20 L/min
    d. may produce gastric distention due to the high pressure of the oxygen being delivered

33. A major problem associated with the use of a bag-valve-mask is:
    a. difficulty maintaining a good seal with the mask
    b. inability to deliver an adequate concentration of oxygen
    c. an inability to see if the patient has vomited
    d. that it is difficult for two operators to use

34. If a patient with an oral airway in place becomes conscious and regains a gag reflex:
    a. restrain the patient and keep the airway in place
    b. remove the airway and suction the patient if necessary
    c. remove the airway and insert a smaller one
    d. replace the oral airway with an endotracheal tube

35. A suction unit should provide a vacuum of:
    a. no more than 100 mm Hg of negative pressure
    b. no more than 200 mm Hg of negative pressure
    c. no less than 300 mm Hg of negative pressure
    d. no less than 400 mm Hg of negative pressure

36. Two common types of suction catheters used by EMTs are:
    a. hard and rigid
    b. French and soft
    c. hard and soft
    d. English and tonsil tip

37. When suctioning a patient, the EMT should:
    a. insert the catheter without suction
    b. suction only while advancing the catheter
    c. not be concerned with wearing gloves as there should be no physical contact with the patient
    d. be careful not to rotate the catheter

38. The maximum length of time the EMT should suction an adult patient is:
    a. 5 seconds at a time
    b. 15 seconds at a time
    c. 20 seconds at a time
    d. 25 seconds at a time

39. A soft suction catheter should not be inserted farther than the:
    a. larynx
    b. first set of molars
    c. trachea
    d. base of the tongue

✳ ENRICHMENT QUESTIONS

40. A hydrostatic test should be conducted on a steel oxygen tank every:
    a. 2 years
    b. 5 years
    c. 8 years
    d. 12 years

41. An oxygen regulator:
    a. increases pressure to 100 psi
    b. provides a constant flow rate of 25 L/min
    c. is needed only on oxygen tanks larger than "E" size
    d. reduces pressure to 40 to 70 psi

42. Generally the pressure in an oxygen cylinder should not be allowed to drop below:
    a. 50 psi
    b. 200 psi
    c. 500 psi
    d. 1,000 psi

43. Inspiration takes place when the:
    a. diaphragm relaxes and the accessory muscles lift the sternum and upper ribs
    b. diaphragm contracts and the intercostal muscles lift the ribs upward and outward
    c. intercostal muscles relax and the diaphragm moves upward
    d. accessory muscles relax and the diaphragm moves downward

44. When a patient breathes:
    a. exhalation is an active process whereas inhalation is a passive process
    b. both inhalation and exhalation are primarily active processes
    c. inhalation is an active process whereas exhalation is a passive process
    d. both inhalation and exhalation are primarily passive processes

45. A reliable sign that a patient in cardiac arrest is being adequately ventilated is if:
    a. the patient becomes cyanotic
    b. breath sounds are heard over the epigastric area
    c. the pupils become dilated
    d. the patient's chest rises and falls as each ventilation is delivered

■ ENDOTRACHEAL INTUBATION

46. The leaf-shaped, flexible cartilage that hangs over the larynx to protect the trachea is the:
    a. pharynx
    b. carina
    c. epiglottis
    d. vallecula

47. A potential complication that may occur during intubation is:
    a. bradycardia
    b. tachycardia
    c. tachypnea
    d. hyperpyrexia

48. The laryngoscope should be held in:
    a. the left hand
    b. the EMT's dominant hand
    c. the right hand
    d. either hand

49. To raise the epiglottis out of the way, the tip of a curved laryngoscope blade should be inserted into the:
    a. glottic opening
    b. vallecula
    c. carotid sinus
    d. carina

50. The type of laryngoscope blade that should be positioned under the epiglottis to expose the glottic opening is the:
    a. curved blade
    b. MacIntosh blade
    c. straight blade
    d. curved or MacIntosh blade

51. When immediate placement of an endotracheal tube is required, the most common size of tube used for an adult is:
    a. 6.5 mm
    b. 7.0 mm
    c. 7.5 mm
    d. 8.0 mm

52. After placing an endotracheal tube, the cuff should usually be filled with:
    a. 3 to 5 mL of air
    b. 5 to 10 mL of air
    c. 10 to 15 mL of air
    d. 15 to 20 mL of air

53. The advantage of the endotracheal tube over an EOA or dual-lumen airway is that the endotracheal tube:
    a. protects the airway from aspiration of gastric contents
    b. is easier to place
    c. can be placed without the use of special instruments
    d. works well in semiconscious patients

54. One way to confirm proper placement of an endotracheal tube is to:
    a. listen for sounds in the lower abdomen
    b. observe for fluid in the tube
    c. note the numerical markings on the tube
    d. attach an end-tidal CO_2 detector to the tube

55. The most critical complication of endotracheal intubation is:
    a. right mainstem bronchus placement
    b. unrecognized esophageal placement
    c. broken teeth
    d. traumatic injuries to the tongue

56. When intubating a non-trauma patient, the head should be:
    a. hyperflexed
    b. placed in a neutral position
    c. tilted slightly forward
    d. placed in the sniffing position

57. When intubating a trauma patient, the head should be:
    a. placed in the sniffing position
    b. hyperflexed
    c. in a neutral, in-line position
    d. slightly hyperextended

58. When properly placed in an endotracheal tube, the tip of the stylet should:
    a. not protrude from the end of the airway
    b. extend no more than ½" out the end of the airway
    c. not extend past the middle of the airway
    d. extend approximately 1" out the end of the airway

59. When inserting the laryngoscope blade into the patient's mouth:
    a. insert the blade into the middle of the mouth and allow the tongue to wrap around both sides of the blade
    b. insert the blade into the right side of the mouth and displace the tongue to the left
    c. insert the blade into the left side of the mouth and displace the tongue to the right
    d. insert the blade into the middle of the mouth and displace the tongue to the right

60. If after inserting an endotracheal tube and listening to lung sounds, sounds are heard only on the right side, the EMT should:
    a. deflate the cuff, pull the airway out, and reattempt intubation
    b. deflate the cuff and push the airway in slightly
    c. leave the airway in place and ventilate at a faster rate
    d. deflate the cuff and pull the airway back slightly

61. Most adult patients can be intubated using a:
    a. size 0 straight blade
    b. size 1 curved blade
    c. size 2 straight blade
    d. size 3 curved blade

62. Uncuffed endotracheal tubes should generally be used:
    a. only for infants below the age of 1 year
    b. for children between the age of 1 and 10 years
    c. for children over the age of 5 years
    d. for children under the age of 8 years

63. A technique for deciding what size endotracheal tube to insert in an infant or child is to match the tube size to the:
    a. diameter of the patient's little finger
    b. diameter of the patient's thumb
    c. diameter of the laryngoscope blade being used
    d. patient's age in years

64. While one EMT attempts to intubate the patient, a second EMT can assist by:
    a. performing chest compressions
    b. performing the Heimlich maneuver
    c. holding the laryngoscope
    d. performing the Sellick's maneuver

■ **Additional Points for Discussion** ■

1. At what point does your service refill or replace its portable or on-board oxygen tanks?

2. What is your department's procedure for refilling or replacing oxygen tanks?

3. How would you handle a situation in which multiple patients require mass oxygen administration?

4. Review the operation of your department's on-board and portable suction units.

ANSWERS TO CHAPTER 3 REVIEW QUESTIONS

1. **b.** An "E" tank will hold approximately 625 L of oxygen. A "D" tank will hold 350 L, and an "M" tank 3,000 L.

2. **c.** The pressure in a full oxygen tank is approximately 2,000 psi.

3. **d.** The date circled is the date of the last hydrostatic test.

4. **c.** The tank's safe working pressure is 2,015 psi. This corresponds to the last four digits of the first line stamped on the tank in Figure 3-1.

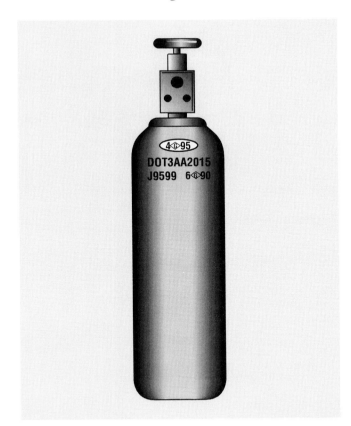

Figure 3-1

5. **d.** "D" and "E" tanks are most commonly used in portable oxygen units. "M" and "G" tanks are commonly used for on-board ambulance oxygen systems.

6. **a.** To "crack" the valve of an oxygen tank, quickly open and close the valve before attaching the regulator to the tank. This blows any dust or dirt out of the valve, thereby protecting the regulator from foreign material that could compromise its operation.

7. **d.** When using supplemental oxygen with a pocket mask or bag-valve-mask, the flowmeter should be set at 15 L/min. If a pocket mask without oxygen inlet is all that is available, a nasal cannula may be worn by the rescuer performing ventilations to increase the concentration of delivered oxygen.

8. **a.** A nasal cannula will oxygenate a patient who is breathing through the mouth provided the nasopharynx is patent. This is because the oropharynx acts a reservoir for the oxygen being delivered, thereby enriching the concentration of oxygen of the air breathed through the mouth. Patients with nasal obstructions, however, will not benefit much from use of a nasal cannula.

9. **c.** A child- or infant-size mask may be placed over the stoma of a laryngectomy patient to provide supplemental oxygen. The use of a humidifier is recommended because the oxygen bypasses the normal structures of the nose and throat, which would naturally humidify it.

10. **b.** Any patient in shock, especially due to trauma, should receive high-flow oxygen via a nonrebreather mask. This is true even if the patient has a history of breathing problems such as emphysema. Early administration is important. Do not wait for victim removal to start giving oxygen.

11. **d.** The proper flow rate when using a nonrebreather mask is 15 L/min in all cases.

12. **b.** The reservoir of a nonrebreather mask allows delivery of high concentrations of oxygen. The reservoir should be filled with oxygen prior to placing the mask on the patient. If the reservoir deflates completely with each patient breath, the oxygen flow rate to the mask is too low and should be increased. There are no circumstances under which the reservoir should be removed.

13. **a.** The nasal cannula should only be used when a patient will not tolerate a nonrebreather mask despite reassurances from EMTs that adequate oxygen is being delivered.

14. **c.** When using a nasal cannula, flow rates greater than 6 L/min are of little value.

15. **b.** A Bourdon gauge flowmeter is shown in Figure 3-2.

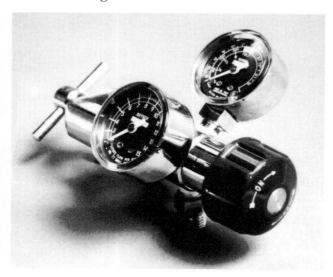

Figure 3-2

16. **d.** A pressure-compensated flowmeter is shown in Figure 3-3.

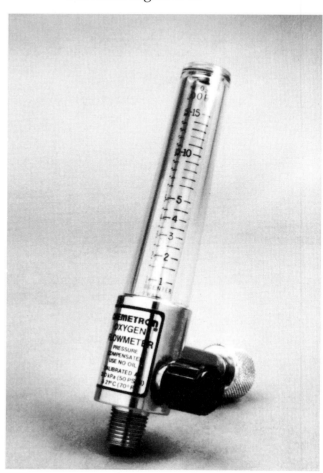

Figure 3-3

17. **a.** Figure 3-4 shows an example of a constant-flow selector valve. This type of valve allows for the adjustment of flow in stepped increments.

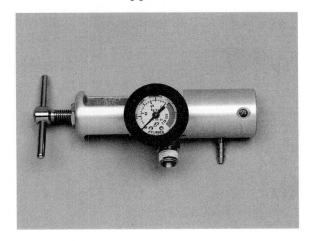

Figure 3-4

18. **c.** The flowmeter in Figure 3-2 does not compensate for backpressure. It is, however, commonly used on portable oxygen systems since it provides high flow rates and is easy to use.

19. **a.** The disadvantage with the flowmeter in Figure 3-3 is it is affected by gravity. It must be used in an upright position and is very accurate when used correctly. Although this type of flowmeter is not good for use with portable oxygen systems, it does work well with on-board systems.

20. **b.** To administer oxygen to a conscious child who will not tolerate a mask, use a blow-by technique. This may be accomplished through various methods. Oxygen tubing can be held about 2" from the patient's face, or it may be inserted into a paper cup held near the child's face. Or, an oxygen mask may be held near the child's face. The objective is to increase the concentration of oxygen in the surrounding air. A good indication of how badly the child needs oxygen is whether he or she will accept it. Seriously ill or injured infants or children usually do not fight the oxygen mask.

21. **b.** A nasopharyngeal airway, although often overlooked by EMTs, is better tolerated in a semiconscious patient with a gag reflex. Oral airways, dual-lumen airways, and endotracheal tubes can only be used when the gag reflex is absent or deeply depressed.

22. **c.** If the patient will tolerate it, an adjunctive airway should always be used when ventilating a patient with a flow-restricted, oxygen-powered ventilation device or when a single rescuer is using a bag-valve-mask. Various airways are available for use with patients of all ages.

23. **d.** Measuring from the bottom of the patient's earlobe to the corner of the mouth will provide a useful guide for sizing an oral airway. The EMT can also measure from the corner of the patient's mouth to the angle of the jaw.

24. **a.** To place an oral airway in an adult, insert it upside-down and then rotate it 180 degrees. An alternate method is to use a tongue depressor to manage the tongue while inserting the airway right-side up.

25. **b.** To determine the proper size of a nasopharyngeal airway to be inserted, measure from the tip of the nose to the earlobe or to the angle of the jaw.

26. **d.** Prior to inserting a nasopharyngeal airway, lubricate it with a water-based lubricant. Do not use petroleum jelly. Since the bevel should be toward the septum, most nasopharyngeal airways are designed to be placed in the right nostril, but if resistance is met, the other nostril can be attempted.

27. **a.** If a patient is not breathing, the EMT should immediately begin ventilating with an appropriate ventilation device. Although an airway and oxygen should be used as soon as possible with such patients, the EMT should not delay ventilations to wait for either. The ventilation rate does not have to be limited to 12 times a minute. Patients in need of oxygen should be hyperventilated in the early stages of ventilatory management.

28. **a.** As a general rule, if a patient's breathing rate falls below 8 breaths a minute, the EMT should assist breathing. Some patients with higher breathing rates may also need assistance. Decisions should be based on the patient's overall condition, not simply the breathing rate.

29. **d.** Although a bag-valve-mask can be used with room air, supplemental oxygen should be connected to the device whenever it is available. Also, an oxygen reservoir should always be attached. In essence, the bag-valve-mask should be considered a multi-part system, and all its parts (i.e., the bag-valve-mask, oxygen reservoir, and tubing) should be stored together.

30. **c.** The advantage to using a flow-restricted, oxygen-powered ventilation device over a bag-valve-mask is that it is easier for a single rescuer to use. The device uses the same type of mask as a bag-valve-mask, and an airway should be used. EMTs need training to properly use the device.

31. **a.** Flow-restricted, oxygen-powered ventilation devices should not be used on infants or small children (consult local protocols for exact age criteria). They can be used on some trauma patients and in patients without a gag reflex. The devices may be used to support ventilations in a patient who is breathing.

32. **d.** The pressure generated with a flow-restricted, oxygen-powered ventilation device may cause gastric distention. They deliver 100% oxygen at flow rates of 40 L/min. Such devices will not operate if the oxygen tank becomes empty.

33. **a.** The major problem associated with a bag-valve-mask, especially when it is used by one rescuer, is an inability to maintain a good seal with the mask to adequately ventilate the patient. This problem can be decreased if two EMT-Basics use the device, with one maintaining a mask seal and the other squeezing the bag. Bag-valve-masks are capable of delivering high concentrations of oxygen. Clear facemasks should be used so the EMT can see if the patient vomits.

34. **b.** If a gag reflex develops in a patient with an oral airway in place, remove the airway and suction the patient if necessary.

35. **c.** Suction units should provide no less than 300 mm Hg of negative pressure.

36. **c.** The hard suction catheter (also known as a rigid catheter, tonsil tip, tonsil sucker, or Yankauer) and soft suction catheter (also known as a French catheter) are commonly used by EMTs.

37. **a.** When suctioning a patient, insert the catheter without suction. Suction should be applied only while withdrawing the catheter. Rotating the catheter between the fingers with a twirling motion will keep the tip from sticking to the tissue and will cover all areas being suctioned. The EMT should wear gloves while suctioning.

38. **b.** An adult patient should not be suctioned for longer than 15 seconds at a time. The goal of suctioning a patient's airway is to clear the airway. But remember, while suctioning fluids the EMT is also suctioning oxygen. It may be necessary to suction the patient a number of times to thoroughly clear the airway. Oxygenate the patient between each suctioning period.

39. **d.** A soft suction catheter should not be inserted farther than the base of the patient's tongue.

✸ **ENRICHMENT QUESTIONS**

40. **b.** Steel oxygen tanks should be hydrostatically tested every 5 years. Although some sources say aluminum oxygen tanks need only be tested every 10 years, it is recommended that aluminum tanks also be tested every 5 years.

41. **d.** The first stage of an oxygen regulator reduces the pressure of the oxygen coming from the cylinder to 40 to 70 psi.

42. **b.** Generally, the pressure of an oxygen tank should not be allowed to fall below 200 psi. This is called the safe residual pressure. Allowing the pressure to drop below this point may allow moisture and dirt to enter the tank, which may cause rust in steel tanks. Many departments refill portable oxygen tanks long before reaching the safe residual pressure so as to ensure an adequate supply of oxygen at an emergency scene. Always follow department policy.

43. **b.** During inspiration, the diaphragm contracts as it moves downward. At the same time, intercostal muscles lift the ribs upward and outward and accessory muscles lift the sternum and upper ribs. All this enlarges the thoracic cavity, thereby reducing pressure within the chest and allowing air to enter the lungs.

44. **c.** During inspiration, the diaphragm and other muscles must contract. Therefore, inhalation is considered an active process. In contrast, exhalation is considered a passive process since it occurs when the muscles simply relax.

45. **d.** A reliable sign that a patient in cardiac arrest is being adequately ventilated is if the chest rises and falls as each ventilation is delivered. Cyanosis is a sign of inadequate oxygenation, and breath sounds heard over the epigastric area indicate air is entering the stomach. Pupils can be expected to become dilated the longer the patient is in cardiac arrest.

■ ENDOTRACHEAL INTUBATION

46. **c.** The epiglottis is the leaf-shaped, flexible cartilage that hangs over the larynx and keeps liquids and solids from entering the trachea. The pharynx is the area directly posterior to the mouth and nose, the carina is the lower end of the trachea where the right and left mainstem bronchi branch, and the vallecula is a groove-like structure anterior to the epiglottis.

47. **a.** When intubating a patient, the patient's heart rate may slow (bradycardia). This can result from stimulation of the nerves that regulate the heart rate, as well as from hypoxia.

48. **a.** The laryngoscope should be held in EMT's left hand regardless of whether he or she is left- or right-handed.

49. **b.** To raise the epiglottis out of the way, the tip of a curved laryngoscope blade should be inserted into the vallecula. The epiglottis is then indirectly lifted.

50. **c.** A straight blade is used to directly lift the epiglottis, thereby exposing the glottic opening. A MacIntosh blade is a type of curved blade.

51. **c.** When immediate placement of an endotracheal tube is required, the most common size tube used for an adult is the 7.5 mm. As a general rule, adult females require a 7.0- to 8.0-mm tube and males require an 8.0- to 8.5-mm tube.

52. **b.** After placing an endotracheal tube, the cuff should be filled with 5 to 10 mL of air.

53. **a.** Although it is more complicated to perform and requires special instruments, the advantage of the endotracheal over an EOA or dual-lumen airway is that the endotracheal tube protects the airway from aspiration of gastric contents. Endotracheal intubation should not be performed on a semiconscious patient with a gag reflex.

54. **d.** Proper placement of an endotracheal tube can be verified by attaching an end-tidal CO_2 detector to the tube. The detector senses the presence of carbon dioxide in the exhaled breath. An esophageal intubation detector device may also be used. Although the numerical markings show how deep the tube is, they do not indicate whether the tube is in the trachea or esophagus.

55. **b.** The most critical complication of endotracheal intubation is unrecognized esophageal placement, which can be fatal. Right mainstem bronchus placement, broken teeth, and tongue injuries are also potential complications, but they are not usually fatal.

56. **d.** When intubating a non-trauma patient, the head should be placed in the sniffing position. To accomplish this, the neck is flexed and the head is extended at the base of the skull. A towel may be placed under the supine patient's occiput to help accomplish this.

57. **c.** When intubating a non-trauma patient, the head should be placed in a neutral, in-line position.

58. **a.** When properly placed in an endotracheal tube, the tip of the stylet should not protrude from the end of the airway. It is best if it does not extend past the proximal end of the Murphy's eye.

59. **b.** When inserting the laryngoscope blade into the patient's mouth, insert the blade into the right side of the mouth and displace the tongue to the left.

60. **d.** If lung sounds are only heard on the right side, remove air from the cuff and pull the airway back slightly.

61. **d.** Most adults can be intubated using a size 3 curved or straight blade.

62. **d.** Uncuffed endotracheal tubes are generally used for children less than 8 years old.

63. **a.** A technique for deciding what size endotracheal tube to insert in an infant or child is to match the tube size to the diameter of the patient's little finger or nasal opening.

64. **d.** While one EMT attempts to intubate the patient, a second EMT can perform the Sellick's maneuver, that is, provide cricoid pressure. This Sellick's maneuver helps to compress the esophagus, thereby reducing the risk of the patient regurgitating. Chest compressions should be discontinued during intubation attempts, and the EMT performing the intubation should hold both the laryngoscope and the endotracheal tube. The Heimlich maneuver is abdominal compressions used to relieve an obstructed airway and is not performed when attempting intubation.

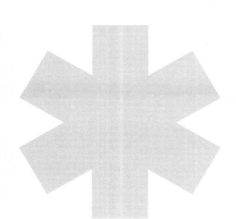

4

Patient Assessment

CHAPTER 4 REVIEW QUESTIONS

1. Scene size up:
   a. includes taking appropriate body substance isolation measures
   b. is only necessary when approaching a trauma scene
   c. should be performed immediately following the initial patient assessment
   d. is the responsibility of the senior EMT on the crew

2. If a scene is not safe and the EMT cannot make it safe:
   a. enter only if the patient's life is in immediate danger
   b. do not enter
   c. one EMT should enter while another stands by for assistance to arrive
   d. return to the station until the scene becomes safe

3. Match the following injuries with their likely mechanism of injury:
   chest injury
   head/cervical spine injury
   hip injury

   _____ windshield broken in a "spiderweb" pattern

   _____ broken car dashboard

   _____ accident in the shallow end of a swimming pool

   _____ bent steering wheel or steering column

4. The initial assessment includes the EMT's general impression of the patient and evaluating, in order, the patient's:
   a. mental status, airway, breathing, and circulation
   b. level of consciousness, blood pressure, and pulse
   c. airway, pulse, blood pressure, and responsiveness
   d. pulse, bleeding, airway, and family history

5. When a life-threatening condition is discovered during the initial assessment:
   a. immediately skip to a focused trauma history
   b. note it and correct it during the appropriate part of the detailed physical exam
   c. manage the problem immediately
   d. note the condition on the run report and let the hospital deal with it

6. Cervical spine stabilization should first be accomplished:
   a. while the secondary survey is being performed
   b. after the patient is log-rolled onto the backboard
   c. when the patient's mental status is being assessed
   d. after the vital signs have been checked

7. When using the AVPU scale for noting a patient's level of consciousness, *V* would signify that the patient:
   a. is "vocal" and able to speak
   b. responds to "verbal" stimuli
   c. responds to "visual" stimuli
   d. has spontaneous "ventilations"

8. The letter *P* in AVPU refers to whether the patient:
   a. is oriented to "place"
   b. is a "priority" patient
   c. has a "pulse"
   d. responds to "painful" stimuli

9. When assessing and reassessing mental status, it is important to note:
   a. precisely how the patient answers the questions
   b. whether the EMT thinks the patient is intoxicated
   c. any changes for the better or worse
   d. all of the above

10. To open the airway of an unresponsive trauma patient, use the:
    a. chin lift
    b. head tilt
    c. modified jaw thrust
    d. neck lift

11. Part of maintaining adequate oxygenation in a trauma patient involves:
    a. placing the patient in a pneumatic antishock garment (PASG)
    b. placing the patient in the shock position
    c. sealing open chest wounds
    d. sitting the patient upright

12. When examining a severely injured or unconscious multisystem trauma patient, it is important to:
    a. remove as little of the patient's clothing as possible
    b. remove all the patient's clothing
    c. remove clothing only around areas of obvious injury or pain
    d. remove no clothing, as this may cause hypothermia

13. For the EMT-Basic, an important part of assessing circulation in all patients includes:
    a. checking a pedal pulse
    b. examining the pupils
    c. checking capillary refill time
    d. checking for major bleeding

14. Fill in each blank of the following list with *Y* (for yes) or *N* (for no) regarding whether the patient would be considered a priority patient.

    _____ Unresponsive patient without a gag reflex

    _____ Pregnant female in labor with no complications

    _____ Elderly male patient complaining of feeling tired

    _____ 48-year-old male patient with chest pain and a blood pressure of 90/60 mm Hg

    _____ 19-year-old female patient with a severe leg laceration that is bleeding uncontrollably

    _____ 16-year-old female patient who experienced chest pain an hour ago but has no pain now

    _____ Patient having severe difficulty breathing

    _____ Patient experiencing signs of hypoperfusion

    _____ Pregnant female patient with breech birth presentation

    _____ Patient with an isolated painful, swollen, deformed extremity with good distal pulses

    _____ Patient experiencing severe abdominal pain

    _____ Conscious patient who is disoriented and does not follow commands

    _____ 28-year-old male patient complaining of nausea and vomiting

    _____ Diabetic patient who was weak and lightheaded but claims to feel fine after drinking sweetened orange juice

    _____ Driver of a vehicle struck from the rear by another vehicle at low speed complaining of upper back and neck pain

15. When a priority patient is identified, the EMT should:
    a. call for Advanced Life Support assistance and wait at the scene
    b. expedite transport to an appropriate medical facility
    c. call medical control and request further instructions for on-scene management
    d. transport the patient to the hospital that he or she has requested

16. When an EMT encounters a patient from a vehicle where an airbag was deployed:
    a. there is little chance of the patient receiving significant injury
    b. the patient has no serious injuries if they appear stable after the first 5 to 10 minutes
    c. check the patient for steam burns
    d. lift the airbag and check the steering wheel for damage

17. A rapid trauma assessment should be performed on:
    a. any unresponsive trauma patient
    b. all trauma patients
    c. any patient complaining of neck pain
    d. any patient with a painful, swollen, deformed extremity

18. A rapid trauma assessment is a:
    a. rapid evaluation of the patient's airway and cervical spine
    b. methodical examination limited to the area of injury
    c. rapid examination of the mechanism of injury and scene
    d. quick head-to-toe examination

19. Ideally, a rapid trauma assessment should be performed in:
    a. 10 to 30 seconds
    b. 30 to 60 seconds
    c. 60 to 90 seconds
    d. 90 to 120 seconds

20. When a multisystem trauma patient is encountered:
    a. deal with life-threatening conditions first
    b. focus on the patient's most painful injury first
    c. focus on the injury that appears to be most serious first
    d. do not manage any injuries until the rapid trauma assessment is complete

Questions 21 through 28 refer to the acronym DCAP-BTLS as it relates to assessment.

21. The letter *D* refers to:
    a. "dizziness"
    b. "deformities"
    c. "difficulty" breathing
    d. "distal" pulses

22. During the *C* portion, check the patient for:
    a. "cardiac" problems
    b. "chest" injuries
    c. "contusions"
    d. "carotid" pulses

23. *A* refers to the presence of:
    a. "airway" problems
    b. "avulsions"
    c. "allergies"
    d. "abrasions"

24. The letter *P* is connected with:
    a. "penetrations or punctures"
    b. "pain"
    c. checking the patient's "pulse"
    d. if the patient is female, whether she is "pregnant"

25. *B* relates to:
    a. checking the patient's "back"
    b. "backboarding" the patient
    c. assessing the patient's "breathing"
    d. checking for "burns"

26. *T* reminds the EMT to:
    a. assess the patient's "trachea"
    b. check for loose "teeth"
    c. look for "tenderness"
    d. question the patient about "time"

27. The letter *L* refers to the presence of:
    a. "lightheadedness"
    b. "lacerations"
    c. "lethargy"
    d. "liquids" coming from the ears or nose

28. *S* represents:
    a. "sweating"
    b. "skin" color
    c. "swelling"
    d. "severity" of injuries

29. When assessing the patient's neck, the EMT should look for:
    a. carotid artery distention
    b. laryngospasms
    c. jugular vein distention
    d. tracheal enlargement

30. If, as a patient breathes, a section of the chest wall moves the opposite direction from the rest of the chest, this is referred to as:
    a. paroxysmal movement
    b. oppositional motion
    c. paradoxical motion
    d. inordinate movement

31. If a conscious trauma patient is complaining of severe pain in the pelvic region:
    a. do not flex or compress the pelvic girdle
    b. compress the pelvic region to see if compression elicits further pain
    c. log-roll the patient onto his or her side and assess the posterior pelvis
    d. have the patient move his or her legs into a position that relieves the pain

32. Evaluation of the adult patient's extremities involves checking for DCAP-BTLS and:
    a. capillary refill, sensation, and circulation
    b. circulation, motor function, and sensation
    c. reflexes, pulses, and color
    d. blood pressure, reflexes, and motor function

33. An often overlooked but important part of the focused history and physical exam of the trauma patient is checking the patient's:
    a. posterior body
    b. airway
    c. reflexes
    d. mental status

34. If only one EMT is present, the rapid trauma assessment should be performed:
    a. before the initial assessment
    b. after baseline vital signs and history are obtained
    c. before any cervical spine precautions are taken
    d. after an initial assessment is done

35. When managing a patient with single-system trauma, such as a lacerated arm, the focused history and physical exam should:
    a. start at the head, then work toward the injury
    b. start at the site of the injury
    c. begin with reevaluation of the airway
    d. begin with cervical immobilization

36. When the EMT encounters an unresponsive medical patient, the next step after the initial assessment is:
    a. an assessment of the chest to evaluate the lungs and heart
    b. a detailed physical exam
    c. a rapid head-to-toe assessment similar to the rapid trauma assessment
    d. an abbreviated focused history

37. The assessment of a responsive medical patient:
    a. emphasizes the patient's vital signs
    b. is not as critical as that of an unresponsive patient if there is no history of medical problems
    c. can usually wait until the patient is moved to the ambulance
    d. is normally based on the patient's chief complaint

Questions 38 through 43 refer to the acronym O-P-Q-R-S-T.

38. The letter *O* refers to:
    a. the patient's last "oral" intake
    b. whether the patient is "oriented"
    c. the time of "onset" of the problem
    d. performing an "ongoing" assessment

39. The letter *P* relates to:
    a. severity of "pain"
    b. "provocation"
    c. what the main "problem" is
    d. the "primary" complaint

40. The letter *Q* refers to:
    a. how "quickly" the problem started
    b. the "quality" of the pain
    c. the "quantity" of medications regularly taken by the patient
    d. whether the patient "qualifies" as a priority patient

41. The letter *R* component involves asking the patient if:
    a. anything provides "relief" of the pain
    b. this is a "regular" problem
    c. the onset of the problem was "rapid"
    d. the pain "radiates" to other areas

42. The letter *S* is associated with:
    a. "symptoms"
    b. "severity"
    c. "signs"
    d. "sensation"

43. *T* refers to:
   a. "time"
   b. the patient's "temperature"
   c. whether the problem involves "trauma"
   d. the "type" of problem

44. When an unresponsive patient is encountered:
   a. O-P-Q-R-S-T information cannot be obtained
   b. it is not important to gain O-P-Q-R-S-T information
   c. O-P-Q-R-S-T information may be obtained from family, friends, or bystanders
   d. accurate O-P-Q-R-S-T information can only be obtained if the patient regains consciousness

45. The detailed physical exam is a:
   a. rapid neurological examination
   b. breathing and pulse check
   c. 15 minute thorough examination limited to the injured body system
   d. a methodical head-to-toe examination

46. The primary purpose of the detailed physical exam is to:
   a. check for signs of abuse or drug use
   b. find less serious hidden injuries or medical problems
   c. confirm a medical problem exists
   d. help the EMT diagnose the patient's problem

47. Of the following patients, the patient who would not need a complete and thorough detailed physical exam is:
   a. an unresponsive medical patient
   b. a trauma patient with an altered mental status
   c. a patient with a history of heart problems who is complaining of mild chest pain
   d. a patient who was ejected from a vehicle but is complaining only of shoulder pain

48. A major part of the detailed physical exam assesses:
   a. O-P-Q-R-S-T
   b. S-A-M-P-L-E history
   c. DCAP-BTLS
   d. A-B-Cs

49. When checking the patient's ears, the EMT should be alert for the presence of blood mixed with:
   a. vitreous humor
   b. cerebrospinal fluid
   c. synovial fluid
   d. lacrimal fluid

50. When assessing the patient's chest:
   a. look for paradoxical movement
   b. check breath sounds
   c. feel for crepitation
   d. all of the above

51. When palpating a patient's abdomen, it is generally considered to be normal if it is:
   a. hard
   b. soft
   c. distended
   d. rigid

52. Ideally, the detailed physical exam should be performed:
   a. while still in the house
   b. prior to leaving for the hospital
   c. after Advanced Life Support personnel arrive
   d. while en route to the hospital

53. When performing the ongoing assessment:
   a. ensure adequacy of oxygen delivery and artificial ventilations, and the adequacy of EMT interventions
   b. repeat a head-to-toe exam
   c. record the vital signs and S-A-M-P-L-E history every 10 minutes
   d. perform a detailed physical exam

54. A stable patient should receive an ongoing assessment every:
    a. 5 minutes
    b. 10 minutes
    c. 15 minutes
    d. 20 minutes

55. In essence, the ongoing assessment repeats all the components of the:
    a. detailed physical exam
    b. initial assessment
    c. rapid trauma assessment
    d. S-A-M-P-L-E history

56. An important component of patient assessment that must not be neglected is:
    a. providing emotional reassurance to the patient
    b. obtaining insurance information for billing purposes
    c. passing information on to law enforcement officers
    d. assuring the patient everything will be all right

✳ Enrichment Questions

57. When an injured patient is found at a crime scene:
    a. have the police bring the patient to the EMTs to provide patient care
    b. wait to begin patient care until law enforcement officials have completed their investigation
    c. try to disturb the scene as little as possible while providing patient care
    d. immediately move the patient to the ambulance prior to providing any care

58. The problem with asking a patient involved in a vehicle crash, "Where are you?" when checking their level of consciousness is:
    a. the patient really may not know where he or she is
    b. street signs may be missing
    c. the EMTs may not know where they are
    d. it does not stimulate enough thinking

59. When checking a patient's orientation to person, place, time, and purpose, the last thing the patient will normally forget is:
    a. place
    b. person
    c. purpose
    d. time

60. A legitimate reason for an EMT to search the wallet of an unconscious patient is:
    a. to look for pertinent medical information, such as a medic alert card
    b. to look for illegal drugs that may have been taken by the patient
    c. to remove money for safekeeping
    d. all of the above

61. When palpating a patient's neck and upper chest, you note it appears swollen and you feel a crackling sensation such as when you pop bubble wrap. This condition is known as:
    a. rales
    b. ischemia
    c. subcutaneous emphysema
    d. parenchyma

62. Wheezing can be described as a:
    a. harsh, raspy sound created by fluid in the lungs
    b. crowing sound heard on inspiration
    c. fine, crackling sound indicating the presence of fluid in the small airways
    d. high-pitched, whistling sound created as air flows through narrowed airways

63. When assessing the abdomen:
    a. inform the patient prior to starting palpation
    b. palpate using only one finger
    c. palpate only in the area of discomfort
    d. press as deeply as possible

64. When a vehicle with a deployed airbag is encountered:
    a. lift the airbag and check for damage to the steering wheel
    b. disconnect the battery before assessing the patient
    c. do not enter the vehicle if a haze is present
    d. cut the airbag with a sharp instrument to prevent it from re-inflating

If your training includes the use of the Glasgow Coma Scale when assessing patients, complete questions 65 through 67. Refer to the Glasgow Coma Scale in Figure 4-1.

1. **Eye opening**	Points	
● Spontaneous	4	
● To voice	3	
● To pain	2	
● None	1	_____
2. **Verbal response**	Points	
● Oriented	5	
● Confused	4	
● Inappropriate words	3	
● Incomprehensible sounds	2	
● None	1	_____
3. **Motor response**	Points	
● Obeys commands	6	
● Localizes pain	5	
● Withdraws (pain)	4	
● Flexion (pain)	3	
● Extension (pain)	2	
● None	1	_____
Total (1 + 2 + 3)		_____

Figure 4-1

65. Your patient is a 30-year-old male who is lying on the sidewalk. His eyes are closed and he opens them only on voice command. He can speak, but his answers are inaccurate. During the examination, he reacts to pain by attempting to push your hand away from the painful area. His Glasgow Coma Scale score is:
    a. 11
    b. 12
    c. 13
    d. 14

66. A hit-and-run patient is found lying next to the road. She does not open her eyes in response to any stimulus. She does respond to painful stimuli by groaning and moving her arms away from the source of pain. Her Glasgow Coma Scale score is:
    a. 5
    b. 6
    c. 7
    d. 8

67. A Glasgow Coma Scale score that would be considered normal is:
    a. 9 to 10
    b. 11 to 12
    c. 14 to 15
    d. 17 to 18

■ Additional Points for Discussion ■

1. Many Emergency Medical Services have a number of hospitals to which they may transport their patients. Some of these medical facilities are specially equipped and staffed to handle certain types of emergencies. It is important for EMTs to be aware of the special skills or limitations of each hospital they use. To what hospitals or medical facilities in your area would you normally transport the following type of patient?

  • Multi-system trauma:

  • Critical burns:

  • Major head injury or neurological problem:

  • Unstable cardiac problems:

  • Critical obstetrical emergency:

  • Contamination with hazardous materials or radiation:

  • Amputation or severe avulsion that may possibly be surgically reattached:

2. If your service is a Basic Life Support service, is Advanced Life Support available from another service? When would you call for Advanced Life Support assistance?

ANSWERS TO CHAPTER 4 REVIEW QUESTIONS

1. **a.** Scene size-up includes taking appropriate body substance isolation measures. It should be done on all calls. The EMT must determine if scene is safe prior to assessing patient. Everyone on the crew is responsible for looking for unsafe situations.

2. **b.** If a scene is not safe and the EMT cannot make it safe, do not enter the scene. Remember, dead EMTs don't save lives.

3.

head/cervical spine injury	windshield broken in a "spiderweb" pattern
hip injury	broken car dashboard
head/cervical spine injury	accident in the shallow end of a swimming pool
chest injury	bent steering wheel or steering column

4. **a.** The initial assessment includes the EMT's general impressions of the patient and assessing the patient's mental status, airway, breathing, and circulation.

5. **c.** When a life-threatening condition is discovered during the initial assessment, it should be managed immediately.

6. **c.** Cervical spine stabilization should take place while the patient's mental status is being assessed.

7. **b.** The letter *V* signifies the patient responds to "verbal" stimuli, *A* corresponds to "alert," and *U* means the patient is "unresponsive" to any stimuli.

8. **d.** The letter *P* refers to whether the patient responds only to "painful" stimuli.

9. **c.** When assessing and reassessing mental status, it is important to note any changes for the better or worse. Changes are important because they act as a baseline for comparison. The patient's answers do not need to be written verbatim. Although a patient may appear to be intoxicated, even someone who has been drinking may have underlying trauma or a medical problem affecting their mental status.

10. **c.** Use the modified jaw thrust to open the airway of an unresponsive trauma patient.

11. **c.** Open chest wounds compromise the lungs' ability to function, therefore, they must be sealed with an occlusive dressing to maintain adequate oxygenation. Placing a trauma patient upright is contraindicated due to the possibility of cervical spine injury. Placing the patient in a PASG or the shock position will not ensure a patent airway.

12. **b.** It is generally recommended that the EMT remove all clothing from a seriously injured multisystem trauma patient, especially if the patient is unconscious and cannot verbally communicate. In many cases, it is not the injuries you see that will kill the patient, but rather the injuries you don't see. Discretion should be exercised to keep embarrassment to a minimum. Because it can be avoided by using blankets, hypothermia is not a valid reason to leave clothing in place.

13. **d.** While assessing circulation, the EMT should check for and correct major bleeding.

14. Fill in each blank of the following list with a *Y* (for yes) or *N* (for no) regarding whether the patient would be considered a priority patient.

   __Y__ Unresponsive patient without a gag reflex

   __N__ Pregnant female in labor with no complications

   __N__ Elderly male patient complaining of feeling tired

   __Y__ 48-year-old male patient with chest pain and a blood pressure of 90/60 mm Hg

   __Y__ 19-year-old female patient with a severe leg laceration that is bleeding uncontrollably

   __N__ 16-year-old female patient who experienced chest pain an hour ago but has no pain now

   __Y__ Patient having severe difficulty breathing

   __Y__ Patient experiencing signs of hypoperfusion

   __Y__ Pregnant female patient with breech birth presentation

   __N__ Patient with an isolated painful, swollen, deformed extremity with good distal pulses

   __Y__ Patient experiencing severe abdominal pain

   __Y__ Conscious patient who is disoriented and does not follow commands

   __N__ 28-year-old male patient complaining of nausea and vomiting

   __N__ Diabetic patient who was weak and lightheaded but claims to feel fine after drinking sweetened orange juice

   __N__ Driver of a vehicle struck from the rear by another vehicle at low speed complaining of upper back and neck pain

15. **b.** When a priority patient is identified, expedite transport to an appropriate medical facility. If Advanced Life Support is available, it should be requested. However, do not delay transport for the arrival of an Advanced Life Support unit.

16. **d.** Although airbags can reduce the incidence of injuries from vehicle crashes, they can be misleading. A patient may sustain an injury yet not show immediate signs of the injury. If an airbag has been deployed, lift the airbag and check the steering wheel for deformity or damage. If either is noted, suspect injury to the patient.

17. **a.** A rapid trauma assessment should be performed on any unresponsive trauma patient as well as any trauma patient who has a significant mechanism of injury.

18. **d.** A rapid trauma assessment is a quick head-to-toe examination.

19. **c.** A rapid trauma assessment should be performed in 60 to 90 seconds

20. **a.** When a multisystem trauma patient is encountered, deal with life-threatening conditions first. Do not be fooled into focusing on the patient's most painful injury or the worst-appearing injury first.

21. **b.** The letter *D* refers to deformities.

22. **c.** *C* involves checking for contusions.

23. **d.** *A* refers to abrasions.

24. **a.** *P* is connected with penetrations or punctures.

25. **d.** *B* relates to checking for burns.

26. **c.** *T* should remind the EMT to look for tenderness.

27. **b.** *L* refers to lacerations.

28. **c.** *S* represents swelling.

29. **c.** When examining the neck, look for jugular vein distention. The veins in the neck will be abnormally enlarged.

30. **c.** Paradoxical motion refers to the unusual, opposite motion of a section of chest wall that may be seen when a patient sustains serious blunt force to the chest. The section of chest wall will move inward as the rest of the chest moves outward on inspiration, and outward as the rest of the chest moves inward on exhalation.

31. **a.** If a conscious trauma patient is complaining of severe pain in the pelvic region, do not flex or compress the pelvic girdle as this may cause further injury. If the patient is unconscious, checking the stability of the pelvis is warranted. Do not log-roll or move the legs of a patient with a suspected pelvic injury.

32. **b.** Evaluation of the patient's extremities includes checking circulation (distal pulses), motor function, and sensation.

33. **a.** Many EMTs often forget to check a patient's posterior body during the trauma assessment. Life-threatening injuries may be missed if this important part of the patient examination is forgotten. The patient's mental status and airway are checked during the initial assessment. Reflexes are not checked by EMTs.

34. **d.** If only one EMT is present, the rapid trauma assessment should be performed after an initial assessment is done. Vital signs and history are taken after the rapid assessment. Although it may be difficult when only one EMT is present, cervical spine precautions should still be taken to the best extent possible before the rapid trauma assessment is performed. If two EMTs are present, some procedures can be performed at the same time.

35. **b.** When managing a patient with single-system trauma, such as a lacerated arm, the focused history and physical exam should begin at the site of the injury. However, if the patient appears confused or there is a significant mechanism of injury, a complete head-to-toe examination is necessary.

36. **c.** When the EMT encounters an unresponsive medical patient, a rapid head-to-toe assessment similar to the rapid trauma assessment should be done after the initial assessment.

37. **d.** The assessment of a responsive medical patient is normally based on the patient's chief complaint. Do not delay assessment until the patient is in the ambulance. If assessment is delayed, then management of the patient such as assisting with medications may also be delayed.

38. **c.** The letter *O* refers to the time of "onset" of the problem. This is when the medical problem first started; the interval between onset and when EMS was called may be short or long.

39. **b.** The letter *P* stands for "provocation," that is, what made the pain start or what makes it worse.

40. **b.** The letter *Q* refers to the "quality" of the pain. This is a description of the characteristics of the discomfort, such as whether the pain is sharp, dull, or stabbing, or whether it is a constant or intermittent pressure.

41. **d.** The *R* involves asking the patient if the pain "radiates" to other areas of the body. However, if the patient is complaining of pain it may not radiate, but rather just stay in one place.

42. **b.** The letter *S* is associated with "severity."

43. **a.** The letter *T* refers to "time." Time primarily relates to duration of the pain, such as if pain has been going on for some time, or if it has increased or decreased. It is also important to note if there was a particular time when the problem got worse, prompting the patient to call EMS.

44. **c.** When an unresponsive patient is encountered, O-P-Q-R-S-T information may be obtained from family, friends, or bystanders.

45. **d.** The detailed physical exam is a methodical head-to-toe examination. Although it covers many items that were checked in the rapid trauma assessment, the detailed exam is slower, methodical, and more comprehensive. It expands upon the assessment steps in the focused history and physical exam.

46. **b.** The primary purpose of the detailed physical exam is to find less serious hidden injuries or medical problems.

47. **c.** A patient with a history of heart problems who is complaining of mild chest pain would not need a detailed physical exam because little information is likely to be gained from palpating every body part of this patient. This would also be true of a patient with minor single-system trauma such as a foot laceration. A detailed physical exam should be performed on any unresponsive medical and trauma patient, patients with altered mental status, or patients with a significant mechanism of injury involved.

48. **c.** A major part of the detailed physical exam assesses DCAP-BTLS.

49. **b.** Check for cerebrospinal fluid when checking the ears. If blood is also present, place some on a 4 × 4 gauze pad. If cerebrospinal fluid is mixed with the blood, it will form a halo-like ring of fluid around the blood in the middle. Vitreous humor is fluid within the eye, synovial fluid lubricates joints, and lacrimal fluid is tears.

50. **d.** All of the above. Check breath sounds when assessing the patient's chest. Note whether they are present or absent, and equal or unequal. Also, look for paradoxical movement and feel for crepitation.

51. **b.** When palpating a patient's abdomen, it is generally considered to be normal if it is soft. A hard, rigid, or distended abdomen is indicative of underlying abdominal problems including internal bleeding.

52. **d.** Ideally, the detailed physical exam should be performed in the back of the ambulance while en route to the hospital.

53. **a.** During the ongoing assessment, ensure adequacy of oxygen delivery and artificial ventilations, as well as the adequacy of EMT interventions, such as checking dressings and splints.

54. **c.** A stable patient should receive an ongoing assessment every 15 minutes. An unstable patient should be reassessed every 5 minutes or less.

55. **b.** In essence, the ongoing assessment repeats all the components of the initial assessment.

56. **a.** An important component of patient assessment that must not be neglected is providing emotional reassurance to the patient. Often, patients are distraught and worried about their condition. The EMT can help to alleviate some of the anxiety. However, do not tell the patient everything will be all right, as this may not be the case.

✻ Enrichment Questions

57. **c.** An injured patient at a crime scene still needs medical attention. However, try to disturb the scene as little as possible. The EMT must be careful not to be in such a hurry to move the patient that further harm is done.

58. **a.** The problem with asking a patient in a vehicle crash, "Where are you?" or "Do you know where you are?" is that many times the patient may be alert and yet not know where he or she is. A better question to ask, especially the elderly, is "Do you know where you were going?"

59. **b.** Normally the last thing patients forget is "person," that is, who they are. That is because this information is stored in long-term memory. Short-term memory, such as where they are (place), time, and what they were doing (purpose) immediately prior to the event, will be forgotten first.

60. **a.** Looking for pertinent medical information is the only legitimate reason for an EMT to search a patient's wallet.

61. **c.** Subcutaneous emphysema is a collection of air in the soft tissue. This often is associated with some type of disruption of the tracheobronchial tree and is a serious finding. Rales refers to an abnormal lung sound, parenchyma is the substance of a gland or solid organ, and ischemia involves inadequate blood flow to a tissue.

62. **d.** Wheezing can be described as a high-pitched, whistling sound created as air flows through narrowed airways.

63. **a.** When assessing the abdomen, inform the patient prior to palpating. Otherwise, the patient may be surprised and tighten the abdominal muscles. Do not begin in the immediate area of pain, if there is any. The EMT does not need to press deeply to note whether the abdomen is soft, firm, or distended.

64. **a.** When a vehicle is encountered with a deployed airbag, lift the airbag and check for damage to the steering wheel. A bent steering wheel indicates the patient may have sustained chest trauma. Although disconnecting the battery is a good idea, it is not always practical to accomplish this prior to patient assessment. The haze present after a deployment is a non-toxic powder that is used to lubricate the bag.

If your training includes the use of the Glasgow Coma Scale when assessing patients, complete questions 65 through 67. Refer to the Glasgow Coma Scale in Figure 4-1.

Eye opening	Points	
● Spontaneous	4	
● To voice	3	
● To pain	2	
● None	1	_____
Verbal response	Points	
● Oriented	5	
● Confused	4	
● Inappropriate words	3	
● Incomprehensible sounds	2	
● None	1	_____
Motor response	Points	
● Obeys commands	6	
● Localizes pain	5	
● Withdraws (pain)	4	
● Flexion (pain)	3	
● Extension (pain)	2	
● None	1	_____
Total (1 + 2 + 3)		_____

Figure 4-1

65. **b.** The patient's score is 12:
        eye opening = 3
        verbal response = 4
        motor response = 5

66. **c.** The patient's score is 7:
        eye opening = 1
        verbal response = 2
        motor response = 4

67. **c.** A normal total score is 14 to 15. A patient's condition would be considered serious if the score were less than 13.

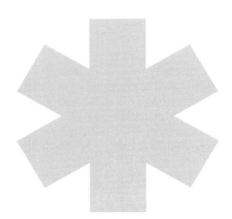

5

Medical Emergencies I

*General Pharmacology, Respiratory Emergencies,
Cardiac Emergencies, and Stroke*

CHAPTER 5 REVIEW QUESTIONS

■ GENERAL PHARMACOLOGY

1. Four routes by which an EMT-Basic administers or assists the patient in administering a medication are:
    a. oral, sublingual, intravenous injection, and subcutaneous injection
    b. oral, sublingual, inhalation, and intramuscular injection
    c. absorption, ingestion, inhalation, and exhalation
    d. intramuscular injection, intravenous injection, intraosseous injection, and intradermal injection

2. Before administering or assisting with the administration of a medication:
    a. ascertain if it was prescribed by a local physician
    b. note what pharmacy filled the prescription
    c. check the medication's expiration date
    d. all of the above

3. The difference between generic names and trade names is that:
    a. a generic name is the same as a brand name, but a trade name is assigned by the government
    b. a medication can have only one generic name but several trade names
    c. generic names are given to a medication by the company that makes it, but trade names are assigned by the government
    d. generic names are generally simple sounding, but trade names are a form of the medication's chemical name

4. The amount of medication to be administered is known as the:
    a. dose
    b. concentration
    c. form
    d. action

5. A situation in which a medication should not be administered to a patient because it may cause harm is:
    a. a contraindication
    b. an untoward effect
    c. a dosing regimen
    d. a specification

6. The method by which a medication affects the human body is the:
    a. mode of operation
    b. mechanism of action
    c. symbiotic effect
    d. standard reaction

7. From the list below, match the medication with its common form.
   fine powder
   gas
   gel
   liquid
   suspension
   tables

   _____ activated charcoal

   _____ epinephrine

   _____ nitroglycerin

   _____ oral glucose

   _____ oxygen

   _____ prescribed inhaler

8. The term "side effect" refers to:
   a. an undesirable action of a drug
   b. a life-threatening reaction to a drug
   c. a reason not to administer a drug to a patient
   d. the way a drug affects the body

9. An example of off-line medical direction is:
   a. a physician on the scene who guides delivery of medical care
   b. receiving an order over the telephone from medical command
   c. a written protocol or standing order for the use of a medication
   d. a radio consultation with a paramedic unit responding to assist an EMT-Basic unit

10. Before assisting a patient with taking a prescribed medication, ask whether the medication was:
    a. prescribed to a family member with a similar problem
    b. purchased at a pharmacy in your service area
    c. prescribed to the patient for the current problem
    d. prescribed by a physician in your service area

11. After administering a medication, the EMT should document on the patient care report:
    a. the time the medication was given
    b. the amount of medication given
    c. any response to the medication
    d. all of the above

12. The disadvantage of using the oral route of medication administration is:
    a. the medication is absorbed faster than when it is injected
    b. very few medications may be given orally
    c. absorption rates are slower than when the medication is injected
    d. oral medications carried on an ambulance cannot be given to children

13. An advantage of using the inhaled route of medication administration is:
    a. any liquid medication can be inhaled
    b. medications can be administered to unresponsive patients through this route
    c. the medication is slowly absorbed into the bloodstream
    d. absorption rates into the bloodstream are rapid

■ **RESPIRATORY EMERGENCIES**

14. Another term for difficulty breathing is:
    a. dysphasia
    b. dysarthria
    c. dysrhythmia
    d. dyspnea

15. The body's normal stimulus to breathe is the blood level of:
    a. oxygen
    b. carbon monoxide
    c. nitrogen
    d. carbon dioxide

16. Signs of difficulty breathing may include all of the following *except*:
    a. wheezing
    b. distended neck veins
    c. an inability to sit upright
    d. extreme anxiety

17. The first priority when caring for a patient experiencing respiratory distress is to:
    a. make the patient comfortable
    b. help the patient take the necessary medication
    c. obtain a thorough medical history
    d. establish an airway and deliver oxygen

18. Generally, a patient having breathing difficulty should be given oxygen:
    a. by cannula at 4 L/min
    b. by nonrebreather mask at 15 L/min
    c. by simple mask at 10 L/min
    d. by cannula at 8 L/min

19. When listening to the lungs of a patient having difficulty breathing, EMTs should be concerned if they hear:
    a. unusual heart sounds
    b. normal breath sounds
    c. wheezing
    d. ascites

20. When wheezing is heard, it means:
    a. the patient must have asthma
    b. the patient might have pulmonary edema or chronic obstructive pulmonary disease (COPD)
    c. the patient does not have pneumonia
    d. the patient has a pulmonary embolus

21. To make breathing easier, patients having difficulty breathing should be placed:
    a. in a position of comfort
    b. flat on their back
    c. on their left side
    d. in Trendelenburg position

22. Unlike treatment of an adult patient, when dealing with a child having breathing problems, the EMT must remember:
    a. as long as the child's color is good he or she is getting enough air
    b. retractions are more commonly seen in children than adults
    c. handheld inhalers should be used only for adults, not children
    d. children seldom experience breathing difficulty as a primary problem

23. A patient with respiratory distress frequently exhibits all of the following *except*:
    a. anxiety and restlessness
    b. increased respiratory rate
    c. the ability to speak in a relaxed, conversational manner
    d. an upright posture (to improve ventilations)

24. The EMT should not assist a patient in using a prescribed inhaler if the patient:
    a. has already used the inhaler once
    b. is wheezing
    c. seems very anxious
    d. has already taken the maximum prescribed dose

25. Prior to helping a patient to use a prescribed inhaler:
    a. chill the inhaler
    b. clean the mouthpiece with alcohol
    c. attach the inhaler to an oxygen or compressed air source
    d. shake the inhaler vigorously

26. While activating the handheld inhaler, the patient should be instructed to:
    a. inhale deeply
    b. exhale forcefully
    c. swallow
    d. breathe normally

27. Immediately after the medication has been delivered, instruct the patient to:
    a. exhale forcefully
    b. cough vigorously
    c. hold his or her breath
    d. swallow

28. The actions and effects of albuterol include all of the following *except*:
    a. slowing of the heart rate
    b. dilation of the bronchioles
    c. speeding up the heart rate
    d. tremors of the hands

29. A common side effect that may be noted after using a prescribed inhaler is:
    a. slow pulse
    b. rapid pulse
    c. hives and itching
    d. cyanosis

30. If after using a prescribed inhaler, the patient has little to no relief, the EMT may be instructed by medical direction to:
    a. administer a second dose
    b. administer epinephrine
    c. place the patient on oxygen by cannula at 2 L/min
    d. discontinue oxygen administration

✳ **ENRICHMENT QUESTIONS**

31. The breath sound characterized as having a musical quality that fluctuates in tone and intensity with respiratory effort is called:
    a. wheezing
    b. rhonchi
    c. rales
    d. crackles

32. The breath sound characterized as resembling the sound of crunching dry leaves and that is heard in patients with emphysema is called:
    a. wheezing
    b. rhonchi
    c. rales
    d. crackles

33. The breath sound characterized as the noise made by air bubbling through water that is frequently heard in pulmonary edema is called:
    a. wheezing
    b. rhonchi
    c. rales
    d. crackles

34. The breath sound caused by the movement of mucus and congestion in the chest is called:
    a. wheezing
    b. rhonchi
    c. rales
    d. crackles

35. Patients with chronic obstructive pulmonary disease (COPD):
    a. tend to have unusually low carbon dioxide levels in the blood
    b. are often borderline hypoxic
    c. often have high carbon monoxide levels in the blood
    d. have abnormally high blood nitrogen levels

36. The two illnesses classified as chronic obstructive pulmonary disease (COPD) are:
    a. asthma and emphysema
    b. chronic bronchitis and pneumonia
    c. croup and asthma
    d. emphysema and chronic bronchitis

37. Destruction of the alveoli and decreased elasticity of lung tissues is characteristic of:
    a. pneumonia
    b. emphysema
    c. asthma
    d. chronic bronchitis

38. Chronic bronchitis is characterized by all of the following *except*:
    a. inflammation of the airways
    b. excessive mucus production
    c. blood clots in the pulmonary arteries
    d. productive cough

39. Regarding COPD, all of the following are true *except*:
    a. wheezing is common
    b. patients with chronic bronchitis are frequently termed "blue bloaters" because cyanosis is common
    c. "pink puffer" is the term often used for patients with emphysema
    d. fever is common

40. Respiratory difficulty experienced by patients with COPD is related to:
    a. a diminished inspiratory and expiratory capacity of the lungs
    b. the blood supply to the lungs being diminished
    c. the lungs not producing enough mucus to lubricate the airways
    d. the patient's lungs becoming more elastic and pliable, thereby inhibiting their ability to expand

41. When listening to the lungs of a patient with COPD, the EMT would expect to hear:
    a. absent breath sounds on one side
    b. normal breath sounds
    c. wheezing
    d. ascites

42. If a patient with COPD is not experiencing severe respiratory distress, oxygen can be delivered:
    a. by nasal cannula at 10 L/min
    b. by nonrebreather mask at 6 L/min
    c. by nasal cannula at 1 to 4 L/min
    d. by nonrebreather mask at 12 to 15 L/min

43. When administering oxygen to a patient with COPD who is in severe shock due to trauma, the EMT should:
    a. always use a nasal cannula
    b. administer low-flow oxygen
    c. administer high-flow oxygen via a mask
    d. only use a Venturi mask

44. When treating a patient with asthma, the EMT should remember that:
    a. asthma is not the same as COPD
    b. asthma is a form of COPD
    c. people with asthma always develop COPD
    d. patients with asthma cannot suffer from COPD

45. Asthma attacks may be precipitated by:
    a. an infection
    b. an allergic reaction
    c. emotional stress
    d. all of the above

46. When an asthma attack occurs, the patient will normally have:
    a. less difficulty exhaling than inhaling
    b. the same amount of difficulty inhaling as exhaling
    c. more difficulty exhaling than inhaling
    d. more difficulty inhaling than exhaling

47. Bronchospasm during an asthma attack causes wheezes to be first noticed during:
    a. inspiration when the bronchioles expand
    b. expiration when the bronchioles contract
    c. between inspiration and expiration
    d. at the end of inspiration

48. The absence of wheezing during a severe asthma attack indicates:
    a. the patient is getting better
    b. the medications are working
    c. the patient is not moving enough air to generate a wheeze
    d. the patient has pneumonia

49. A patient having a severe asthma attack starts to become confused and irritable. The most likely reason for this is that:
    a. the patient's medication is causing anxiety
    b. there is another medical problem present in addition to the asthma attack
    c. the asthma attack has caused the patient to become hypoglycemic
    d. the patient is becoming hypoxic

50. Respiratory difficulty experienced by asthmatics is associated with:
    a. a sudden dilation of the bronchi coupled with an increase in mucus production
    b. a sudden constriction of the bronchi coupled with an decrease in mucus production
    c. a sudden constriction of the bronchi coupled with an increase in mucus production
    d. a sudden dilation of the bronchi coupled with an decrease in mucus production

51. Status asthmaticus is the term used to refer to:
    a. an asthma attack brought on by an allergic reaction
    b. a severe asthma attack unrelieved by oxygen and medication
    c. an asthma attack complicated by an accompanying infection
    d. the period following an asthma attack when the patient has returned to their normal status

52. A patient with a pulmonary embolism would be most likely to:
    a. complain of a gradual development of difficulty breathing
    b. complain of sudden onset of unexplained dyspnea, cyanosis, and sharp stabbing chest pain
    c. have a slow heart rate
    d. complain of crushing left-sided chest pressure

53. A history of fever and chills, productive cough, and an ill appearance are most consistent with:
    a. COPD
    b. asthma
    c. pulmonary embolus
    d. pneumonia

54. Hyperventilation syndrome:
    a. occurs because the patient has too much carbon dioxide in the lungs
    b. is caused by anxiety and should be routinely treated by having the patient breathe into a brown paper bag
    c. may cause carpopedal spasm, which is characterized by a "drawing up" of the hand and wrist with cramped and flexed fingers
    d. may be controlled by using a bag-valve-mask to assist the patient's respirations

■ **CARDIOVASCULAR EMERGENCIES**

55. Factors that put a person at risk of developing coronary artery disease include all of the following *except*:
    a. low blood pressure
    b. smoking
    c. high cholesterol
    d. obesity

56. The pain commonly associated with cardiac emergencies is usually described as a:
    a. crushing or pressure type of pain
    b. pain that becomes worse when the patient inhales deeply
    c. sharp, stabbing pain
    d. cramping, intermittent pain

57. Chest pain associated with a cardiac emergency may radiate:
    a. to the jaw
    b. to the shoulder
    c. to either arm
    d. all of the above

58. Persons experiencing chest pain frequently will:
    a. summon the local EMS
    b. drive to the nearest hospital
    c. deny they may be having a heart attack
    d. immediately call the family doctor

59. A patient experiencing a cardiac emergency will often:
    a. sweat profusely
    b. feel dry to the touch
    c. appear flushed
    d. appear jaundiced

60. A patient experiencing chest pain should be placed on oxygen:
    a. using a cannula at 15 L/min
    b. immediately using a nonrebreather mask
    c. only after the EMT has assisted with nitroglycerin
    d. only if the pain is accompanied by difficulty breathing

61. A patient experiencing cardiac compromise should usually be transported:
    a. in a supine position
    b. in a prone position
    c. in a position of comfort, preferably semi-sitting
    d. on his or her left side

62. An important aspect of caring for patients with cardiac compromise involves:
    a. explaining they may have died if they waited to summon help
    b. waiting at the scene to see if oxygen reduces the pain
    c. transporting the patient to their hospital of choice
    d. reassuring the patient

63. The EMT may assist a patient in taking his prescribed nitroglycerin if the patient has:
    a. substernal chest pain and a history of heart problems
    b. weakness on one side of the body
    c. difficulty breathing and dizziness
    d. difficulty breathing and stabbing pain associated with taking a deep breath

64. The two common forms of nitroglycerin are:
    a. capsule and tablet
    b. elixir and capsule
    c. tablet and spray
    d. spray and elixir

65. Nitroglycerin works by:
    a. increasing the workload of the heart
    b. dilating the bronchial passages
    c. dilating the body's blood vessels
    d. constricting the coronary arteries

66. Nitroglycerin should be:
    a. administered under the tongue
    b. swallowed
    c. administered intramuscularly
    d. inhaled

67. Before a patient takes nitroglycerin, the blood pressure should be:
    a. less than 70 mm Hg diastolic
    b. greater than 80 mm Hg diastolic
    c. greater than 100 mm Hg systolic
    d. less than 120 mm Hg systolic

68. If a cardiac patient has no relief of pain, medical control may direct the EMT to assist with additional doses of nitroglycerin:
    a. every 10 minutes until reaching the hospital
    b. one additional time in 5 minutes
    c. every 8 to 10 minutes up to a maximum of two doses
    d. every 3 to 5 minutes up to a maximum of three doses

69. After administering each dose of nitroglycerin, the EMT should:
    a. reassess the patient's blood pressure
    b. check breath sounds
    c. reassess the patient's Glasgow Coma Scale score
    d. check the expiration date of the drug

70. Automated external defibrillation should be performed:
    a. after beginning CPR
    b. immediately after reaching the patient
    c. only if bystander CPR was being performed prior to the EMT's arrival
    d. after placing the patient on oxygen

71. An automated external defibrillator (AED) should not be used on patients:
    a. who have drowned
    b. over 190 pounds in weight
    c. with known cardiac disease history
    d. under the age of 8 years

72. Automated external defibrillators:
    a. advise the EMT whether or not to administer a shock
    b. operate without action on the part of the EMT
    c. use paddles to deliver shocks
    d. will automatically deliver an appropriate shock

73. While the automated external defibrillator is analyzing the patient's cardiac rhythm:
    a. continue CPR
    b. perform ventilations only
    c. discontinue all contact with the patient
    d. check the patient's blood pressure

74. While an automated external defibrillator is delivering a shock:
    a. continue ventilating the patient
    b. do not touch the patient
    c. secure the patient to prevent jerking and possible injury
    d. continue CPR

75. The patient's pulse should be checked after delivery of:
    a. the first shock only
    b. the second and fourth shocks
    c. the third and sixth shocks
    d. each shock

76. Between delivery of the first series and second series of shocks on a pulseless patient:
    a. do not touch the patient
    b. ventilate the patient only
    c. assess the patient's blood pressure
    d. perform CPR for 1 minute

77. If on-scene ALS is not available, the patient should be transported:
    a. after six shocks are delivered
    b. after delivery of the third shock
    c. immediately once the automated external defibrillator indicates that no shock is advised
    d. prior to attaching the automated external defibrillator

78. If, after delivery of a shock, the patient's pulse returns:
    a. remove the automated external defibrillator from the patient
    b. transport with the automated external defibrillator attached to the patient
    c. continue CPR
    d. continue administering shocks until six shocks are delivered

79. If a patient needs to be defibrillated in the ambulance:
    a. bring the ambulance to a safe stop prior to analyzing the rhythm
    b. continue transporting while defibrillating
    c. stop the ambulance only when the automated external defibrillator is ready to deliver the shock
    d. turn off the ambulance engine to reduce vibration

80. Delivery of inappropriate shocks by an automated external defibrillator is most often a result of:
    a. automated external defibrillator computer error
    b. misplaced electrodes
    c. operator error
    d. roughly moving the patient

81. You have delivered a shock with the automated external defibrillator and the machine is prompting you to check a pulse. You do so and find one. You should:
    a. assist the patient in taking their nitroglycerin if they have it available
    b. continue CPR until you get to the hospital since the heart is probably failing
    c. apply oxygen by nasal cannula and transport
    d. assess the adequacy of breathing and assist ventilations with a bag-valve-mask if respirations are slow or shallow

✳ **ENRICHMENT QUESTIONS**

82. Common signs and symptoms of a heart attack include all of the following *except*:
    a. sweating
    b. drooping of one side of the face
    c. chest pain that radiates to the arm
    d. difficulty breathing

83. A heart attack is commonly referred to as a:
    a. cerebrovascular accident
    b. myocardial infarction
    c. transient ischemic attack
    d. anginal episode

84. When assessing a patient with chest pain:
    a. if the pain is relieved with oxygen, the patient only has angina and is not having a heart attack
    b. the pain may be referred to as a pressure rather than a pain
    c. if the pain is on the right side of the chest the patient does not have angina
    d. apply oxygen only if the patient complains of shortness of breath

85. Myocardial infarction occurs:
    a. because the patient did not take an aspirin a day
    b. when an area of the heart muscle is deprived of oxygen and dies
    c. when the heart stops beating
    d. when the blood becomes too thick to move through the blood vessels

86. The term *myocardial ischemia* means that heart tissue is:
    a. not receiving enough oxygen
    b. fibrillating
    c. turning into scar tissue
    d. receiving too much blood

87. Angina pectoris is caused by:
    a. an inflammation of the heart muscle
    b. a problem with the valves of the heart
    c. inadequate blood flow to an area of the heart
    d. an accumulation of blood in the sac surrounding the heart

88. The pain of angina pectoris is usually relieved by:
    a. doing mild exercises
    b. taking aspirin
    c. applying cold compresses to the left side of the chest
    d. taking nitroglycerin

89. Complications of a myocardial infarction (heart attack) include all the following *except*:
    a. abnormal electrical rhythms (dysrhythmias) caused by an irritable heart
    b. cardiogenic shock due to damage of the ventricles
    c. congestive heart failure
    d. pneumonia secondary to poor ventilation

90. Nitroglycerin is helpful in relieving cardiac related chest pain because it:
    a. makes the blood cells "slippery" so they can travel through the heart more easily
    b. slows the heart rate down and decreases myocardial workload
    c. calms the patient's anxiety
    d. dilates the coronary arteries to allow more blood flow to the ischemic heart muscle

91. Nitroglycerin taken by a patient experiencing chest pain:
    a. prevents the patient from having a heart attack
    b. improves delivery of oxygen to the heart by making the heart beat slower
    c. may cause hypotension
    d. is explosive and should only be handled by trained professionals

92. Oxygen is given to the patient experiencing chest pain because:
    a. it reduces anxiety and therefore the heart rate
    b. it opens the blocked coronary arteries
    c. it improves blood pressure, which is often high in heart attacks
    d. angina is caused by ischemia, which is a condition of low oxygen levels in the heart muscle

93. A rapid heart rate is called:
    a. bradycardia
    b. tachycardia
    c. tachypnea
    d. bradyasystole

94. Bradycardia is characterized by:
    a. an irregular heart rate
    b. a heart rate less than 60 beats per minute
    c. a heart rate more than 100 beats per minute
    d. a heart rate between 80 and 100 beats per minute

95. Referring to Figure 5-1, the correct pad placement is shown in:
    a. part A
    b. part B
    c. part C
    d. part D

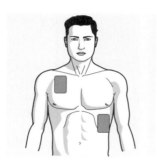
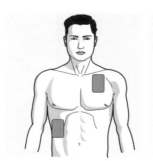

A   B

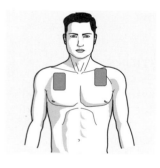
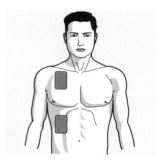

C   D

Figure 5-1

96. Using the list of arrhythmias below, label
the four ECG strips shown in Figure 5-2.
asystole
normal sinus
ventricular fibrillation
ventricular tachycardia

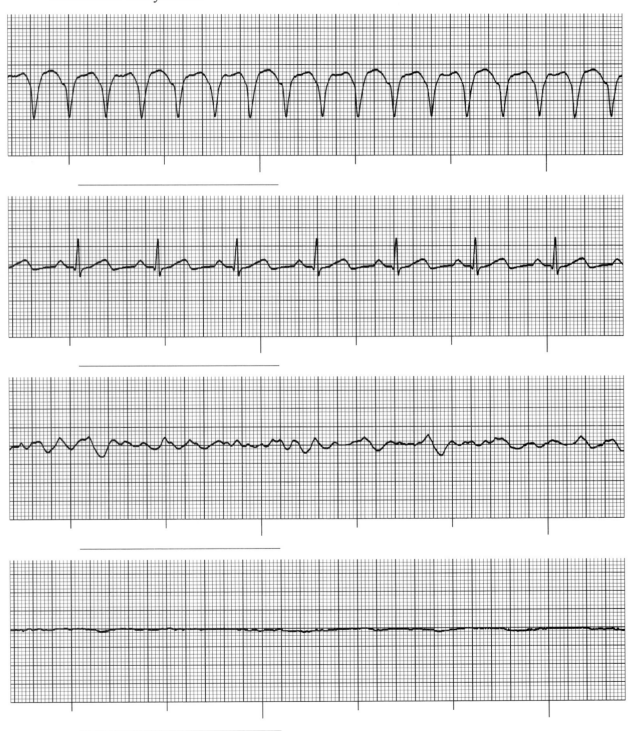

Figure 5-2

97. Congestive heart failure (CHF) may be simply described as:
    a. a heart attack
    b. an accumulation of fluid in the sac surrounding the heart
    c. a blockage of the coronary arteries
    d. a condition in which the heart is not pumping blood adequately

98. The signs and symptoms of CHF include all the following *except*:
    a. swelling of the lower extremities
    b. difficulty lying flat
    c. fever
    d. distended neck veins

99. A patient experiencing congestive heart failure will often present with:
    a. sharp chest pain that is worse when taking a deep breath
    b. thin, spindly looking lower legs and ankles
    c. serious respiratory difficulty
    d. severe, crushing chest pain with no accompanying shortness of breath

100. Congestive heart failure patients should be transported:
    a. lying flat while receiving high-concentration oxygen
    b. sitting upright while receiving low-concentration oxygen
    c. lying flat while receiving low-concentration oxygen
    d. sitting upright while receiving high-concentration oxygen

✳ **ENRICHMENT QUESTIONS**

The following Enrichment Questions deal with stroke.

101. Basically speaking, a stroke involves:
    a. a brief lack of oxygen to brain tissue with little accompanying damage
    b. a widespread dilation of cerebral arteries
    c. lowered cardiac output
    d. an interruption of blood supply to part of the brain causing tissue damage

102. A stroke is most commonly referred to as a:
    a. cerebrovascular accident
    b. subdural hematoma
    c. epidural bleed
    d. concussion

103. Strokes are caused by all of the following *except*:
    a. a clot or thrombus that forms in a cerebral artery
    b. a clot that travels from the heart and lodges in a cerebral artery
    c. a cerebral artery that bursts
    d. not giving an unconscious patient enough oxygen

104. A stroke should be suspected if the patient presents with a sudden onset of:
    a. weakness or paralysis of one side of the body
    b. chest pain that radiates down the left arm
    c. pain on one side of the body
    d. respiratory difficulty and wheezing

105. A stroke occurring on the left side of the brain results in weakness:
    a. on the left side of the body
    b. on the right side of the body
    c. in the arms more than the legs
    d. in the legs more than the arms

106. An unconscious stroke patient should be transported:
    a. on their side with the affected side down
    b. sitting upright
    c. in the Trendelenburg position
    d. prone

107. The conscious stroke patient should be transported:
    a. in the prone position to allow saliva to drain
    b. flat to equalize the pressure in the brain and heart
    c. with the head elevated about 30 degrees to help lower intracranial pressure
    d. in a position of comfort on their side

108. A transient ischemic attack (TIA) is:
  a. an indication that the patient is improving and will recover from their stroke
  b. caused by a spasm in the coronary blood flow to the heart
  c. a brief episode of stroke-like symptoms that are not permanent
  d. an indication that the patient is at low risk for the possibility of more serious strokes

■ Additional Points for Discussion ■

Hospitals now use drugs that can dissolve clots in a coronary artery, restoring blood flow to the heart muscle. These drugs are known as thrombolytics. Early administration of these drugs can make a major difference in patient outcome and quality of life. The EMT is a vital first link in the chain of care for heart attack patients, as the drug must be administered within a certain amount of time after onset of a cardiac emergency. In addition, certain criteria must be met by the patient for the drugs to be used. Some patients may not be given the medication and may undergo angioplasty or cardiac bypass surgery instead.

1. What criteria must a patient meet to be considered as a candidate for drug administration?

2. Which hospitals in your area are capable of performing angioplasty or cardiac bypass surgery?

3. How will knowing the criteria and which hospitals may perform angioplasty or cardiac bypass surgery, affect the following?

  • Your patient management:

  • Your decision on where to transport a cardiac emergency patient:

4. Review the operation of your department's automated external defibrillator.

5. Does your department use off-line medical direction, on-line medical direction, or both?

  • What medications can you use with off-line medical direction?

  • What medications require on-line medical direction to use?

ANSWERS TO CHAPTER 5 REVIEW QUESTIONS

■ GENERAL PHARMACOLOGY

1. **b.** The routes by which an EMT can administer or assist a patient with medications are oral (glucose), sublingual (nitroglycerin), inhalation (prescribed inhalers such as albuterol, Alupent, Bronkosol and Proventil), and intramuscular injection (epinephrine).

2. **c.** Before administering or assisting in the administration of a medication, the EMT should check the medication's expiration date. Checking what pharmacy filled the prescription is not important, nor is it necessary that the medication was prescribed by a local physician.

3. **b.** The difference between generic and trade names is that a medication can have only one generic name but several trade names. A generic name is assigned by the government and is usually a simple form of the medication's complex chemical name. A trade name, or brand name, is given to a medication by the company that sells the medication.

4. **a.** The dose is the amount of medication that should be administered to a patient. The correct dose can vary based on the patient's weight and age. Concentration refers to the quantity of a specified substance in a unit amount of another substance (i.e., number of milligrams of a medication in a milliliter of liquid).

5. **a.** A contraindication is a situation in which a medication should not be administered to a patient. In such situations, the medication may cause harm or it may provide no effect to improve the patient's condition or illness. An untoward effect is a side effect that proves harmful to the patient.

6. **b.** The mechanism of action is the way a medication affects the human body.

7.

suspension	activated charcoal
liquid	epinephrine
tablet	nitroglycerin
gel	oral glucose
gas	oxygen
fine powder	prescribed inhaler

8. **a.** A side effect is an undesirable action of a medication. It is not the same as a contraindication. Side effects may or may not be serious, but they are still unwanted. Knowing the potential side effects of a medication can help prepare the EMT to deal with them if they occur.

9. **c.** A written protocol or standing order for the use of a medication is an example of off-line medical direction. On-line medical direction refers to a situation in which the EMT speaks directly to medical command via a telephone or radio.

10. **c.** Be sure the medication was prescribed to the patient for the current problem before assisting with its administration. Caution must be exercised because family members often want to be helpful and will give their medication to other family members who appear to have the same problem. The medication does not have to be from a local pharmacy or prescribed by a local doctor as long as it was prescribed for the patient.

11. **d.** All of the above. On the patient care report, note the time the medication was given, the dose given, and any response (or unusual response) to the medication. Also, note the route by which the medication was administered.

12. **c.** Although many different medications may be given orally, including ones used by the EMT-Basic, the disadvantage of using the oral route of administration for a medication is absorption rates are slower than when the medication is injected. Other disadvantages are that oral medications cannot be given to semi-responsive or unresponsive patients, and some medications are not absorbed well from the stomach. Activated charcoal, carried on EMT-Basic units, can be given to children.

13. **d.** An advantage of using the inhaled route of administration for a medication is the drug is rapidly absorbed into the bloodstream. However, patients must be alert to use an inhaler and only certain medications can be administered by this route. Another advantage to using an inhaler is that small amounts of the medication are applied directly to the site of action. This minimizes the systemic effects that can occur if higher doses of medication are absorbed into the blood.

■ RESPIRATORY EMERGENCIES

14. **d.** A patient having breathing difficulty is said to be experiencing dyspnea. Dysphasia and dysarthria refer to speech impairments, and a dysrhythmia is an abnormal heart rhythm.

15. **d.** The body's normal stimulus to breathe is the blood level of carbon dioxide.

16. **c.** Patients experiencing breathing difficulty may present sitting upright and leaning forward, or using accessory muscles to try to breathe. Also, wheezing, distended neck veins, use of accessory muscles, and bulging eyes may be noted.

17. **d.** Airway and oxygen delivery are the most important factors in caring for the patient with respiratory distress. It should not be delayed to perform any of the other listed actions.

18. **b.** Generally, patients having breathing difficulty should be given oxygen by nonrebreather mask at 15 L/min. Although patients with certain respiratory diseases may develop problems if too much oxygen is given, this is rarely a concern during the short time EMTs treat the patient. EMTs must be careful, however, not to withhold oxygen from a truly hypoxic patient. Remember, if a patient stops breathing because too much oxygen was administered, the EMT can ventilate the patient and sustain life. There are many places worse than the back of an ambulance for this to happen. However, if a patient stops breathing because oxygen was withheld and severe hypoxia developed, the chances of resuscitation are slim.

19. **c.** The EMT should be concerned if wheezing is heard when listening to a patient's lungs. Note the presence of wheezing on the patient care report and report its presence to medical command. Ascites is an abnormal pooling of fluid in the abdominal cavity.

20. **b.** All that wheezes is not asthma. Fluid or congestion in the lung may constrict the airway and cause wheezes to be heard.

21. **a.** To make breathing easier, patients with breathing difficulty should be transported in a position of comfort. Allow the patient to tell you which position makes it easiest to breathe, and try to transport him or her in that position.

22. **b.** When dealing with children experiencing breathing difficulty, retractions (the use of accessory muscles) are more commonly seen than in adults. In infants, a "seesaw" breathing pattern, where the abdomen and chest move in opposite directions, may be noted. Don't be fooled because the child's color is good. Cyanosis is a late sign of breathing distress in children.

23. **c.** During respiratory distress, the patient is gasping for air and the work of breathing is tiring and difficult. Speaking is often difficult, and the patient may not even be able to speak in complete sentences. Anxiety and restlessness are common because of fear and hypoxia, and patients often breathe rapidly and shallowly. An upright posture helps the patient breathe by allowing the abdominal contents to drop by gravity, thereby allowing the diaphragm to work more easily.

24. **d.** If the patient has used an inhaler prior to the arrival of EMS and has reached the maximum prescribed dose, do not give additional medication. Patients having difficulty breathing may present with wheezing and anxiety, both of which may be alleviated after taking their medication.

25. **d.** Shake the inhaler vigorously several times prior to administering the medication. The inhaler should be at room temperature. Inhalers are already under pressure and do not need an external compressed gas source for power.

26. **a.** Instruct the patient to inhale deeply while activating the handheld inhaler to deliver the medication.

27. **c.** Immediately after the patient inhales the medication, have the patient hold his or her breath for as long as comfortably possible. This will allow more of the medication to be absorbed.

28. **a.** Albuterol, the active ingredient in most prescribed inhalers, acts by reducing bronchospasm of the bronchioles, thereby resulting in improved ventilation. Having some characteristics similar to epinephrine, it causes an increase in heart rate and can cause the hands to tremble.

29. **b.** After using the prescribed inhaler, the patient may experience a rapid pulse; however, this is usually not of great concern. If the medication does its job, the patient should experience some relief from the breathing difficulty.

30. **a.** If the first dose does not produce the desired results, medical direction may authorize a second dose. Oxygen is still of critical importance as the patient's blood oxygen level may have dropped markedly during the episode. It is most appropriately administered via nonrebreather mask.

✳ **ENRICHMENT QUESTIONS**

31. **a.** Wheezing is caused by air moving through a tight constriction in the airway. It will have a pitch or tone that varies with the force of breathing and the severity of the constriction.

32. **d.** The alveoli of the emphysema patient are stiff, and the bronchioles frequently collapse and open. This opening and closing of the small airways results in the crackling sound.

33. **c.** Pulmonary edema is the presence of fluid in the alveoli and bronchioles. As the patient breathes, they must move air through this liquid, causing a bubbling sound called rales.

34. **b.** Congestion in the chest from bronchitis or pneumonia occludes the airways and rattles back and forth during breathing. As the obstruction clears, a hoarse sound called rhonchi is heard.

35. **b.** Patients with COPD tend to be somewhat hypoxic. They may also have somewhat elevated blood levels of carbon dioxide.

36. **d.** COPD is a combination of emphysema and/or chronic bronchitis. It differs from asthma and pneumonia in that there is permanent damage to the lungs. Asthma and pneumonia are reversible conditions.

37. **b.** Emphysema results from destruction of the alveoli and decreased elasticity of the lung resulting in air trapping. Pneumonia is an infection in the lungs caused by bacteria or viruses. Asthma is caused by constriction of the bronchioles secondary to exposure to an allergen. Chronic bronchitis is caused by excessive production of mucus, which plugs the airways.

38. **c.** Chronic bronchitis is characterized by inflammation of the airways, excessive mucus production, and a productive cough. A blood clot in the pulmonary artery is called a pulmonary embolus.

39. **d.** Due to loss of lung elasticity and mucus plugging, the airways become constricted and cause wheezing. People with chronic bronchitis are called "blue bloaters" because they are often cyanotic. Emphysema patients are called "pink puffers" because they tend to have skinny chests and breathe through pursed lips to keep their airways open. Fever occurs during an infection, which may precipitate a worsening of COPD but is not a common feature.

40. **a.** A patient with COPD has a diminished inspiratory and expiratory capacity of the lungs. Although the blood supply to the lungs is still adequate, emphysema causes the walls of the alveoli to break down and a loss of elasticity of the lung tissue. Additionally, in chronic bronchitis, excess mucus is formed, which interferes with normal respiratory function.

41. **c.** Wheezing is commonly associated with COPD. Ascites is an accumulation of fluid in the abdominal cavity and is not associated with COPD.

42. **c.** If a patient with COPD is not experiencing severe respiratory distress, oxygen should be delivered at low concentrations, such as by nasal cannula at 1 to 4 L/min. However, if a patient with COPD is experiencing severe respiratory distress, oxygen should given at a high flow rate by nonrebreather mask.

43. **c.** Any patient in hypovolemic shock should be given high-flow oxygen, regardless of medical history.

44. **a.** Asthma is not a form of COPD. This must be remembered when dealing with a patient with an acute asthma attack.

45. **d.** All of the above. With asthma, the airways are oversensitive to stimuli in the environment and to emotional stress. Therefore, infections, allergic reactions, and emotional stress may all precipitate an acute attack.

46. **c.** Asthma patients normally have little difficulty with inspiration, but great difficulty with expiration.

47. **b.** Normally, when the chest enlarges during inspiration, the bronchioles expand. During expiration, they contract. When bronchospasm occurs it will first be detected during expiration when the bronchioles are naturally at their smallest. Wheezing heard during both inspiration and expiration signifies a severe attack.

48. **c.** Air flow must be of sufficient velocity to cause the wheezing sound. As the asthma attack worsens, the patient grows tired and respirations become shallow and the wheezing diminishes. Patients with pneumonia may or may not have wheezes, but more often have rhonchi due to the congestion in their lungs.

49. **d.** A patient having a severe asthma attack who starts to become confused and irritable is probably becoming hypoxic. There is a shortage of oxygen at the cellular level. These patients can quickly deteriorate into respiratory arrest followed by cardiac arrest.

50. **c.** Respiratory difficulty experienced by asthmatics is associated with a sudden constriction of the bronchi (bronchospasm), coupled with an increase in mucus production, which restricts air flow in the lungs.

51. **b.** Unlike a simple asthma attack where one or two inhalations of albuterol eliminate the bronchospasm, status asthmaticus does not respond to initial doses of bronchodilators. It represents a dire emergency during which shock, cyanosis, and respiratory arrest may occur. Rapid transport by EMT-Basics while administering oxygen is necessary so the patient can be treated aggressively at a hospital.

52. **b.** Pulmonary embolism refers to blockage of a pulmonary artery by a blood clot or other foreign material that has traveled there from another place of origin, commonly the lower extremities. It is associated with a sudden onset of unexplained dyspnea, cyanosis, and sharp stabbing chest pain (pleuritic chest pain) that is usually aggravated by a deep breath. The pain may occur anywhere in the chest, not just the left side. A pulmonary embolus keeps oxygen-poor blood from reaching the lungs to be oxygenated, and if large enough, can cause hypoxia to develop.

53. **d.** Pneumonia is caused by an infection that is frequently associated with fever and chills, cough, and illness. Although COPD may cause a chronic cough, it does not cause a fever. Asthma is caused by bronchospasm and a pulmonary embolus is a blood clot in the lung.

54. **c.** Hyperventilation results in a decrease in carbon dioxide (CO_2) in the body, which is called respiratory alkalosis. The alkalosis causes irritation of the nerves resulting in spasms of the fingers and wrists and tingling around the lips and fingers. Having a patient breathe into a paper bag may worsen hypoxia and should not be performed. Aside from attempting to calm the patient, no active measures should be taken to control respiratory rate other than administering oxygen.

■ **CARDIOVASCULAR EMERGENCIES**

55. **a.** There are a number of factors that put a person at greater risk of developing coronary artery disease. Some of these cannot be controlled, such as one's gender and family history. Other risk factors can be modified. High blood pressure, smoking, obesity, high cholesterol levels, and lack of exercise are some of these modifiable risk factors.

56. **a.** A crushing pain or heavy pressure that radiates into other parts of the body is most often associated with a cardiac emergency. The pain is seldom described as sharp or stabbing and is usually not affected by inhaling deeply.

57. **d.** All of the above. The chest pain most commonly radiates to the left arm but may radiate to either arm, the jaw, either shoulder, the back, or abdomen.

58. **c.** People having chest pain commonly deny they may be having a heart problem such as a heart attack. These patients will wait an average of 3 hours to call for help.

59. **a.** A patient experiencing a cardiac emergency often sweats profusely (is diaphoretic) and is pale.

60. **b.** Oxygen should immediately be administered to the cardiac emergency patient since a lack of oxygen to the heart muscle can cause permanent damage. Use a nonrebreather mask at 15 L/min.

61. **c.** Patients experiencing cardiac compromise should usually be transported in a position of comfort. Generally, they are most comfortable in a semi-sitting position.

62. **d.** The patient should be constantly reassured. He or she may now realize the seriousness of the situation and start to worry about death. Do not ridicule or counsel the patient. To reduce the risk of sudden death from an abnormal cardiac rhythm, the patient should be transported to the closest appropriate hospital.

63. **a.** If a patient who is experiencing chest pain has a history of heart problems and has a personal prescription for nitroglycerin, the EMT may receive permission to assist the patient in taking this medication.

64. **c.** The nitroglycerin an EMT may assist in administering commonly comes in a tablet or spray form.

65. **c.** Nitroglycerin dilates the body's blood vessels, thereby decreasing the workload of the heart.

66. **a.** Regardless of whether the medicine is in tablet or spray form, nitroglycerin is administered sublingually, that is, under the patient's tongue. Make sure the patient understands this. Although the medication was prescribed to the patient, some do not understand that the medication should not be swallowed or chewed. Nitroglycerin spray should not be inhaled.

67. **c.** The patient's blood pressure should be greater than 100 mm Hg systolic before nitroglycerin is given. If the patient's blood pressure is lower, medical direction may be consulted.

68. **d.** If the pain is not relieved, the EMT may be permitted to give nitroglycerin every 3 to 5 minutes for a total of three doses (including the initial dose).

69. **a.** Reassess the patient's blood pressure after each dose of nitroglycerin. This should be performed about 2 minutes after the patient takes the medication.

70. **b.** If an automated external defibrillator is immediately available, automated external defibrillation should be performed immediately after reaching the patient, even before starting CPR.

71. **d.** An automated external defibrillator should not be used on patients under the age of 8 years or who weigh less than 55 pounds.

72. **a.** An automated external defibrillator advises the EMT whether to shock or not. The EMT must then activate the shock. This means there is a risk of not delivering an appropriate shock if the EMT does not activate the unit.

73. **c.** While the automated external defibrillator is analyzing the patient's cardiac rhythm, EMTs should discontinue all contact with the patient, including CPR. This allows the unit to properly analyze the cardiac rhythm.

74. **b.** While an automated external defibrillator is delivering a shock, EMTs should not touch the patient. There is a risk of accidental shock to the rescuers if they come in contact with the patient.

75. **c.** Shocks are delivered in series of three. Check the patient's pulse after the third and sixth shocks.

76. **d.** If the first series of shocks does not convert the patient to a normal rhythm, perform CPR for 1 minute, then deliver the second series of shocks.

77. **a.** If on-scene ALS is not available, it is generally recommended that the EMT transport the patient after six shocks are delivered or the automated external defibrillator gives three consecutive messages (separated by 1 minute of CPR) that a shock is not advised. Because guidelines regarding when to transport may vary from area to area, local protocols should be followed.

78. **b.** If the patient's pulse returns after delivery of a shock, discontinue CPR, load the patient, and transport. Since the patient may go into cardiac arrest again, leave the automated external defibrillator pads attached to the patient.

79. **a.** Bring the ambulance to a safe stop before attempting defibrillation. Although defibrillation can be performed in an ambulance, the automated external defibrillator cannot adequately analyze the patient's cardiac rhythm in a bouncing vehicle. Also, there is more risk of an EMT being accidentally shocked in a moving ambulance.

80. **c.** Delivery of inappropriate shocks by an automated external defibrillator is most often a result of operator error.

81. **d.** After successful resuscitation, cardiac arrest victims frequently will not be breathing. The EMT must assess the adequacy of ventilations and assist with a bag-valve-mask when appropriate. CPR is not indicated if the patient has a pulse. If the patient is breathing, apply 100% oxygen via nonrebreather mask since cardiac arrest victims are usually hypoxic.

✳ ENRICHMENT QUESTIONS

82. **b.** Substernal chest pain that radiates to the arms or jaw, difficulty breathing, and cool and sweaty skin are all signs and symptoms commonly associated with a heart attack. Drooping of one side of the face is more commonly associated with a stroke.

83. **b.** Another term for heart attack is *myocardial infarction.*

84. **b.** The heart has many nerves connected to it. Some carry the sensation of pain. Some carry the sensation of pressure or tightness. This is why patients experiencing cardiac-related chest pain often complain of a crushing pressure rather than a stabbing or sharp pain. The pain may also radiate to the jaw, neck, or arm. However, not every patient experiencing ischemia will complain of chest pain.

85. **b.** Myocardial (heart) muscle requires a great deal of oxygen to operate, just like any organ in the body. When a myocardial infarction (heart attack) occurs, an area of the heart muscle is deprived of oxygen. If the supply of oxygen is cut off, the muscle will reach a point at which it cannot produce energy by any means and will die.

86. **a.** Ischemia refers to a decreased supply of oxygenated blood to a body organ. Myocardial (heart) muscle requires a great deal of oxygen to operate, so when it becomes starved of oxygen, there is often accompanying pain. However, if perfusion with oxygenated blood can be restored quickly, no harm comes to the muscle.

87. **c.** The pain of angina pectoris is the result an inadequate flow of blood to an area of the heart that results in ischemia to that area. The pain is often brought on by exertion or exercise.

88. **d.** The pain associated with angina is usually relieved by rest or, if not by rest alone, nitroglycerin.

89. **d.** When a heart attack occurs, the ischemic muscle is prone to erratic electrical activity that can result in dysrhythmias such as ventricular tachycardia and fibrillation. Also, the muscle fails to work efficiently, which can lead to congestive heart failure. If the failure progresses, the heart may be unable to maintain an adequate blood pressure and shock will occur.

90. **d.** Nitroglycerin acts directly on the coronary arteries to dilate them. This dilation results in an increased blood flow to the heart muscle (myocardium) supplying it with more oxygen. Nitroglycerin has no direct effect on heart rate, anxiety, or the blood cells.

91. **c.** Nitroglycerin dilates not only the coronary arteries but all the arteries in the body. This dilation may cause hypotension (a drop in blood pressure). The EMT should be prepared to treat this by placing the patient in a supine position and elevating the legs. While nitroglycerin promotes increased blood flow to the heart muscle, it will not remove the obstruction in the coronary artery. Therefore, it does not prevent the patient from having a heart attack. Also, it does not act directly on the heart rate, and in pill form it is safe to handle since it is not explosive.

92. **d.** The cause of angina and myocardial infarction is low levels of oxygen (ischemia) in the heart muscle. Supplemental oxygen will increase these levels but will not reduce any coronary obstruction. Oxygen has no effect on blood pressure and does not directly reduce anxiety.

93. **b.** A rapid heart rate is called tachycardia. Tachypnea is rapid breathing, and bradyasystole refers to a type of cardiac arrest.

94. **b.** A heart rate less than 60 beats per minute is called bradycardia. Bradycardic heart rates may be regular or irregular.

95. **b.** Part B of Figure 5-1 shows the correct location to place the automated external defibrillator pads.

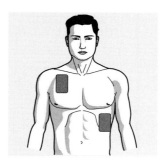

Figure 5-1

96. Using the list of arrhythmias below, label the four ECG strips shown in Figure 5-2.
asystole
normal sinus
ventricular fibrillation
ventricular tachycardia

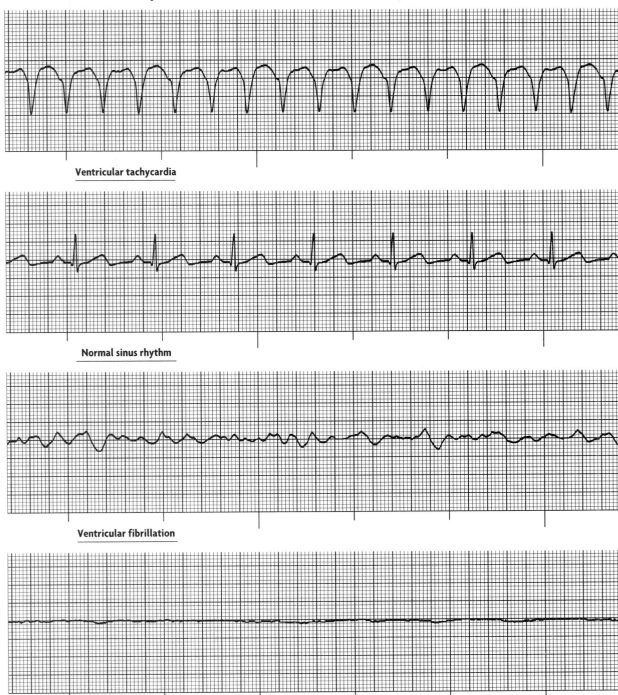

Ventricular tachycardia

Normal sinus rhythm

Ventricular fibrillation

Asystole

Figure 5-2

97. d. Congestive heart failure occurs when the heart muscle weakens and is unable to pump blood adequately. The weakening may be due to damage, disease, or age. Heart attacks or blockage of coronary arteries may damage the heart and eventually lead to congestive heart failure. An accumulation of fluid in the sac surrounding the heart is called pericardial tamponade.

98. c. Patients with CHF may having swelling of the lower extremities (referred to as edema) and distended neck veins. They often have difficulty lying flat due to fluid in the lungs. Fever is not a sign of CHF.

99. c. Patients with CHF often present with serious respiratory difficulty caused when fluid accumulates in the lungs. They often also have swelling of the lower legs and ankles, and may have distended neck veins. Although damage to the heart muscle may have been caused by a heart attack at one time, the patient may present with little or no chest pain.

100. d. Transport the patient sitting upright and administer high-concentration oxygen via a nonrebreather mask. Patients in congestive heart failure will have great difficulty breathing lying flat or with their legs elevated since this will deliver more blood to the heart muscle than it can pump out. Oxygen should always be administered since the condition is due to an ailing heart whose myocardium requires more oxygen to operate. The patient should be transported to the nearest hospital for stabilization.

101. d. A stroke involves an interruption of the blood supply to an area of the brain, causing tissue damage.

102. a. A stroke is also known as a cerebrovascular accident. Subdural hematomas and epidural bleeds are specific types of intracranial bleeds that may present with stroke-like symptoms. A simple concussion does not involve bleeding into the head and is not a type of stroke.

103. d. Strokes may be caused by compression, hemorrhage, or obstruction of a cerebral blood vessel. This can be related to a thrombus forming in the artery, a clot or embolus traveling to the brain, or a hemorrhage of the cerebral artery. While lack of oxygen may cause brain damage, the damage is diffuse and affects the entire brain rather than a particular area that is supplied by a single artery.

104. a. A stroke interferes with the connection between the brain and the part of the body it controls. Weakness or paralysis will occur, usually on one side of the body. Strokes generally affect motor function and do not cause pain of any kind. Breathing is controlled by reflexes and generally not affected by a stroke unless it is severe.

105. b. Each side of the brain controls the opposite side of the body. It controls the legs and arms equally, and a stroke occurring on one side of the brain will affect the arm and leg on the opposite side of the body.

106. **a.** The unconscious victim should be transported lying on their side to maintain an airway and guard against aspiration in the event of vomiting. The side affected by the stroke should be down so that the patient may use the good side as much as possible to assist you in providing care.

107. **c.** Strokes can be caused by the hemorrhage of a blood vessel from hypertension. Increased pressure in the brain will reduce blood flow to the brain, worsening the stroke. The awake patient with an intact airway should be transported with the head elevated so that the pressure in the brain can be reduced.

108. **c.** A transient ischemic attack often has the same signs and symptoms as a stroke. However, after it occurs the cerebral artery occlusion clears and the area of the brain affected recovers within a few minutes or hours of the onset. It is often referred to as a "mini-stroke" and is a warning sign for the potential of more and possibly worse strokes to come.

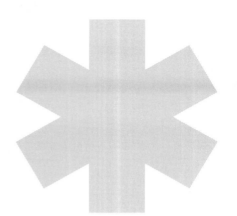

6

Medical Emergencies II

Altered Mental Status, Diabetic Emergencies, Seizures, and Allergic Reactions

D.O.T. Curriculum Objectives Covered in This Chapter:

Lesson 4-4
Lesson 4-5

CHAPTER 6 REVIEW QUESTIONS

■ ALTERED MENTAL STATUS AND DIABETIC EMERGENCIES

1. Common causes of altered mental status include:
   a. poisoning
   b. infection
   c. decreased oxygen levels
   d. all of the above

2. The first priority in treating a patient with altered mental status is to:
   a. administer sugar
   b. ensure an adequate airway
   c. perform a focused exam
   d. assess baseline vital signs

3. Of particular importance to the EMT who has encountered a patient with altered mental status is:
   a. the age and weight of the patient
   b. whether the patient used nitroglycerin
   c. the patient's history
   d. whether the patient has a prescribed inhaler

4. Diabetes mellitus is a condition in which:
   a. there is not enough sugar in the bloodstream
   b. the body is unable to use glucose normally
   c. the body produces too much insulin
   d. the cells produce too much sugar

5. Hypoglycemia is characterized by:
   a. low blood sugar
   b. high blood sugar
   c. low insulin levels
   d. slow metabolism

6. A hypoglycemic patient may:
   a. appear intoxicated
   b. have flushed, warm skin
   c. have a slow, strong pulse
   d. have dry, cool skin

7. Two questions a diabetic patient should be asked are:
   a. "Have you eaten today?" and "Do you know where you are?"
   b. "Have you eaten today" and "Have you taken your medication today?"
   c. "Do you know where you are?" and "What day is today?"
   d. "Have you taken your medication today?" and "What day is today?"

8. A medication commonly taken by diabetic patients is:
   a. nitroglycerin
   b. antihistamines
   c. aspirin
   d. insulin

9. Hypoglycemia may be caused by:
   a. an unusual strenuous period of exercise or physical work
   b. eating too much
   c. not taking enough insulin
   d. all of the above

10. Oral glucose should be given to a patient with altered mental status and a history of:
    a. heart problems
    b. diabetes mellitus
    c. asthma
    d. seizures

11. Oral glucose comes in the form of a:
    a. liquid suspension
    b. powder
    c. gel
    d. tablet

12. Oral glucose should not be given to patients who:
    a. already drank a solution containing sugar
    b. are unable to protect their airway
    c. have vomited
    d. are confused

13. The normal initial dose of oral glucose is:
    a. ¼ tube
    b. ½ tube
    c. 1 tube
    d. 2 tubes

14. Oral glucose should be placed:
    a. on the patient's tongue
    b. between the patient's cheek and gums
    c. at the back of the patient's throat
    d. on the patient's teeth

15. The greatest danger associated with the use of oral glucose is:
    a. allergic reactions
    b. low blood pressure
    c. hyperglycemia
    d. aspiration

✳ **ENRICHMENT QUESTIONS**

16. Diabetic ketoacidosis (DKA) is associated with:
    a. hyperglycemia
    b. a decreased need for insulin
    c. a decreased production of ketone bodies
    d. taking too much insulin

17. The respirations commonly associated with hyperglycemia are known as:
    a. sonorous respirations
    b. Cheyne-Stokes respirations
    c. Kussmaul respirations
    d. agonal respirations

18. A common problem associated with hyperglycemia is:
    a. hypovolemia
    b. hypertension
    c. a slow respiratory rate
    d. a slow pulse rate

19. The normal blood glucose level is:
    a. 10 to 50 mg/dL
    b. 50 to 100 mg/dL
    c. 80 to 120 mg/dL
    d. 200 to 250 mg/dL

20. Mark the following signs and symptoms as being associated with either *hypoglycemia* or *hyperglycemia*.

_____ sudden onset

_____ dry mouth and thirst

_____ rapid, deep respirations

_____ dizziness

_____ abdominal pain and vomiting

_____ pale, cool, and moist skin

_____ full, rapid pulse

_____ faintness or fainting spells

_____ sweet, fruity odor to breath

_____ dry, flushed skin

_____ weak, normal to rapid pulse

_____ extreme or general weakness

_____ gradual onset

_____ headache

_____ frequent urination

■ SEIZURES

21. Apatient who experiences a seizure has:
    a. diabetes mellitus
    b. violent muscular activity
    c. status epilepticus
    d. abnormal electrical activity in the brain

22. The EMT should remember that seizures:
    a. are always life-threatening
    b. signify the patient has epilepsy
    c. have many causes
    d. are always associated with a medical history of neurological problems

23. In children, a seizure associated with a rapid increase in body temperature is known as a:
    a. focal seizure
    b. febrile seizure
    c. hypothermic seizure
    d. petit mal seizure

24. EMTs should be aware that seizures may be caused by:
    a. increased oxygen levels in the body
    b. head trauma
    c. psychotic behavior
    d. all of the above

25. The movement associated with a seizure:
    a. may range from violent jerking to simple staring episodes
    b. always affects the entire body
    c. generally starts in one area then moves to another
    d. should be considered combative or purposeful behavior

26. When treating a patient who is actively seizing:
    a. physically restrain the patient
    b. protect the patient from further injury
    c. place an oral airway in the patient's mouth
    d. administer glucose under the tongue

27. During the period immediately following a generalized seizure, the patient is likely to be:
    a. alert and oriented to place and time
    b. sleepy but aware of what has happened
    c. unresponsive or difficult to arouse
    d. hyperactive and unable to stay still

28. If there is no cervical spine trauma suspected, the patient who has had a seizure should be placed in:
    a. a prone position
    b. a supine position
    c. the shock position
    d. the recovery position

✳ ENRICHMENT QUESTIONS

29. The EMT should be particularly concerned if a patient experiences:
    a. the same type of seizure that he or she has had in the past
    b. repeated, uncontrolled seizures with no return of consciousness between episodes
    c. a seizure involving one limb
    d. a full-body seizure with no loss of consciousness

30. An adult patient with a history of epilepsy has experienced a seizure but is now alert and oriented. He does not want to go to the hospital. The EMT should:
    a. restrain the patient and take him to the hospital
    b. thoroughly document the incident and have the patient sign a refusal form
    c. have the patient take an extra dose of his antiseizure medicine
    d. suggest the patient drive himself to his family doctor

31. Full-body convulsive activity is characteristic of a:
    a. petit mal seizure
    b. grand mal seizure
    c. temporal lobe seizure
    d. psychomotor seizure

32. The best way to describe the tonic and clonic phases some seizure patients experience is that:
    a. during the tonic phase the patient experiences sensations warning of an impending seizure; during the clonic phase the body becomes stiff
    b. during the tonic phase the body jerks about violently; during the clonic phase the patient is very lethargic and sleepy
    c. during the tonic phase the body becomes rigid and stiff; during the clonic phase the patient is confused and drowsy
    d. during the tonic phase the body becomes rigid and stiff; during the clonic phase the body jerks about violently

33. Status epilepticus may be defined as:
    a. the type of seizure experienced by a person with epilepsy
    b. repeated, uncontrolled seizures with no return of consciousness in between
    c. a series of mini seizures
    d. a full-body seizure with no loss of consciousness

34. Simple partial seizures are best described as:
    a. seizures that start in the hand or foot and then spread to the entire side of the body
    b. brief periods of unconsciousness without accompanying loss of motor tone
    c. generalized convulsive activity
    d. seizures in which the patient experiences no loss of consciousness

35. The peculiar sensation experienced by some patients that may precede and warn of an impending seizure is known as:
    a. an aura
    b. a mantra
    c. a pre-seizure
    d. an absence seizure

■ ALLERGIC REACTIONS

36. A patient with an allergic reaction may present with:
    a. hives and itching
    b. difficulty breathing
    c. a tight feeling in the throat
    d. all of the above

37. The most serious complication in a severe allergic reaction is:
    a. hives and itching
    b. slow heart rate
    c. difficulty breathing
    d. increased blood pressure

38. Concerning allergic reactions, it must be remembered that:
    a. the reaction may affect many parts of the body
    b. all reactions occur to the same extent
    c. all patients react the same way to an allergen
    d. the reaction is limited to the immediate area of the exposure to the allergen

39. The difficulty breathing experienced during an allergic reaction may be caused by:
    a. widespread dilation of the bronchial passages
    b. swelling of the throat and respiratory tract
    c. bacteria in the throat
    d. the diaphragm not contracting properly

40. The altered mental status exhibited by some patients having a severe allergic reaction is due to:
    a. constriction of blood vessels in the brain
    b. increased blood pressure
    c. low blood sugar
    d. hypoperfusion and hypoxia

41. The use of epinephrine is indicated:
    a. if a patient is having a severe allergic reaction accompanied by difficulty breathing or hypoperfusion
    b. anytime a patient experiences an allergic reaction
    c. whenever a patient is having an allergic reaction accompanied by hives and itching
    d. whenever a patient with an epinephrine prescription has been stung by a bee

42. The effects of epinephrine on the respiratory and circulatory systems include:
    a. dilating bronchioles and dilating blood vessels
    b. constricting bronchioles and dilating blood vessels
    c. dilating bronchioles and constricting blood vessels
    d. constricting bronchioles and constricting blood vessels

43. A contraindication for administering epinephrine to a patient experiencing a severe allergic reaction is:
    a. hypersensitivity to bee stings
    b. a history of asthma
    c. a patient under the age of 16
    d. there is no contraindication

44. Epinephrine used to manage an allergic reaction is usually administered:
    a. intravenously
    b. intramuscularly
    c. subcutaneously
    d. intradermally

45. The adult dose of epinephrine for allergic reactions is:
    a. 0.1 mg
    b. 0.2 mg
    c. 0.3 mg
    d. 0.4 mg

46. The usual autoinjector dose of epinephrine for infants or children experiencing an allergic reaction is:
    a. 0.05 mg
    b. 0.15 mg
    c. 0.25 mg
    d. 0.35 mg

47. The preferred anatomic location for administering epinephrine is:
    a. the lateral portion of the thigh midway between the waist and the knee
    b. the buttocks
    c. the abdomen, immediately below the navel
    d. the medial portion of the forearm, midway between the elbow and the wrist

48. For the epinephrine autoinjector to work:
    a. it is preferable but not always necessary to remove the clothing over the injection site
    b. the clothing over the injection site must be removed
    c. the injector must be filled with medication by the EMT
    d. a needle must be attached to the injector by the EMT

49. After the epinephrine autoinjector activates:
    a. immediately remove it from the patient's skin
    b. move it to an alternate spot on the patient and activate it again
    c. reset it for use on the next patient
    d. hold it in place for 10 seconds

50. Side effects of epinephrine include:
    a. decreased pulse rate and pale skin
    b. decreased pulse rate and flushed skin
    c. increased pulse rate and flushed skin
    d. increased pulse rate and pale skin

51. If a patient's condition continues to deteriorate after epinephrine is administered:
    a. the patient is most likely experiencing a reaction to the epinephrine itself
    b. half the original dose should be administered
    c. an additional dose may be ordered
    d. defibrillate the patient using an automated external defibrillator

■ **MISCELLANEOUS MEDICAL EMERGENCIES**

✳ **ENRICHMENT QUESTIONS**

52. An aneurysm is a:
    a. large varicose vein
    b. section of artery clogged with plaque
    c. deformed section of vein
    d. ballooning out of a weak spot in a blood vessel

53. An aortic aneurysm should be suspected if a patient displays any of the following signs or symptoms *except*:
    a. unequal or absent pulses in some or all extremities
    b. sudden onset of shortness of breath
    c. sharp, tearing pain in the midline or back
    d. a pulsating mass in the abdomen

54. A patient suffering from kidney stones may complain of pain radiating:
    a. from the flank to the groin
    b. from the umbilicus to the shoulder
    c. from the groin down both legs
    d. from the back to the neck

55. If a kidney stone is suspected, the EMT may:
    a. attempt to secure a urine specimen
    b. refer the patient to a urologist
    c. place cold packs over the affected area
    d. ask the patient if he or she has been experiencing any difficulty or pain with urination

56. A patient with a kidney stone will usually:
    a. assume one position and not move
    b. complain of mild pain
    c. be calm and relaxed
    d. be unable to find a position of comfort

57. In most cases, anytime a female patient is encountered who complains of abdominal pain, the EMT should suspect the patient may be:
    a. having a heart attack
    b. suffering from kidney stones
    c. pregnant
    d experiencing a diabetic emergency

■ **Additional Points for Discussion** ■

1. What brand or brands of oral glucose is carried on your ambulance? Review the directions for administration.

2. Familiarize yourself with the names of common antiseizure medications that patients may take.

3. Is your service allowed to assist an anaphylaxis patient with the use of an AnaKit? If so, review its use.

ANSWERS TO CHAPTER 6 REVIEW QUESTIONS

■ ALTERED MENTAL STATUS AND DIABETIC EMERGENCIES

1. **d.** All of the above. Altered mental status may be caused by poisoning, infection, or decreased oxygen levels. It may also be caused by head trauma or hypoglycemia, or may be seen after a seizure.

2. **b.** Ensuring an adequate airway is the first concern when treating a patient with an altered mental status.

3. **c.** The patient history is of particular importance when a patient with an altered mental status is encountered. The history enables the EMT to determine whether the condition is related to an ongoing medical problem or is a new occurrence.

4. **b.** Diabetes mellitus is a condition in which the body is unable to utilize glucose normally.

5. **a.** Hypoglycemia is characterized by low blood sugar.

6. **a.** A hypoglycemic patient may seem intoxicated. Because of this, the EMT must use caution when assessing a patient who is believed to be drunk. Misdiagnosis could be deadly. The hypoglycemic patient normally presents with pale, moist skin and a rapid pulse.

7. **b.** Diabetic patients should be asked if they have eaten today and taken their insulin today. If the patient is unconscious, ask a family member these questions.

8. **d.** Diabetic patients may take insulin. Insulin allows glucose to cross the cell membrane.

9. **a.** Hypoglycemia may occur after an unusually strenuous period of exercise or physical work. It may also occur if the patient eats too little or vomits after eating, or if the patient has taken too much insulin.

10. **b.** A patient with altered mental status and a history of diabetes should be given oral glucose.

11. **c.** Oral glucose comes in the form of a gel.

12. **b.** Oral glucose should not be given to a patient who is unable to protect his or her airway. It should not be given to unconscious patients or those who are unable to swallow.

13. **c.** The normal initial dose of oral glucose is one tube.

14. **b.** Oral glucose should be placed between the patient's cheek and gums.

15. **d.** The greatest danger associated with administering oral glucose is aspiration into the lungs.

❋ ENRICHMENT QUESTIONS

16. **a.** Diabetic ketoacidosis (DKA) is associated with hyperglycemia, or high blood glucose. This can occur if a patient has a lack of adequate insulin or if a patient on insulin stops taking it. In DKA, there is an increase in the production of ketone bodies, some of which are acidic and lead to acidosis.

17. **c.** Patients in diabetic coma may exhibit rapid, deep sighing respirations known as Kussmaul respirations. The patient is attempting to lower the acidity of the blood by blowing off carbon dioxide.

18. **a.** A common problem associated with hyperglycemia is hypovolemia. Volume depletion can be severe enough to result in low blood pressure.

19. **c.** A normal range for blood glucose is 80 to 120 mg/dL.

20. Mark the following signs and symptoms as being associated with either hypoglycemia or hyperglycemia.

<u>hypoglycemia</u>   sudden onset

<u>hyperglycemia</u>   dry mouth and thirst

<u>hyperglycemia</u>   rapid, deep respirations

<u>hypoglycemia</u>   dizziness

<u>hyperglycemia</u>   abdominal pain and vomiting

<u>hypoglycemia</u>   pale, cool, and moist skin

<u>hypoglycemia</u>   full, rapid pulse

<u>hypoglycemia</u>   faintness or fainting spells

<u>hyperglycemia</u>   sweet, fruity odor to breath

<u>hyperglycemia</u>   dry, flushed skin

<u>hyperglycemia</u>   weak, normal to rapid pulse

<u>hypoglycemia</u>   extreme or general weakness

<u>hyperglycemia</u>   gradual onset

<u>hypoglycemia</u>   headache

<u>hyperglycemia</u>   frequent urination

■ **SEIZURES**

21. **d.** Abnormal electrical activity in the brain is associated with seizures. Not all patients with seizures have epilepsy, and seizures do not always involve violent muscular activity.

22. **c.** There are many causes of seizures. Seizures normally are not life-threatening, although they can be frightening. The patient does not always have an associated medical history of epilepsy.

23. **b.** A febrile seizure is a seizure associated with a high temperature and is normally seen in infants and children. It is related more to the rapid increase in body temperature rather than the temperature itself.

24. **b.** When a patient is encountered who has had a seizure, the EMT should consider the presence of head trauma.

25. **a.** Seizures may be characterized by violent jerking of parts of the body or may be as simple as a staring episode. The EMT should carefully note on the run report the area of the body involved and how it was affected.

26. **b.** An EMT should protect an actively seizing patient from further injury and, if possible, from embarrassment. The only time a patient should be physically restrained is if the patient is in danger of physically harming himself or herself. Bite blocks are not recommended in most EMS systems; however, if they are used, they should not be placed while the patient is actively seizing. Do not put glucose in the patient's mouth during the seizure, as it may be aspirated into the lungs.

27. **c.** During the period immediately following a generalized seizure, the patient will most likely be unresponsive or difficult to arouse. This is known as the postictal phase or period. As time passes, the patient will become more oriented to person, place, and time, but may not remember having a seizure.

28. **d.** After a patient has experienced a seizure, he or she should be placed in the recovery position if there is no associated cervical spine trauma.

✳ **ENRICHMENT QUESTIONS**

29. **b.** Repeated, uncontrolled seizures with no return of consciousness between seizures is a true emergency. This is referred to as status epilepticus.

30. **b.** An adult patient with a history of seizures who is alert and oriented has the right to refuse transport, even if he or she has recently had a seizure. The EMTs should thoroughly document the incident and explain to the patient their concern about not transporting and their willingness to do so. If he or she still does not want to go, have the patient sign a refusal.

31. **b.** Grand mal seizures are full-body convulsions. They are also known as generalized motor seizures. Repetition of inappropriate acts is characteristic of psychomotor seizures or temporal lobe seizures.

32. **d.** During the tonic phase the body becomes rigid and stiff. During the clonic phase the body jerks about violently. With this type of activity, the patient may lose bladder and bowel control, and drool and foam at the mouth.

33. **b.** Repeated, uncontrolled seizures with no return of consciousness between seizures is status epilepticus. This is a true emergency.

34. **d.** Patients who experience simple seizures have no accompanying loss of consciousness. However, motor activity may be present. One form of partial seizure activity is the Jacksonian seizure, which is usually characterized by seizure activity starting in the hand or foot and spreading to the entire side of the body.

35. **a.** An aura may warn a patient of an impending seizure. It may be an unusual smell, taste, visual disturbance, or sensation the patient experiences prior to the seizure. Petit mal seizures are sometimes referred to as absence seizures.

■ **ALLERGIC REACTIONS**

36. **d.** All of the above. Signs and symptoms of an allergic reaction may include itching and hives, difficulty breathing, a tight feeling in the throat. Also, wheezing, increased heart rate, decreased blood pressure, and a variety of other signs and symptoms may be present.

37. **c.** Breathing difficulty is the most serious complication of an allergic reaction. The patient may also experience severe hypoperfusion and eventual death.

38. **a.** Although the allergic reaction may result from something happening in a particular area of the body, such as a bite or sting, the reaction may affect other parts of the body. Reactions can vary, depending on the patient.

39. **b.** The difficulty breathing experienced by a person having an allergic reaction may be related to swelling of the throat and respiratory tract.

40. **d.** The altered mental status exhibited by some patients having a severe allergic reaction is due to hypoperfusion and hypoxia.

41. **a.** Epinephrine should be administered to a patient who has been prescribed the medication and is experiencing a severe allergic reaction accompanied by difficulty breathing or hypoperfusion. Use of the medication is not indicated simply because the patient has been stung by a bee or is experiencing a mild allergic reaction.

42. **c.** Epinephrine dilates bronchioles and constricts blood vessels. Bronchiole dilation enables the patient to breathe easier, and blood vessel constriction increases blood pressure, thereby improving perfusion to the brain.

43. **d.** There is no contraindication for using epinephrine when a person is experiencing a severe allergic reaction. Epinephrine can even be given to infants and children.

44. **b.** The epinephrine autoinjector used to manage an allergic reaction injects the medication intramuscularly.

45. **c.** The adult dose of epinephrine for an allergic reaction is 0.3 mg.

46. **b.** The usual autoinjector dose of epinephrine for infants and children experiencing an allergic reaction is 0.15 mg.

47. **a.** The preferred location for administering epinephrine is the lateral portion of the thigh, midway between the waist and the knee. Some areas allow the fleshy portion of upper arm to be used also. Consult local protocols.

48. a. For the autoinjector to work it is preferable to remove the clothing over the site. However, if clothing is thin enough, the injection can be performed through it. The injector comes prefilled with the medication and with a needle attached.

49. d. After the injector activates, hold it in place for 10 seconds to allow the medication to be injected. Dispose of the autoinjector in an approved sharps container.

50. d. Side effects of epinephrine include increased pulse and pale skin. The patient may also complain of dizziness, chest pain, headache, and may become nauseated and vomit.

51. c. If a patient's condition continues to deteriorate after epinephrine is administered, an additional dose may be ordered by medical control.

■ MISCELLANEOUS MEDICAL EMERGENCIES

✳ ENRICHMENT QUESTIONS

52. d. A ballooning out of a weak spot in a blood vessel is an aneurysm. Aneurysms, especially aortic aneurysms, are extreme emergency situations.

53. b. A patient with an aortic aneurysm may present with unequal or absent pulses in some or all extremities; sharp, tearing pain in the midline or back; or a pulsating mass in the abdomen. The EMT may also note a difference in blood pressure readings in the arms, or a sudden loss of circulation in the legs. Aortic aneurysms may also be located in the thorax. A patient with an aortic aneurysm should be promptly, but gently, transported to a hospital with surgical capabilities if possible.

54. a. Pain accompanying kidney stones may radiate from the flank to the groin.

55. d. A patient with a suspected kidney stone may be questioned concerning any urinary difficulty or pain, and this should be noted on the patient report.

56. d. A patient with a kidney stone will typically be unable to find a comfortable position. This is considered one of the most severe forms of pain.

57. c. In most cases, the EMT should suspect a gynecologic problem if a female patient complains of abdominal pain. Also, unless a female patient is very young or very old, the EMT should suspect the patient may be pregnant.

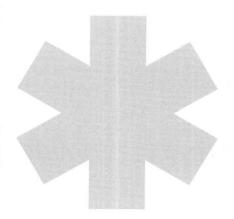

7

Poisoning, Overdose, and Environmental Emergencies

D.O.T. Curriculum Objectives Covered in This Chapter:

Lesson 4-6
Lesson 4-7

CHAPTER 7 REVIEW QUESTIONS

■ POISONING AND OVERDOSE

1. Four main ways poisons enter the body are:
   a. injection, inhalation, ingestion, and insect stings
   b. unintentional, absorption, accidental, and intentional
   c. ingestion, inhalation, injection, and absorption
   d. direct, inhalation, indirect, and ingestion

2. Most poisonings in children are related to:
   a. drug abuse
   b. surface contact
   c. accidental ingestion
   d. child abuse

3. Poisoning should be suspected if a patient displayed:
   a. discoloration around the mouth and lips
   b. burning or pain in the mouth, throat, or stomach
   c. difficulty talking or swallowing
   d. all of the above

4. With orders from medical command, management of a patient who has ingested poison may include:
   a. degrading the poison
   b. making the patient vomit
   c. attempting to locate a specific antidote for the poison
   d. administering activated charcoal

5. An important piece of information to obtain when managing a poisoning incident that is less critical when managing most other medical emergencies is the patient's:
   a. date of birth
   b. weight
   c. medical history
   d. allergy history

6. Any containers, bottles, or labels found at the scene of a poisoning emergency should be:
   a. taken to the receiving hospital
   b. decontaminated and given to fire department personnel
   c. given to law enforcement officers
   d. destroyed immediately to prevent further contamination of personnel and the scene

7. When managing a patient who has ingested poison, the EMT should try to determine:
   a. what the substance tasted like
   b. how much of the substance was ingested
   c. where the substance was obtained
   d. the age of the substance

8. The EMT should attempt to determine exactly when a substance was ingested because:
   a. the information may affect the treatment of the patient
   b. many substances lose their potency after a certain period
   c. if no ill effects are noted after 2 or 3 hours, the patient probably is not in danger
   d. antidotes administered at a hospital usually must be given within an hour of ingestion

9. The first step in treating a victim who has inhaled poison gas is to:
   a. apply oxygen
   b. determine the type of gas involved
   c. open the airway and assess breathing
   d. remove the patient from the toxic environment

10. Early signs and symptoms of carbon monoxide poisoning include:
    a. cherry-red skin color
    b. headache, nausea, and vomiting
    c. unconsciousness
    d. chest pain radiating to the left arm

11. During an incident involving a poisonous gas, the EMT must remember:
    a. poisonous gases have distinct odors that make them readily identifiable
    b. poisonous gases are lighter than air and rapidly dissipate
    c. the poisonous gas may still be present but undetectable by the EMTs
    d. the patient will improve once he or she is out of the toxic environment

12. Insect and spider bites are examples of poisons that enter the body through:
    a. absorption
    b. subjection
    c. trajection
    d. injection

13. Dry fertilizer is an example of a poison that enters the body through:
    a. injection
    b. absorption
    c. osmosis
    d. digestion

14. Management of a patient who has been poisoned by contact with a powdered chemical includes:
    a. brushing away as much chemical as possible, then washing away the rest with water
    b. leaving the chemical on the patient so it can be identified at the hospital
    c. diluting the chemical with a light mist of water
    d. wrapping the patient in a sheet to prevent spread of the chemical

15. When liquid toxins have contacted the skin, the site should be irrigated:
    a. with sterile water
    b. until an odor is no longer present
    c. for at least 20 minutes
    d. until the site looks clean

16. Activated charcoal may be useful in managing poisons that enter the body:
    a. intravenously
    b. through the lungs
    c. over a prolonged time
    d. through ingestion

17. Activated charcoal is useful in cases involving poisonings because it:
    a. causes vomiting
    b. decreases stomach motility
    c. prevents the body from absorbing a poison
    d. is a direct antidote for most poisons

18. Activated charcoal used by EMTs normally comes:
    a. as a powder
    b. as a gel
    c. in tablet form
    d. premixed in water

19. Contraindications for using activated charcoal include all of the following *except*:
    a. an inability to swallow
    b. ingestion of detergents
    c. altered mental status
    d. ingestion of acids and alkalis

20. The usual adult dose of activated charcoal is:
    a. 5 to 12.5 g
    b. 12.5 to 25 g
    c. 25 to 50 g
    d. 50 to 75 g

21. The usual dose of activated charcoal for infants and children is:
    a. 5 to 12.5 g
    b. 12.5 to 25 g
    c. 25 to 50 g
    d. 50 to 75 g

22. When basing the dose of activated charcoal on a patient's weight, the dose is:
    a. 1 g/kg of body weight for both children and adults
    b. 1 g/kg of body weight for adults and 0.5 g/kg of body weight for children
    c. 0.5 g/kg of body weight for both children and adults
    d. 2 g/kg of body weight for adults and 1 g/kg of body weight for children

23. Before administering activated charcoal:
    a. shake the container vigorously
    b. mix the charcoal with water
    c. avoid agitating the container
    d. have the patient drink a large glass of water or milk

24. A normal side effect that is associated with taking activated charcoal is:
    a. diarrhea
    b. abdominal cramps
    c. heartburn
    d. black stools

25. If the patient vomits shortly after taking activated charcoal:
    a. repeat the activated charcoal at twice the initial dose
    b. administer syrup of ipecac
    c. repeat the initial dose one time
    d. do not give any more activated charcoal

✳ ENRICHMENT QUESTIONS

26. Ingested poisons most commonly affect the:
    a. respiratory system
    b. cardiovascular system
    c. gastrointestinal tract
    d. nervous system

27. A major concern when dealing with inhaled poisons is that they:
    a. are often exhaled by the patient and may contaminate the EMT
    b. may also damage the lining of the patient's airway
    c. take longer to enter the bloodstream
    d. all of the above

28. If poisoning was caused by an animal bite or sting:
    a. be careful not to also become a victim
    b. take whatever means are necessary to catch the animal for identification
    c. transport the patient to a rabies control center
    d. the effects are generally local in nature

29. If a child has handled a corrosive substance, the EMT should:
    a. wash the child's hands and fingers
    b. administer syrup of ipecac
    c. bandage the hands
    d. wear utility gloves and a mask

30. Your patient is a known narcotics user and has apparently overdosed. The greatest risk to a patient associated with this type of overdose is:
    a. hypertensive crisis
    b. rapid heart rate
    c. respiratory depression or arrest
    d. hypoglycemia

31. Common signs and symptoms of a narcotics overdose include:
    a. constricted or pinpoint pupils
    b. rapid respiratory rates
    c. Kussmaul breathing
    d. hyperactivity

32. Common narcotics include all of the following *except*:
    a. heroin
    b. morphine
    c. cocaine
    d. codeine

33. A teenage patient presents with a fast pulse rate, dilated pupils, and flushed skin. He can speak but is making no sense, and he keeps wanting you to kill the "spiders and bugs" on the floor that aren't there. Friends say he took some unknown pills they got from an acquaintance at school. You suspect he has taken:
    a. heroin
    b. downers
    c. narcotics
    d. hallucinogens

34. A patient who has taken amphetamine or methamphetamine would be expected to display:
    a. a rapid pulse, rapid breathing, and dilated pupils
    b. a slow pulse, constricted pupils, and excitement
    c. drowsiness, slow breathing, and constricted pupils
    d. excessive salivation, rapid breathing rate, and drowsiness

■ ENVIRONMENTAL EMERGENCIES

35. A direct transfer of heat from a warm body to a cooler object, such as would occur if a person was immersed in cold water, is:
    a. conduction
    b. evaporation
    c. convection
    d. radiation

36. A medical condition that could predispose a patient to hypothermia is:
    a. asthma
    b. obesity
    c. spinal injury
    d. high blood pressure

37. Infants and young children are more at risk than adults for hypothermia because they have:
    a. slower breathing rates than adults
    b. more body fat than adults
    c. slower pulse rates than adults
    d. a larger body surface area than adults

38. To assess a suspected hypothermia patient's body temperature, feel the patient's:
    a. abdominal skin
    b. forehead
    c. arms
    d. feet

39. When a patient becomes hypothermic, shivering:
    a. is always present
    b. is not present
    c. may or may not be present
    d. is undesirable

40. In the early stages of hypothermia, a patient's vital signs typically include a:
    a. rapid pulse and slow breathing
    b. slow pulse and rapid breathing
    c. slow pulse and slow breathing
    d. rapid pulse and rapid breathing

41. During management of a hypothermic patient, alcoholic beverages should be avoided because they:
    a. decrease the pulse rate
    b. can cause an allergic reaction
    c. cause vasodilation
    d. increase the patient's breathing rate

42. Management of a hypothermic patient who is alert and responding appropriately would include:
    a. having the patient exercise to generate body heat
    b. rewarming the patient by applying heat packs to the groin, armpits, and neck areas
    c. massaging arms and legs to stimulate circulation
    d. giving the patient hot coffee to drink

43. When managing a severely hypothermic unresponsive patient:
    a. hyperventilate the patient
    b. do not perform chest compressions because they may cause ventricular fibrillation
    c. handle the patient very gently, avoiding rough movements
    d. do not administer oxygen

44. Before starting CPR on an unresponsive hypothermia patient, check the:
    a. radial pulse for 20 seconds
    b. radial pulse for 1 minute
    c. carotid pulse for 15 seconds
    d. carotid pulse for 30 to 45 seconds

45. When an unresponsive hypothermia patient is encountered:
    a. resuscitation should be attempted only on a patient who has been hypothermic less than 20 minutes
    b. the patient is not dead until he or she is warm and dead
    c. a patient with muscle rigidity should not be resuscitated
    d. if the patient appears dead, he or she is probably dead

46. A superficial local cold injury is characterized by:
    a. blanching of the skin
    b. white, waxy skin
    c. the area feeling frozen when it is palpated
    d. blisters

47. A sign of a deep local cold injury is:
    a. soft skin
    b. moist skin
    c. white, waxy skin
    d. tingling in the injured area

48. If an early or superficial local cold injury is noted on an extremity:
    a. splint the extremity
    b. rub or massage the affected area
    c. apply snow to the area if available
    d. leave the area uncovered

49. To manage a late or deep cold injury:
    a. apply heat to the injured area
    b. break any blisters that may have formed to allow cold fluid to escape
    c. cover the injured area with dry dressings
    d. rub or massage the affected area to restore circulation

50. A local cold injury may need to be rewarmed if:
    a. severe pain develops
    b. extremely long or delayed transport is inevitable
    c. the injured area is likely to refreeze
    d. the patient is unresponsive

51. In the field, a local cold injury should be rewarmed:
    a. gradually in cool water
    b. rapidly in very hot water
    c. gradually using rubbing alcohol
    d. rapidly in warm water

52. When dressing hands or feet after rewarming:
    a. place dry, sterile dressings between the fingers or toes
    b. use an occlusive dressing
    c. use moist dressings
    d. wrap them tightly using elastic bandages

53. Climate contributes to the chances of heat emergencies occurring if:
    a. barometric pressure is low
    b. there is high relative humidity
    c. it is warm and dry
    d. ambient temperature is low

54. Elderly patients are particularly at risk for heat emergencies because they:
    a. are very mobile and cannot remove their own clothing
    b. have higher pulse rates and low blood pressure
    c. are less sensitive to heat and have better blood supply to their extremities
    d. have poor thermoregulation and may take many medications

55. After ensuring an adequate airway, the first step in treating a victim of a heat emergency is to:
    a. remove the patient from the hot environment
    b. lay the patient on the left side
    c. loosen the patient's clothing
    d. drench the patient with cold water

56. The muscle cramps that may accompany a heat emergency are believed to be related to:
    a. excessive blood supply to the muscles
    b. a loss of body salts
    c. hypothermia
    d. heat exhaustion

57. A dire emergency exists if a patient has:
    a. moist, pale, normal-temperature skin
    b. moist, pale, cool skin
    c. moist, pink, normal-temperature skin
    d. dry or moist, hot skin

58. Heat emergency patients should be given water to drink if they are:
    a. feeling nauseated
    b. semiresponsive and have dry, hot skin
    c. responsive and have moist, pale, normal-temperature skin or cool skin
    d. complaining of thirst

59. An important early step in treating a patient with skin that is hot to the touch is to:
    a. conserve the patient's body heat so as not to cause rebound hypothermia
    b. wipe down the patient with rubbing alcohol
    c. keep the patient's skin dry
    d. apply cold packs to the neck, groin, and armpits

60. The difference between near-drowning and drowning is:
    a. near-drowning occurs close to shore
    b. near-drowning does not involve aspiration of water into the lungs
    c. near-drowning patients survive at least temporarily after the incident
    d. near-drowning patients have not stopped breathing

61. Early management of the drowning or near-drowning patient primarily involves:
    a. caring for hypovolemic shock
    b. early respiratory and circulatory support
    c. removing water from the patient's lungs
    d. reversing acidosis

62. Any patient found unconscious in a swimming pool should be suspected of having:
    a. spinal injuries
    b. a heart attack
    c. abdominal injuries
    d. extremity fractures

63. When rescuing an unconscious patient from a swimming pool:
    a. wait until the patient is out of the water to start artificial ventilations
    b. move the patient to the side of the pool in the position in which he or she was found
    c. start chest compressions while the patient is still in the water if there is no pulse
    d. roll the patient face up as soon as possible while providing spinal support

64. A cold-water near-drowning patient:
    a. should not be resuscitated if submerged longer than 30 minutes
    b. should be aggressively rewarmed in the back of the ambulance
    c. may survive even after a long submersion time
    d. is likely to have brain damage if resuscitated

65. If spinal injury is not suspected, a near-drowning patient who is breathing should be placed in the:
    a. recovery position
    b. prone position
    c. shock position
    d. Trendelenburg position

66. If gastric distention interferes with performing artificial ventilations on a drowning patient, the EMT should:
    a. discontinue ventilations and perform chest compressions only
    b. place the patient on his or her left side and apply firm pressure over the epigastric area
    c. administer more forceful ventilations
    d. insert a suction catheter as far as possible into the patient's throat to remove stomach contents

67. To remove an insect stinger from a patient, the EMT should:
    a. scrape it off
    b. grasp it with a pair of tweezers and pull gently
    c. freeze the stinger with an ice cube before removing it
    d. coat the stinger with petroleum jelly before removing it

68. If possible, the site of a sting or bite should be:
    a. elevated above the level of the patient's heart
    b. massaged gently during transport
    c. directly rubbed with ice
    d. positioned slightly below the level of the patient's heart

69. When managing a snakebite victim:
    a. apply heat to the bite area
    b. do not apply cold to the bite area
    c. elevate the bite area if an extremity is involved
    d. try to keep the patient active

70. If a snakebite is encountered, a constricting band should be applied:
    a. whenever it is a known pit viper bite
    b. only if the snake can be immediately captured and identified
    c. only after consulting medical direction
    d. if incision and suction are to be performed

71. While managing a patient with an animal sting or bite, the EMT should be alert for the potential development of:
    a. hypoglycemia
    b. cellulitis
    c. an allergic reaction
    d. high blood pressure

■ **Additional Points for Discussion** ■

1. What is the phone number for your local poison information center?

2. What are your local protocols regarding rewarming of the following?

   • Hypothermia patients:

   • Local cold injuries:

3. What venomous animals or insects are common in your area? (NOTE: Many may be found in private collections, not just in the wild.)

4. What medical facilities in your area are best able to treat poisonous animal bites or stings?

5. There is no universal snake antivenin. The snake must be identified, and the specific type of antivenin administered. If a poisonous snakebite is encountered:

   • How would you go about getting a positive identification of the type of snake involved?

   • Where is the closest supply of snake antivenin located, and what specific snakebites could be treated?

6. What are your local protocols regarding management of the following?

   • Poisonous snakebites:

   • Marine life stings:

ANSWERS TO CHAPTER 7 REVIEW QUESTIONS

■ POISONING AND OVERDOSE

1. **c.** The four main ways poisons enter the body are through ingestion, inhalation, injection, and absorption.

2. **c.** Accidental ingestion accounts for most poisonings in children.

3. **d.** All of the above. If a patient displays discoloration around the mouth and lips; has burning or pain in the mouth, throat or stomach; or has difficulty talking or swallowing, suspect poisoning.

4. **d.** With orders from medical command, the EMT may administer activated charcoal to some poisoning patients. Inducing vomiting in the field is no longer indicated. Do not waste time trying to locate a specific antidote for the poison.

5. **b.** The weight of the individual is of particular concern when treating a poisoning patient. The same amount of poison will have greater effects on a person with less body weight than a person with greater body weight.

6. **a.** Any containers, bottles, or labels found at the scene of a poisoning should be taken to the receiving hospital. Take care, however, not to contaminate medical personnel or equipment when collecting or transporting the substance or container.

7. **b.** If possible, try to determine how much of a substance was ingested because this information can affect treatment. This may not always be easy if the poisoning involves a small child or if a patient has accidentally ingested a poison.

8. **a.** Although finding a specific antidote is not important, trying to determine when a poison was ingested since this may affect treatment of the patient. The effects of some poisons may not be noted for several hours after exposure.

9. **d.** Before all else, remove the victim of poison gas inhalation from the toxic environment. This should be done only while wearing protective equipment, such as self-contained breathing apparatus.

10. **b.** Headache, nausea, and vomiting are early signs and symptoms of carbon monoxide poisoning. The headache is caused by widespread dilation of the cerebral arteries. A cherry-red color is a late sign of carbon monoxide poisoning and is often seen only after the patient is dead.

11. **c.** Caution must be exercised when a poison gas inhalation incident is encountered since the gas may still be present but undetectable by the EMTs. Some gases have no odor, color, or taste. The patient's condition may continue to deteriorate even after removal from the toxic environment because the poison is already in the patient's bloodstream.

12. **d.** The poison from insect and spider bites enters the body by injection.

13. **b.** Dry fertilizer is a poison that enters the body through absorption.

14. **a.** Chemicals that have contacted the body should be brushed off if dry, or washed off if liquid. The chemical must be removed to decrease further absorption.

15. **c.** When a patient is contaminated by a liquid toxin, irrigate the contaminated area for at least 20 minutes. Rather than delay transport, irrigation can normally be accomplished en route to the hospital. The water should be clean but need not be sterile. Just because the site looks clean or an odor is no longer present does not mean that all the toxin has been removed.

16. **d.** Activated charcoal is used to treat certain poisons that enter the body through ingestion. Poisons that enter the body over a long period, regardless of the method of entry, tend to be more difficult to treat.

17. **c.** Activated charcoal prevents the poison from being absorbed into the body through the gastrointestinal tract. It works by adsorbing (not absorbing) poisons, that is, it binds with the toxins. This allows them to pass through the patient's digestive system with a minimum of harm.

18. **d.** The activated charcoal carried by EMTs comes premixed in water. Although it is available as a powder, this form is not recommended for use in the field.

19. **b.** Generally, contraindications for the use of activated charcoal include ingestion of acids and alkalis, altered mental status, or an inability to swallow. Always follow local protocols regarding exact contraindications.

20. **c.** The usual adult dose of activated charcoal is 25 to 50 g.

21. **b.** The usual dose of activated charcoal for infants and children is 12.5 to 25 g, approximately one-half the adult dose.

22. **a.** When using the patient's weight as a dosing guideline, administer 1 g of activated charcoal per kilogram of patient body weight.

23. **a.** Before administering the activated charcoal, shake the container vigorously to mix the charcoal with the water. Although it does not have a particularly bad taste, do not tell the patient it tastes good (they may not agree after trying it).

24. **d.** Black stools are a normal side effect of activated charcoal.

25. **c.** If the patient vomits shortly after taking activated charcoal, the EMT may repeat the dose one time.

✳ ENRICHMENT QUESTIONS

26. **c.** Ingested poisons most commonly affect the gastrointestinal tract. The patient may experience nausea, vomiting, abdominal cramps, and diarrhea.

27. **b.** Inhaled poisons may also damage the lining of the patient's airway. In general, these poisons are rapidly absorbed into the bloodstream through the capillaries in the lungs. There usually is no danger that the EMT will be poisoned by the patient's exhaled breath. However, solvents inhaled to get high may be excreted by the lungs and pose a danger to a rescuer doing mouth-to-mask resuscitation.

28. **a.** Because EMTs may not be familiar with methods for handling poisonous insects or animals, be careful not to become a victim also. The capture and identification of such animals should be performed by qualified personnel.

29. **a.** Wash the hands and fingers of a child who has handled or been poisoned by corrosives. This prevents eye damage that may be caused if the child rubs his or her eyes. Wearing rubber gloves may be indicated, but a mask is not necessary and may upset the child. Be careful to avoid being splattered while cleaning the child.

30. **c.** Narcotics cause respiratory depression and arrest. EMTs must be aggressive in managing the airway and ventilations of a narcotics overdose patient.

31. **a.** Signs and symptoms of a narcotics overdose include constricted or pinpoint pupils, depressed mental status, and a slow respiratory rate. Kussmaul breathing, which is characterized by deep, rapid respirations, is not seen.

32. **c.** Heroin, morphine, codeine, opium, and paregoric are just a few examples of narcotics. Cocaine is an upper or stimulant.

33. **d.** These signs and symptoms are consistent with those produced by hallucinogens. Narcotics (including heroin), and downers are not usually associated with fast pulse rates and hyperactivity.

34. **a.** Amphetamine and methamphetamine are examples of uppers, or stimulants. Patients will usually present with an increased pulse and respiratory rate, dilated pupils, and sweating, and appear very excited.

■ ENVIRONMENTAL EMERGENCIES

35. **a.** Conduction refers to heat transfer through the direct contact of two objects. Convection refers to heat transfer through the movement of liquids or gases.

36. **c.** A patient with a spinal injury may be more at risk for hypothermia because such an injury can affect the body's ability to regulate heat. Any unresponsive patient found in a cool environment should also be checked for hypothermia.

37. **d.** Infants and children are more at risk for hypothermia because they have a larger proportional body surface area and less body fat. Also, they have small muscle mass and therefore cannot shiver as efficiently as adults. Younger children may not be able to put on additional clothes by themselves when they get cold.

38. **a.** Feel the patient's abdominal skin to get a more accurate sense of the patient's core temperature.

39. **c.** Depending on the core temperature of the hypothermic patient, shivering may or may not be present. Shivering ceases after the core temperature drops below 90 degrees. Shivering is usually good since it is one way the body produces heat.

40. **d.** In the early stages of hypothermia, the patient will present with a rapid pulse and rapid breathing.

41. **c.** Alcoholic beverages should never be given to a hypothermic patient. Alcohol will produce vasodilation that, although giving the patient a transient sense of warmth, actually increases heat loss.

42. **b.** Although protocols regarding treatment of hypothermic patients vary, a patient who is alert and responding appropriately can be rewarmed by applying heat packs or hot-water bottles to the groin, armpits, and neck area. These are very vascular areas and the warm blood is pumped to all parts of the body. Use of warm oxygen also helps. Do not massage the patient, have the patient walk, or give stimulants to drink.

43. **c.** Hypothermic patients must be handled gently. A particular danger associated with rough handling or incorrect rewarming procedures is core temperature afterdrop. Cold, stale, highly acidic blood from the extremities may suddenly flood the core, causing cardiac arrest and death. Placement of airway adjuncts or hyperventilation may also cause cardiac arrest. However, if a pulse cannot be felt, chest compressions must be performed.

44. **d.** The pulse of a severely hypothermic patient may be hard to detect. Check the carotid pulse for 30 to 45 seconds before beginning CPR. Avoid the radial pulse because circulation to the extremities will be impaired, making it even more difficult to detect a pulse in these areas.

45. **b.** Hypothermic patients are cold to the touch, may display muscle rigidity, and may appear to be dead. A hypothermic patient is not dead, however, until he or she is warm and dead. Prolonged resuscitation times, which allow for controlled rewarming in the hospital, may be necessary, but the outcome may be positive.

46. **a.** An early or superficial local cold injury may be characterized by blanching of the skin and loss of feeling and sensation in the injured area. The skin remains soft.

47. **c.** When a late or deep local cold injury occurs, the skin is white and waxy in appearance. When palpated, it will feel firm to frozen. Swelling or blisters may be present.

48. **a.** If an extremity suffers a superficial local cold injury, it should be splinted. Cover the injured area. Do not rub or massage the area or allow it to be re-exposed to the cold.

49. **c.** Cover a deep cold injury with dry dressings. Do not break any blisters, rub or massage the area, apply heat to the area, or rewarm it.

50. **b.** A local cold injury may need to be rewarmed if an extremely long or delayed transport time is inevitable. However, it should not be done if the area is likely to refreeze or simply because the patient is unresponsive.

51. **d.** Rewarming should be accomplished rapidly by immersing the injured area in warm water. Continually stir the water to ensure it does not cool due to the temperature of the frozen part. Do not allow the injured area to refreeze. The patient will complain of severe pain.

52. **a.** When dressing hands or feet after rewarming, each finger or toe should be separated with a dry sterile dressing to prevent them from sticking together.

53. **b.** High relative humidity and high ambient temperature reduce the body's ability to dissipate heat.

54. **d.** The elderly are particularly susceptible to heat emergencies because they have poor thermoregulation and may be taking many medications that affect the body's ability to dissipate heat. Although they may be capable of removing their own clothing, since they lack mobility they may not be capable of leaving a hot environment.

55. **a.** After ensuring the patient has a patent airway, the patient should be removed from the hot environment and placed in a cool environment.

56. **b.** Many sources link the muscle cramps that may accompany a heat emergency with a loss of body salts. Dehydration may also be a factor.

57. **d.** A dire emergency exists if a patient has dry or moist, hot skin, since this indicates that the body's temperature-regulating mechanism has malfunctioned. The patient may then suffer rapid brain damage and death.

58. **c.** A responsive patient with moist, pale, normal-temperature to cool skin should be encouraged to drink water. Do not give water simply because the patient is complaining of thirst. Water should not be given if the patient is nauseated or semi-responsive.

59. **d.** A patient with skin that is hot to the touch must be cooled rapidly. Cool packs can be applied to the areas of the neck, groin, and armpits to cool the patient's blood. The patient's clothing should be removed. Wetting the patient's skin with sponges or wet towels also helps dissipate body heat. Do not rub the patient with alcohol.

60. **c.** By definition, near-drowning patients survive at least temporarily after the incident. They may die later, however, usually from respiratory complications. Drowning is defined as death by asphyxia after submersion. In either case, breathing may have ceased. Near-drowning patients may be resuscitated. Only after sufficient time has passed to render resuscitation efforts useless can it be said that drowning has truly taken place.

61. **b.** Early respiratory and circulatory support are of utmost importance when managing a drowning or near-drowning patient.

62. **a.** Patients who are found unconscious in swimming pools should be suspected of having spinal injuries caused by diving into the pool.

63. **d.** A patient who is face down in a pool must be rolled face up while spinal support is provided and maintained. Ventilations should be started immediately. Chest compressions should be performed in the water only if the EMT has special training in the technique.

64. **c.** Cold-water near-drowning patients may survive a long period of immersion, far greater than 30 minutes. The EMT should attempt resuscitation. Do not try to rewarm the patient in the field. If properly treated, the patient may experience total recovery with little or no brain damage.

65. **a.** If spinal injury is not suspected, place the breathing near-drowning patient in the recovery position to facilitate drainage of water, vomitus, and other secretions from the upper airways.

66. **b.** If gastric distention interferes with artificial ventilations, have suction ready and place the patient on his or her left side. Apply firm pressure over the epigastric area of the abdomen to relieve distention.

67. **a.** Stingers should be scraped off using something like the edge of a card. Avoid using tweezers or forceps since these can force more venom out of the venom sac and into the patient.

68. **d.** If possible, place the injection site slightly below the level of the patient's heart to help keep the poison from reaching central circulation.

69. **b.** Generally, do not apply cold to the area of a snakebite unless ordered to do so by medical direction. Also, avoid applying heat, elevating an extremity, or allowing the patient to move around since these actions will spread the poison.

70. **c.** When treating a snakebite, constricting bands should be applied only when ordered by medical direction.

71. **c.** The EMT should always be alert for signs and symptoms of an allergic reaction and treat these accordingly.

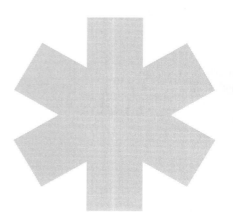

8

Behavioral Emergencies

D.O.T. Curriculum Objectives Covered in This Chapter:

Lesson 4-8

CHAPTER 8 REVIEW QUESTIONS

1. A behavioral emergency can be defined as a situation in which a patient:
   a. is feeling sad and down
   b. exhibits abnormal or unacceptable behavior that is intolerable to the patient, family, or community
   c. is disoriented and unsure of where he or she is or what day it is
   d. is under the influence of alcohol or drugs

2. Common causes for altered behavior include:
   a. traumatic injuries
   b. low blood sugar
   c. acute illness and lack of oxygen
   d. all of the above

3. A behavioral emergency in which a patient has lost touch with reality is referred to as an episode of:
   a. neurotic thinking
   b. narcotic thinking
   c. psychotic thinking
   d. obsessive-compulsive thinking

4. When dealing with a patient who is experiencing a behavioral emergency:
   a. lie to the patient if necessary
   b. tell the patient to "snap out of it"
   c. act in a calm, reassuring manner and always be honest
   d. speak in a commanding, authoritarian tone

5. When performing a scene size-up at a behavioral emergency, the EMT should be particularly alert for the presence of:
   a. clutter or poor housekeeping
   b. uneaten food on the table
   c. a pet or signs of a pet
   d. unsafe objects

6. An EMT may best be able to determine if a patient's behavior is abnormal or if there is a history of violence by talking to:
   a. family members
   b. the patient himself
   c. police officers
   d. medical direction

7. If a patient is displaying disturbed or abnormal thinking, such as verbalizing hallucinations:
   a. continue to treat the patient in a respectful manner
   b. play along with the situation to avoid agitating the patient
   c. explain to the patient that is simply his or her imagination
   d. forcibly restrain the patient before transporting to a hospital

8. When treating a patient who appears to be having a behavioral emergency:
   a. always consider the possibility that the behavior may be the result of a medical or traumatic condition
   b. always consider the patient to be suicidal
   c. always play along with any visual or auditory hallucinations
   d. avoid asking any personal questions about the patient's history

9. Patients threatening suicide are at particular risk if they:
   a. are married
   b. have no history of suicidal behavior
   c. have a vague plan of action
   d. are over 40 years of age

10. When dealing with a suicidal patient, the EMT should remember that:
    a. any suicidal act or gesture should be taken seriously
    b. people who talk about suicide do not carry out the threat
    c. people who really intend to kill themselves cannot be prevented from committing suicide
    d. all of the above

11. When managing a patient who is actively threatening suicide, the course of action may include:
    a. encouraging the patient to think about alternatives and the effects his suicide may have on others
    b. daring the patient to do it to shock him or her into reality
    c. allowing the patient to remain with family members if the suicidal feelings abate
    d. telling the patient he or she doesn't really want to commit suicide

12. Potential signs of violence on the part of an emotionally disturbed patient include:
    a. sitting on the edge of a seat
    b. laying on a bed or couch
    c. exhibiting open hands
    d. using monotone speech

13. To help calm an agitated patient:
    a. put your arm around the patient to provide reassurance
    b. maintain eye contact
    c. give the patient some time alone to regain composure
    d. avoid any slow, deliberate movements

14. Reasonable force is the amount of force it takes to:
    a. punish the patient for his or her behavior
    b. cause injury to the patient
    c. make the patient do what the EMT says
    d. keep the patient from injuring himself or herself or others

15. The amount of reasonable force that an EMT uses depends on the:
    a. patient's vital signs
    b. patient's strength and degree of agitation
    c. amount of vulgarity the patient uses
    d. type of medication the patient is taking

16. If a violent patient is encountered, the best course of action is to:
    a. approach the patient alone to gain his or her confidence
    b. surprise the patient and overpower him or her
    c. approach the patient only with backup assistance
    d. threaten the patient with bodily harm if he or she does not cooperate

17. Restraints should be used on patients who:
    a. pose a danger to themselves or others
    b. have a history of serious behavioral problems
    c. have committed a crime
    d. are intoxicated but refuse to go to the hospital

18. Generally, the minimum number of persons needed to restrain a patient is:
    a. two
    b. three
    c. four
    d. five

19. When approaching the patient who is about to be restrained:
    a. do not speak to the patient during the restraining process
    b. only one rescuer at a time should approach the patient
    c. all the rescuers should approach at the same time
    d. one EMT should carry a weapon to use in case the patient overpowers the other rescuers

20. After restraints are applied, the EMT should:
    a. remove them if the patient agrees not to cause further trouble
    b. not loosen them before reaching the hospital
    c. remove only the wrist restraints if the patient agrees not to cause further trouble
    d. not remove the restraints but frequently reassess circulation

21. If the patient starts spitting on the EMTs:
    a. cover the patient's face with a surgical mask
    b. use surgical tape to tape the patient's mouth closed
    c. place a pillowcase over the patient's face
    d. place the patient in a supine position

22. When transporting a female patient who is experiencing a behavioral emergency:
    a. a male EMT should ride with the patient
    b. the patient should never be restrained
    c. a female EMT should ride with the patient if possible
    d. a police officer should accompany the EMTs

23. When documenting a situation in which restraints were used:
    a. avoid implying the patient was violent, as this could be considered slander
    b. note the techniques used to restrain the patient and what position the patient was placed in
    c. always record word for word any abusive speech directed toward the EMTs
    d. all of the above

✳ **ENRICHMENT QUESTIONS**

24. Patients experiencing a behavioral emergency:
    a. have psychological problems and not physical problems
    b. may have an underlying physical condition causing the abnormal behavior
    c. pose little danger to the EMT if they appear calm
    d. are usually not taking their prescribed medications

25. Types of patients with special communications needs include:
    a. pediatric patients
    b. geriatric patients
    c. the hearing impaired
    d. all of the above

26. Conversation with a suicidal patient may include:
    a. asking why the patient thinks suicide is the only answer
    b. talking specifically about the patient's intentions
    c. asking the patient about any conflicts he or she may feel about committing suicide
    d. all of the above

27. The patient, who has been depressed about the recent loss of his job, called his wife at work and told her he was thinking of suicide. Her call to 9-1-1 is the basis for your response. After talking with the patient, you find he is alert and oriented. He tells you he is "OK now," no longer feels that way, and does not want to go to the hospital. He is very adamant about refusing transport; he states that his wife is on her way home and will be there shortly. Your best course of action is to:
    a. leave the patient alone and advise him to call 9-1-1 if he starts feeling suicidal again
    b. restrain the patient and take him to the hospital
    c. wait for the wife to arrive and advise her to call 9-1-1 if he starts talking of suicide again
    d. call for an ALS unit to take the patient to the hospital

■ Additional Points for Discussion ■

1. What is your local Suicide Prevention phone number?

2. To which hospital(s) would you normally transport a behavioral emergency patient?

3. What are your department's policies regarding transportation of violent patients?

4. What types of restraints are carried on your ambulance? Review the procedure for using each type.

ANSWERS TO CHAPTER 8 REVIEW QUESTIONS

1. **b.** A behavioral emergency exists when a patient exhibits abnormal or unacceptable behavior that is intolerable to the patient, the family, or the community. Some people, such as elderly persons, may normally be disoriented to place and time but may not be experiencing a behavioral emergency.

2. **d.** All of the above. There are a number of common causes for behavioral emergencies, including psychogenic causes or the use of mind-altering substances. Medical causes include traumatic injuries, low blood sugar, lack of oxygen, and various illnesses.

3. **c.** Psychotic thinking is marked by loss of touch with reality and is frequently accompanied by delusions or hallucinations.

4. **c.** Act in a calm, reassuring manner when dealing with behavioral emergencies. Never lie to the patient or speak in an authoritarian manner.

5. **d.** EMTs should be particularly alert for the presence of unsafe objects that could be used as weapons. Such objects may either be in the patient's possession or within the patient's reach.

6. **a.** The family and sometimes bystanders familiar with the patient's history are the best resource for an EMT to determine if a patient's behavior is abnormal. These individuals may also be able to provide information on the patient's potential for violence. The patient may normally display what the EMT would consider to be abnormal behavior—the question is, what is different about the behavior this time that warrants intervention by EMTs? Although police officers may not be familiar with the patient, they may provide helpful information if they have dealt with the patient before.

7. **a.** A patient should always be treated in a respectful manner, even when displaying signs of disturbed or abnormal thinking. Do not go along with the situation or try to argue with the patient. Restraint is usually unnecessary unless the patient is a danger to himself or herself or others.

8. **a.** Anytime a patient is encountered who appears to be having a behavioral emergency, the EMT must consider that the problem may be the result of a medical or traumatic condition and not necessarily psychological in nature. Specific questions about the patient's medical and psychological history need to be asked. If the patient is experiencing visual or auditory hallucinations, do not play along with them.

9. **d.** Patients who are over 40 years of age are at a higher risk for suicide. Other risk factors include being widowed, single, divorced, or having a history of depression or alcoholism. A defined plan of action and easy access to lethal means, and a history of self-destructive behavior also place the patient in a high-risk category for suicide.

10. **a.** Any suicidal act or gesture must be taken seriously. People who talk about suicide do commit suicide. With proper care, the patient may be helped through a suicidal crisis.

11. **a.** A patient may be encouraged to think about other alternatives to suicide. Getting the patient to think about how the suicide will affect others who care may also help. Do not dare the patient to commit suicide. Also, some patients sincerely want to commit suicide. Telling them that they don't may make them think that their feelings are not important.

12. **a.** The patient's posture and actions can do much to alert an EMT to potential violence. The patient may be sitting on the edge of a seat, swearing and yelling, or clenching the fists. Any behavior displayed by the patient that makes the EMT feel uneasy should be taken seriously.

13. **b.** It is important to maintain eye contact when trying to calm a patient. Remain a comfortable distance from the patient when talking, and avoid sudden movements. Do not leave the patient alone.

14. **d.** Reasonable force is the amount of force it takes to keep the patient from injuring himself or herself or others. Force should not be used as a means of telling a patient that the EMT is in control or be used as a form of punishment. Force should be used in a manner that does not injure the patient.

15. **b.** The amount of reasonable force that an EMT uses will be dependent on the patient's strength and size. Other factors to be taken into account include the patient's sex, mental state, the type of abnormal behavior being displayed, and the method of restraint to be used. These patients are often uncooperative and will not allow EMTs to obtain vital signs.

16. **c.** Never approach a violent patient alone. Have backup assistance, preferably that of the police. If a patient has a weapon, let the police handle the situation. Do not surprise or threaten the patient.

17. **a.** The policy for use of restraints varies from area to area. Generally, they should be used if the patient poses a physical threat to himself or herself or others. Once the patient has been restrained, do not remove the restraints until reaching the hospital.

18. **c.** Generally, at least four persons, one assigned to each limb, are needed to restrain a patient. More people can be used if available. Law enforcement personnel and medical direction should be consulted prior to restraining the patient.

19. **c.** Everyone involved in restraining the patient should approach at the same time. One EMT should talk to the patient during the restraining process. EMTs should not use weapons against a patient.

20. **d.** Restraints on the wrists and ankles can impair circulation, so frequently reassess circulation in the hands and feet. Loosen restraints if circulation is impaired, but do not remove them. Once restraints have been applied they should not be released until after reaching the receiving facility.

21. **a.** If the patient is spitting on the rescuers, place a surgical mask over the patient's face. Do not do anything that could interfere with the airway or create a problem in the event that the patient vomits.

22. **c.** It is desirable to have a female EMT ride with a female patient who is experiencing a behavioral emergency. If the patient is violent, restraints may be necessary. Although police may be involved, local protocol will dictate whether a law enforcement officer must accompany the EMTs and the patient.

23. **b.** Documentation is critical when a patient has been restrained. Note the reason restraints were necessary, the type of restraints used, the technique used to restrain the patient, and the position of the patient on the ambulance cot. If the patient was violent, this should be clearly noted as it is part of the reason the patient was restrained. It is not necessary to document the patient's speech word for word. Noting that abusive language was directed toward the EMTs is all that is necessary.

⚕ Enrichment Questions

24. **b.** EMTs must remember that behavioral emergencies may be caused by physical conditions, such as low oxygen or low blood sugar, as well as psychological conditions. In either case, the EMT should use caution because of the potential for harm to the patient if an underlying serious medical condition is overlooked.

25. **d.** All of the above. Types of patients with special communications needs include pediatric, geriatric, and disabled patients, including those with hearing and visual impairments. Non–English-speaking patients may also have special communication needs. These communications problems may be mistaken for behavioral problems by the EMT.

26. **d.** All of the above. Ask the patient why he or she feels suicide is the only recourse. Don't be afraid to talk specifically about the patient's intentions of committing suicide or feelings about it.

27. **c.** Adult patients who are competent have the right to refuse medical treatment. Although it is understandable that an EMT would be concerned about this patient, he cannot be forced to go to the hospital. However, he should also not be left alone. The best course, if he continues to refuse to go to the hospital despite repeated attempts to encourage him to seek medical assistance, is to leave him in the care of a competent family member who can monitor him for any further problems.

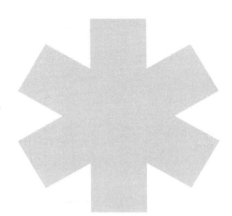

9

Obstetrics and Gynecology

D.O.T. Curriculum Objectives Covered in This Chapter:

Lesson 4-9

CHAPTER 9 REVIEW QUESTIONS

1. The structure in which the fetus grows and develops is the:
   a. fallopian tube
   b. vagina
   c. uterus
   d. ovary

2. The bag of waters that protects the baby is called the:
   a. afterbirth
   b. pericardial sac
   c. meninges
   d. amniotic sac

3. The placenta:
   a. mixes the baby's blood with the mother's blood
   b. exchanges oxygen, nutrients, and waste products between the mother and fetus
   c. is used by the fetus for food
   d. is normally positioned in the uterus over the cervix

4. The cervix is the:
   a. wall of the ovary
   b. neck of the uterus
   c. lower portion of the fallopian tube
   d. distal end of the perineum

5. The area of skin between the vagina and the anus that can tear during delivery is the:
   a. perineum
   b. periosteum
   c. peritoneum
   d. pericardium

6. A pregnant patient should be asked:
   a. when the baby is due
   b. whether she is experiencing any pains or contractions
   c. whether there is any bleeding or discharge, and when it began
   d. all of the above

7. Questions about labor would normally include all of the following *except*:
   a. when labor began
   b. how far apart the contractions are
   c. whether contractions are aggravated by movement
   d. the duration of the contractions

8. If the possibility of splashing is likely, the most appropriate personal protective equipment to wear when delivering a baby is:
   a. gloves and mask
   b. gloves, gown, eye protection, and mask
   c. gown and mask
   d. eye protection, mask, and gloves

9. The first stage of labor covers the period from:
   a. when EMS is called until the EMTs arrive at the scene
   b. when regular contractions begin until the cervix is fully dilated
   c. the patient's first contractions to the delivery of the baby's head
   d. dilation of the cervix to the birth of the baby

10. The second stage of labor covers the period from:
    a. delivery of the baby's head to the delivery of the placenta
    b. arrival of the ambulance to the start of transport
    c. complete dilation of the cervix to the birth of the baby
    d. the end of contractions to the presentation of the baby's head

11. The third stage of labor covers the period:
    a. from dilation of the cervix to delivery of the placenta
    b. from the arrival at the hospital to transfer to the obstetrics ward
    c. following the birth of the baby through delivery of the placenta
    d. following delivery of the baby to arrival at the hospital

12. The EMT should consider delivery imminent when:
    a. contractions are less than 2 minutes apart
    b. contractions last longer than 20 seconds
    c. it is the mother's first pregnancy and contractions are 5 minutes apart
    d. the patient is experiencing lower abdominal pain with no back pain

13. The baby's head bulging against the vaginal opening is known as:
    a. presenting
    b. crowning
    c. birthing
    d. showing

14. During delivery, rotation of the baby's head normally occurs:
    a. when the patient is crowning
    b. after the shoulders deliver
    c. prior to crowning
    d. once the head is delivered

15. The EMT may insert his or her fingers into a pregnant patient's vagina:
    a. to support the baby's head during delivery
    b. only in the case of a breech delivery or prolapsed cord
    c. to assist in delivery of the baby's shoulders
    d. to check the baby's pulse in the case of a limb presentation

16. Immediately following delivery of the baby's head, all of the following should be done *except*:
    a. stimulating breathing
    b. checking if the umbilical cord is around the baby's neck
    c. checking to be sure the amniotic sac is not covering the baby's mouth and nostrils
    d. suctioning the mouth and nostrils

17. When suctioning a newborn, the EMT should:
    a. wait until delivery is complete to begin suctioning
    b. squeeze the bulb syringe after inserting it
    c. insert the tip of the bulb syringe 2" to 3" into the mouth and each nostril
    d. squeeze the bulb syringe before inserting it

18. The first place the EMT should suction the newborn is:
    a. the right nostril
    b. the left nostril
    c. the mouth
    d. either nostril, then the mouth

19. A major concern when caring for newborns is:
    a. starting the mother-infant bonding process
    b. wrapping the newborn in moist towels
    c. guarding against heat loss
    d. a breathing rate greater than 30 breaths per minute

20. To stimulate the newborn to breathe:
    a. hold it upside-down by its feet and ankles
    b. gently rub its back or flick the soles of its feet
    c. slap it sharply on the buttocks
    d. ventilate it with an oxygen-powered resuscitator

21. After delivery is completed but before the cord is cut, the baby should be positioned:
    a. at the same level as the mother's vagina
    b. higher than the mother
    c. with its head slightly elevated
    d. lower than the mother

22. The generally recommended time to cut the umbilical cord is:
    a. after delivery of the placenta
    b. 10 to 15 minutes after delivery
    c. before the infant starts to breathe
    d. after pulsations in the cord cease

23. If a decision is made to cut the umbilical cord, the first clamp should be placed about:
    a. 4" from the baby
    b. 4" from the mother
    c. 10" from the baby
    d. 10" from the mother

24. After cutting the cord, the baby should be positioned:
    a. on its right side
    b. with its head slightly higher than its trunk
    c. in a prone position
    d. with its head slightly lower than its trunk

25. If the newborn is breathing but his or her heart rate is below 100 breaths per minute:
    a. start artificial ventilations
    b. flick the soles of the feet
    c. start chest compressions only
    d. perform CPR

26. The placenta should deliver:
    a. 30 to 45 minutes after birth
    b. immediately after the cord is cut
    c. 1 hour after birth
    d. within 20 minutes of birth

27. After the placenta has been delivered:
    a. wrap it in a towel, place it in a plastic bag, and take it to the hospital with the mother
    b. discard it
    c. have the mother walk to induce uterine contraction
    d. sit the mother in an upright position

28. During childbirth, a patient may normally experience blood loss up to:
    a. 500 cc
    b. 5 cups
    c. 2 pints
    d. 1 L

29. Excessive maternal bleeding after delivery may be managed in all the following ways *except*:
    a. massaging the mother's lower abdomen
    b. packing the vagina with a sterile dressing
    c. having the baby suckle
    d. placing a sterile pad over the vaginal opening

30. A newborn is considered premature if he or she:
    a. is born before the ninth month of pregnancy
    b. weighs more than 6 pounds
    c. delivers before 37 weeks (8 months) gestation
    d. delivers before the expected due date

31. A correct statement regarding premature infants is:
    a. do not give oxygen because it will cause blindness
    b. the head is smaller in proportion than the rest of the body
    c. do not suction the mouth or nose as it can cause excessive drying of the mucous membranes
    d. they are at risk for hypothermia

32. Breech presentation refers to an abnormal delivery in which:
    a. the baby's shoulders are too large to pass through the birth canal
    b. the amniotic sac fails to rupture
    c. the baby's buttocks deliver first
    d. the umbilical cord is wrapped around the baby's neck

33. Management of a breech delivery may include:
    a. pulling on the baby to assist with delivery
    b. placing two gloved fingers in the vagina to form an airway for the baby
    c. having the mother cross her legs to delay delivery
    d. placing one hand over the vaginal orifice to prevent delivery

34. In a situation involving a prolapsed cord, breech presentation, or limb presentation, the mother may be placed:
    a. in a head-down position with her pelvis elevated
    b. on her right side with her legs squeezed together
    c. in a prone position
    d. on her back with her head higher than her feet

35. When examining a patient in labor, if a prolapsed cord is discovered:
    a. do not allow anything to touch the cord
    b. attempt to push the cord back into the vagina and uterus
    c. insert several gloved fingers into the vagina and gently push on the baby's head to take pressure off the cord
    d. pull on the cord to induce delivery

36. If a delivery involving a limb presentation is encountered:
    a. attempt to push the limb back into the uterus
    b. encourage the mother to push
    c. pull on the limb to assist delivery
    d. immediately transport the patient to the hospital

37. The presence of meconium indicates:
    a. a lack of lubricating fluid in the birth canal
    b. possible fetal distress during labor
    c. an abnormal passage of the baby through the birth canal
    d. the probability of a breech presentation

38. The primary problems associated with a meconium emergency are:
    a. cardiac complications
    b. neurological complications
    c. breathing complications
    d. intestinal complications

39. When a pregnant patient with a spinal injury is transported on a backboard, the backboard should:
    a. be tilted to the right side
    b. be tilted to the left side
    c. have the head elevated
    d. be completely flat

40. Vaginal bleeding that occurs late during pregnancy usually indicates:
    a. imminent birth
    b. a problem with the placenta
    c. the possibility that seizures will occur
    d. a probable multiple birth situation

41. Abnormally low blood pressure in a pregnant patient may be caused by:
    a. toxemia of pregnancy
    b. compression of the aorta by the baby
    c. premature uterine contractions
    d. compression of the vena cava by the baby

42. The EMT should be alert for the possibility of seizures when a pregnant patient presents with:
    a. swelling of the face, hands, and feet
    b. abnormally low blood pressure
    c. sudden loss of weight
    d. severe lower abdominal pain

43. After seizures are experienced by a pregnant patient, the patient should be transported:
    a. in a supine position
    b. rapidly using red lights and siren
    c. with her legs and feet elevated
    d. with her shoulders and head elevated

44. Miscarriage refers to:
    a. delivery of the fetus before it can live independently of the mother
    b. self-induced termination of pregnancy
    c. bleeding that occurs before the 37th week of pregnancy
    d. incorrect placement of the placenta on the wall of the uterus

45. An important part of managing a miscarriage includes:
    a. discarding of fetal tissues to avoid disturbing the mother
    b. advising the patient to make an appointment with her obstetrician
    c. rendering emotional support to the mother and father
    d. transporting the patient on her left side with her head elevated if she is in shock

46. The soft areas in a baby's head where the fusion of the bones of the skull is not complete are known as:
    a. fontanelles
    b. varices
    c. follicles
    d. parietes

47. When managing a sexual assault patient, the EMT should:
    a. tell the patient how the assault could have been avoided
    b. reassure the patient that she is now safe
    c. tell the patient that everything will be all right
    d. avoid any physical examination of the patient

48. Appropriate care for a sexual assault patient would include:
    a. being careful to preserve any evidence
    b. encouraging the patient to wash and change clothes
    c. getting as much information as possible about the incident
    d. wearing a gown and mask to avoid possible exposure to a sexually transmitted disease

49. Documentation regarding a sexual assault that should be included on an EMS report includes:
    a. the EMT's personal opinions about the incident
    b. what the patient said and things that are directly observed
    c. theories regarding who the EMT thinks may be involved in the incident
    d. all of the above

✳ **ENRICHMENT QUESTION**

50. An assessment of the APGAR score should be made:
    a. immediately following delivery and upon reaching the hospital
    b. 1 and 5 minutes after birth
    c. 5 and 10 minutes after birth
    d. immediately following delivery and 10 minutes later

For questions 51 and 52, refer to the APGAR scale in Figure 9-1.

Sign	0	1	2
Appearance (Skin color)	bluish or pale	pink or typical newborn color; hands and feet are blue	pink or typical newborn color; entire body
Pulse (Heart rate)	absent	below 100	over 100
Grimace (Irritability)	no response	crying; some motion	crying; vigorous
Activity (Muscle tone)	limp	some flexion— extremities	active; good motion in extremities
Respiratory effort	absent	slow and irregular	normal; crying

Figure 9-1

51. A newborn presents with some pink skin color, a pulse rate of 140, a weak cry, good muscle tone, and a breathing rate of 36 breaths per minute. The APGAR score is:
   a. 6
   b. 7
   c. 8
   d. 9

52. A baby was delivered by its father 3 minutes before your unit's arrival. The baby is cyanotic, has a pulse rate of 106, a weak cry, no muscle tone, and a breathing rate of 18 breaths per minute. The APGAR score is:
   a. 3
   b. 4
   c. 5
   d. 6

53. When taking the vital signs of a pregnant patient, the EMT would expect her:
   a. heart rate to be faster and blood pressure lower
   b. heart rate to be slower and blood pressure higher
   c. heart rate to be slower and blood pressure lower
   d. heart rate to be faster and blood pressure higher

54. Placenta previa refers to a condition in which:
   a. the placenta separates prematurely from the wall of the uterus
   b. the fetus is not connected to the placenta with an umbilical cord
   c. the placenta develops in an abnormal location in the uterus
   d. the placenta does not deliver in one piece

55. When a patient suffers from abruptio placenta, the placenta:
    a. delivers at the same time as the infant
    b. is torn during delivery
    c. delivers in an abrupt, rapid manner
    d. has separated prematurely from the wall of the uterus

56. The abnormal condition that may occur in the last 3 months of pregnancy characterized by sudden, severe, low abdominal pain with or without vaginal bleeding is:
    a. abruptio placentae
    b. uterine inversion
    c. placenta previa
    d. eclampsia

57. When a fertilized egg starts to develop in an area outside the uterus, this is known as:
    a. pelvic inflammatory disease
    b. a spontaneous abortion
    c. an ectopic pregnancy
    d. uterine inversion

58. The most common cause of fetal death is:
    a. maternal death
    b. drug abuse by the mother
    c. strangulation by the umbilical cord
    d. suffocation by the amniotic sac

59. When caring for an injured pregnant patient, the general rule is:
    a. do not waste time packaging the patient if delivery is imminent
    b. the life of the unborn child takes precedence over the life of the mother
    c. the life of the mother takes precedence over the life of the unborn child
    d. there is little concern unless the patient is near term

■ Additional Points for Discussion ■

1. Review the equipment carried in your OB kits and each piece's use.

2. Is there a specific hospital in your area that is designated to treat and examine victims of sexual assault? If so, which?

3. Review with your local law enforcement any special procedures involving patient management and crime scene preservation that should be followed at the scene of a sexual assault.

4. What is your local Rape Crisis Hotline phone number?

ANSWERS TO CHAPTER 9
REVIEW QUESTIONS

1. **c.** The uterus is a muscular organ in which the fetus grows and develops. The ovaries produce sex hormones and ova. Ova are carried from the ovaries to the uterus by the fallopian tubes. The vagina is the lower part of the birth canal.

2. **d.** The amniotic sac protects the infant in the uterus. Afterbirth is another term for the placenta. The pericardial sac encloses the heart, and the meninges are membranes that surround the brain and spinal cord.

3. **b.** The placenta exchanges oxygen, nutrients, and waste products between the mother and the fetus. It is normally positioned high in the uterus and does not allow mixing of the baby's with the mother's blood.

4. **b.** The cervix is the neck of the uterus.

5. **a.** The perineum is the area of skin between the vagina and anus. During delivery, the skin in this area may tear due to the pressure exerted by the fetus as it passes through the birth canal. The periosteum is a fiberlike covering of the bones, the pericardium is the sac around the heart, and the peritoneum is the membrane lining the abdominal cavity.

6. **d.** All of the above. An obstetrics patient should be questioned concerning when the baby is due and if the patient is experiencing any pains or contractions. Ask if she has been experiencing any bleeding or discharge, such as if the water has broken, and if so, when.

7. **c.** Question the patient concerning how far apart her labor pains are and the duration of the pain. It is also helpful to know when the pain started.

8. **b.** When delivering a baby, it is recommended that the EMT wear gloves and a gown due to the amount of blood and fluids present, as well as a mask and protective eyewear if splashing is likely. Since there is generally time to prepare for delivery, the EMT should be more cognizant of taking the proper personal protective precautions.

9. **b.** The first stage of labor encompasses the period from the beginning of regular contractions until the cervix is fully dilated.

10. **c.** The second stage of labor encompasses the period from complete dilation of the cervix to the birth of the baby.

11. **c.** The third stage of labor encompasses the period following the birth of the baby through the delivery of the placenta.

12. **a.** Consider delivery imminent if contractions are less than 2 minutes apart or if crowning occurs. Labor during a first delivery will take longer than subsequent deliveries. Transport unless delivery is expected within 5 minutes. Remember, there are worse places to have a baby than in the back of an ambulance, so don't be afraid to transport.

13. **b.** Crowning is the term used for when the baby's head bulges against the vaginal opening.

14. **d.** Rotation of the baby's head normally occurs once the head is delivered.

15. **b.** There are only two cases in which an EMT should insert fingers into a pregnant patient's vagina: 1) in the case of a breach birth to form an airway for the baby, and 2) in the case of a prolapsed cord to relieve pressure on the cord. Always wear sterile gloves to diminish the risk of infecting the mother.

16. **a.** Immediately following delivery of the baby's head is not the time to stimulate breathing. It is the time to check for the umbilical cord around the baby's neck, check to ensure that the amniotic sac is not in place over the baby's head and face, and to suction the mouth and nose. If the amniotic sac is not broken, puncture it and push it away from the newborn's head and mouth.

17. **d.** Suction should be applied immediately. Always squeeze the bulb before inserting, and insert it only 1" to 1½" into the mouth and nostrils.

18. **c.** The EMT should first suction the mouth of the newborn and then the nostrils. This prevents aspiration of matter in the mouth in the event that spontaneous breathing is stimulated by suctioning the nostrils.

19. **c.** The EMT must guard against heat loss in a newborn. Quickly dry the infant, and wrap it in a warm blanket. Since the infant's head is so large, a covering (such as a stockinette) should always be placed over the head to diminish heat loss. Breathing rates greater than 30 breaths a minute are normal for a newborn.

20. **b.** Breathing may be stimulated by gently rubbing the baby's back or tapping the soles of its feet. Do not hold it upside down, slap it, or use an oxygen-powered breathing device.

21. **a.** Following delivery, the baby should be kept level with the mother's vagina until the cord is clamped and cut. Positioning the baby too high may cause hypovolemia as blood is siphoned back into the placenta. Placing the baby too low may cause fluid overload.

22. **d.** After pulsations in the umbilical cord cease, it may be clamped and cut.

23. **a.** The first umbilical clamp should be placed about 4" or four finger-widths away from the baby. The second clamp is then placed about 2" farther away from the first clamp, toward the placenta. Cut between the clamps.

24 **d.** After the cord is cut, position the baby with its head slightly lower than its trunk to facilitate the drainage of fluids from its mouth and nose.

25. **a.** Start artificial ventilations if the newborn's heart rate drops below 100 beats per minute. Low heart rates are often a result of low oxygenation, so good ventilation can actually increase the infant's heart rate. If the heart rate remains less than 60 beats per minute after 30 seconds of adequate assisted ventilation, start chest compressions.

26. **d.** The placenta should normally deliver in about 20 minutes, but may take up to 30 minutes.

27. **a.** The placenta should be wrapped in a towel, then placed in a plastic bag and taken to the hospital for examination. Do not have the patient squeeze her legs together or walk around.

28. **a.** Blood loss of up to 500 cc (about 4 cups) may be normal during childbirth.

29. **b.** Maternal bleeding may be managed by massaging the patient's abdomen, having the baby suckle, or placing the patient in the shock position with a sterile pad over the vaginal opening. Never pack the vagina.

30. **c.** A baby born before 37 weeks (8 months) gestation or one that weighs less than 5½ pounds is considered premature. Full-term newborns weigh about 7 pounds.

31. **d.** Premature babies are very susceptible to hypothermia. If oxygen is given over a short time, it should not cause complications, but the stream should not be directed at the baby's face. The head is usually larger, and suctioning may need to be repeated frequently as the airways can easily become obstructed.

32. **c.** A breech presentation occurs when the baby's buttocks or lower extremities are low in the uterus and deliver first.

33. **b.** It may be necessary to place two gloved fingers in the mother's vagina to form an airway for the baby. Do not pull on the baby or in any way attempt to delay delivery.

34. **a.** Patients may be placed in a head-down position with the hips elevated when such obstetric emergencies as breech or limb presentation or a prolapsed cord are encountered.

35. **c.** Management of a prolapsed umbilical cord may include inserting several gloved fingers into the vagina and gently pushing on the baby's head to relieve the pressure on the cord. Do not attempt to push the cord back into the vagina. Any exposed portion of cord should be covered with moist, sterile dressings.

36. **d.** In the case of a limb presentation, immediate transportation is of utmost importance.

37. **b.** The presence of meconium (the dark-green contents of the intestines of the fetus) in the amniotic fluid indicates possible fetal distress during labor. The amniotic fluid resembles thick pea soup.

38. **c.** The presence of meconium in the amniotic fluid denotes a true emergency. If the infant aspirates meconium, breathing complications may be serious to fatal. If a meconium emergency exists, rapid transportation to a hospital is warranted. Take extra care to thoroughly suction the infant.

39. **b.** When transporting an injured pregnant female on a backboard, the backboard should be tilted to the left side. This relieves the pressure that the fetus may place on the vena cava, which is a major blood vessel in the abdomen.

40. b. Vaginal bleeding occurring during late pregnancy usually indicates a problem with the placenta. The bleeding may or may not be accompanied by pain.

41. d. Compression of the mother's vena cava (the vein that returns blood from the lower body to the heart) by the baby in the uterus can cause abnormally low blood pressure. If this is suspected, transport the patient on her left side to take pressure off the vessel.

42. a. Swelling of the face, hands, and feet of a pregnant patient should alert the EMT to the possibility of the patient having a seizure. Also, the patient may have an elevated blood pressure and a recent history of sudden weight gain.

43. d. After a pregnant patient has experienced seizures, the patient should be transported with the shoulders and head elevated. Use of the ambulance siren should be avoided as it may precipitate additional seizures.

44. a. Miscarriage refers to the delivery of the fetus before it can live independently of the mother.

45. c. An important part of managing a miscarriage includes providing emotional support to the parents. Tissues should be taken to the hospital for examination. Because the EMT cannot adequately assess the patient's uterus, the patient should be evaluated at a hospital. If the patient displays signs of hypoperfusion, transport her on her back with her legs elevated.

46. a. The fontanelles are soft areas in a baby's head where the cranial bones have not fused together. The EMT must exercise care to avoid pushing on these areas while managing the infant's head during normal or abnormal delivery. Varices are dilated and tortuous blood vessels. Follicles are masses of cells usually containing a cavity, and parietes are walls of a body cavity.

47. b. Always act in a professional, reassuring manner. Do not tell the patient how the assault could have been avoided or that everything will be all right. The patient should be examined, but the examination may have to be altered to fit the situation.

48. a. Be careful to preserve evidence at the scene and on the patient. Although the EMT cannot prohibit it, the patient should be discouraged from changing clothes, washing, or using the bathroom. EMTs are usually not police officers and should not question the patient about specifics relating to the assault.

49. b. An EMT should note only facts on the EMS report. This could include what the patient said as well as what can be directly observed. This document will probably be used in court, so avoid including personal opinions or theories.

✺ ENRICHMENT QUESTIONS

50. b. An assessment of the APGAR score should be made 1 minute and 5 minutes after birth. APGAR is an acronym for: *Appearance, Pulse, Grimace, Activity, Respiratory* effort.

Sign	0	1	2
Appearance (Skin color)	bluish or pale	pink or typical newborn color; hands and feet are blue	pink or typical newborn color; entire body
Pulse (Heart rate)	absent	below 100	over 100
Grimace (Irritability)	no response	crying; some motion	crying; vigorous
Activity (Muscle tone)	limp	some flexion—extremities	active; good motion in extremities
Respiratory effort	absent	slow and irregular	normal; crying

Figure 9-1

51. **c.** The patient's APGAR score is 8: Appearance = 1, Pulse = 2, Grimace = 1, Activity = 2, Respiratory Effort = 2.

52. **b.** The patient's APGAR score is 4: Appearance = 0, Pulse = 2, Grimace = 1, Activity = 0, Respiratory Effort = 1.

53. **a.** When taking the vital signs of a pregnant patient, the EMT would expect her heart rate to be faster and blood pressure lower.

54. **c.** In placenta previa, the placenta develops in an abnormal location low in the uterus and close to or over the cervix. This can interfere with normal delivery. Also, as the cervix dilates, the placenta tears and bleeding occurs.

55. **d.** In abruptio placentae (also called placenta abruptio), the placenta partially or completely separates from the wall of the uterus.

56. **a.** Abruptio placentae is most often characterized by sudden, severe, low abdominal pain. It may or may not be accompanied by bleeding. Placenta previa generally presents with bright red bleeding but may be painless.

57. **c.** In an ectopic pregnancy, the fertilized egg starts to develop in an area outside of the uterus, often within a fallopian tube. The fallopian tube is not large enough to support the growth of the fetus and will eventually rupture. When this occurs, it produces abdominal pain and, more important, massive bleeding that may be fatal if not corrected quickly.

58. **a.** Maternal death is the most common cause of fetal death. If the mother dies from trauma, perform CPR and transport her to a hospital. A physician may be able to perform an emergency cesarean section and save the infant.

59. **c.** The general rule is that the life of the mother takes precedence over the life of the unborn child.

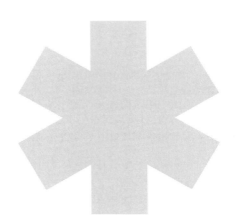

10

Bleeding and Shock

D.O.T. Curriculum Objectives Covered in This Chapter:

Lesson 5-1

CHAPTER 10 REVIEW QUESTIONS

1. Shock may be defined as:
   a. lack of blood in the circulatory system
   b. inadequate perfusion of the body's cells and tissues
   c. an inability of the heart to pump efficiently
   d. a severe allergic reaction causing dilation of the blood vessels

2. Hypoperfusion caused by bleeding is known as:
   a. hemorrhagic shock
   b. anaphylactic shock
   c. cardiogenic shock
   d. circulatory shock

3. Concerning the blood pressure of a patient in shock, the EMT must remember that:
   a. a drop in blood pressure is an early sign of shock
   b. blood pressure is directly proportional to the pulse
   c. blood pressure drops initially and then rises
   d. a drop in blood pressure is a late sign of shock

4. Capillary refill time should be checked on:
   a. all hypoperfusion patients
   b. any patient injured in a vehicle crash
   c. trauma patients only
   d. infants and children only

5. Normal capillary refill time is:
   a. less than 2 seconds
   b. more than 3 seconds
   c. between 2 and 4 seconds
   d. less than 4 seconds

6. An early indicator of shock may be:
   a. constricted pupils
   b. decreased pulse rate
   c. restlessness and anxiety
   d. dry skin

7. The key elements of the circulatory system that are needed to maintain tissue perfusion include all of the following *except*:
   a. a functioning pump (the heart)
   b. a two-way directional system (the valves in veins and the heart)
   c. adequate fluid in the system (the blood)
   d. intact pipes (the blood vessels)

8. When caring for a patient in shock:
   a. administer oxygen after splinting fractures
   b. control bleeding after ensuring an airway and breathing
   c. apply warm packs or hot water bottles to warm the patient
   d. check vital signs every 15 minutes

9. To place a patient in the shock position:
   a. elevate the entire body with the head higher than the feet
   b. place the patient in Trendelenburg position if no spinal injury is suspected
   c. elevate the lower extremities if no spinal injury is suspected
   d. elevate only the upper torso and head

10. Ideally, the vital signs of a patient in shock should be checked:
    a. every 5 minutes
    b. every 10 minutes
    c. every 15 minutes
    d. every 20 minutes

11. When managing a patient with severe external blood loss:
    a. control the bleeding prior to donning gloves
    b. only gloves and eye protection are needed
    c. determine whether the patient has a communicable disease prior to donning personal protective equipment
    d. use gloves, eye protection, gown, and mask when possible

12. A serious amount of sudden blood loss in an adult is:
    a. 1 U
    b. 500 cc
    c. 1 L
    d. 2 cups

13. Venous bleeding is best described as:
    a. a slow flow of bright red blood
    b. a steady ooze of blood from a wound
    c. a steady flow of dark-red blood
    d. difficult to control with direct pressure

14. Bleeding from an artery:
    a. is bright red and spurts with each heartbeat
    b. is not life-threatening
    c. can be easily controlled with direct pressure
    d. can only be controlled with a tourniquet

15. Capillary bleeding is:
    a. associated with long clotting times
    b. slow, oozing, and dark red
    c. bright red and steady
    d. normally controlled with use of pressure points

16. After personal protective equipment is donned, the first step to control bleeding is:
    a. applying direct pressure
    b. placing the patient in shock position
    c. applying digital pressure to an artery
    d. applying a cold pack

17. To provide pressure to control bleeding, all of the following may be used *except*:
    a. a gauze bandage
    b. the hand
    c. an air splint
    d. a narrow cravat

18. Along with using direct pressure to control bleeding from an extremity:
    a. immerse the extremity in cold water
    b. lower the extremity
    c. apply ice to the area of the wound
    d. elevate the extremity

19. The pressure point of choice for controlling bleeding from a forearm injury is the:
    a. temporal artery
    b. popliteal artery
    c. brachial artery
    d. tibial artery

20. To manage uncontrolled bleeding from a leg injury, the pressure point of choice is the:
    a. subclavian artery
    b. radial artery
    c. brachial artery
    d. femoral artery

21. A tourniquet should be used:
    a. on all crush injuries involving an extremity
    b. only as a last resort
    c. when direct pressure alone will not control bleeding
    d. whenever an amputation is encountered

22. When a bandage is used as a tourniquet, it should be:
    a. wrapped around an extremity twice
    b. loosened every 20 minutes to resupply the distal area with blood
    c. between 1 and 2 inches wide
    d. applied as far from the wound as possible

23. Tighten a tourniquet:
    a. just enough to occlude venous blood flow
    b. enough to occlude arterial blood flow
    c. as much as possible
    d. until pain below the wound is relieved

24. After applying a tourniquet:
    a. document its use and the time it was applied on the EMS report
    b. cover the wound and tourniquet with sterile dressings and bandages
    c. lower the extremity below the level of the heart
    d. apply digital pressure to the appropriate pressure point

25. A potential problem with using a blood pressure cuff as a tourniquet is:
    a. it is not wide enough
    b. it cannot occlude arterial blood flow
    c. there is a greater likelihood of damaging underlying structures
    d. pressure in the cuff may gradually be lost

26. Another term for nosebleed is:
    a. epinephrine
    b. epiphysial
    c. epistaxis
    d. epidural

27. To manage a nosebleed when there is no associated cervical spinal injury:
    a. apply direct pressure to the facial artery
    b. have the patient lean forward
    c. pack the nostril with gauze
    d. have the patient lie on his or her back

28. When managing a patient with a head injury accompanied by a nosebleed:
    a. pack the nose with gauze
    b. pinch the nostrils and tip the head back
    c. do not attempt to stop bleeding
    d. place the patient in a sitting position

29. Vomiting of coffee-ground emesis may indicate:
    a. appendicitis
    b. bleeding from the colon
    c. diverticulitis
    d. bleeding in the stomach

30. Tarry-looking stool is indicative of:
    a. an abdominal aneurysm
    b. appendicitis
    c. bleeding in the upper intestinal tract
    d. gastritis

31. Signs of internal bleeding may include all of the following *except*:
    a. bright-red blood in the stool or vomitus
    b. a lack of thirst
    c. an enlarging, tender, rigid abdomen
    d. a rapid, weak pulse

32. If internal bleeding is suspected, be alert for the possibility of:
    a. a severe allergic reaction
    b. an increase in blood pressure
    c. nausea and vomiting
    d. fever

33. If signs of shock are present, use of the pneumatic anti-shock garment (PASG) would be indicated in the event of:
    a. a pelvic injury with signs of abdominal bleeding
    b. an open wound to the chest with severe external bleeding
    c. blunt trauma to the chest with signs of internal bleeding
    d. an isolated, open head injury accompanied by severe external bleeding

34. A contraindication to applying the PASG is:
    a. a diminished level of consciousness
    b. a rapid pulse
    c. signs of fluid in the lungs
    d. dropping blood pressure

35. When properly placed, the top of the PASG should lie:
    a. below the last pair of ribs
    b. at the nipple line
    c. at the level of the umbilicus
    d. at the level of the sixth rib

36. When applying the PASG, inflate it until the:
    a. patient states he or she feels better
    b. patient's blood pressure reaches 120 mm Hg systolic
    c. hook-and-loop tape starts to crackle
    d. pressure gauges reach 90 mm Hg

37. Deflation of the PASG should be accomplished:
    a. in the field after IVs are started
    b. by first deflating the leg chambers, then the abdominal chamber
    c. slowly, stopping deflation after each blood pressure drop of 10 to 15 mm Hg to stabilize the patient with fluids
    d. only by trained personnel in a clinical setting

✳ **ENRICHMENT QUESTIONS**

38. When using digital pressure on an arterial pressure point:
    a. continue to apply direct pressure to the wound
    b. alternate between 2 minutes of pressure on the artery and then 2 minutes with no pressure
    c. do not apply any pressure to the wound
    d. the artery chosen should be distal to the wound

39. Match each bone injury with its associated blood loss.
    femur
    humerus
    pelvis
    rib
    tibia

    _____ 125 cc (¼ unit)

    _____ 250 cc (½ unit)

    _____ 500 to 750 cc (1 to 1½ units)

    _____ 1,000 cc (2 units)

    _____ 1,000 to 10,000 cc (2 to 20 units)

40. Bilateral femur fractures may be accompanied by:
    a. brachial nerve damage
    b. shock, but only if associated with other internal injuries
    c. moderate to severe shock
    d. spasms of the Achilles tendons

41. In trauma care, the "golden hour" begins when:
    a. the EMT assesses the patient
    b. the patient arrives at the hospital
    c. EMS personnel begin treatment
    d. the injury occurs

42. Two types of shock that are associated with widespread vasodilation are:
    a. neurogenic and hypovolemic
    b. cardiogenic and psychogenic
    c. hypovolemic and anaphylactic
    d. septic and neurogenic

43. The type of shock associated with a severe infection that causes toxins to be released into the bloodstream is:
    a. septic shock
    b. oligemic shock
    c. neurogenic shock
    d. metabolic shock

44. The type of shock that is usually self-correcting and is associated with simple fainting is:
    a. septic shock
    b. anaphylactic shock
    c. psychogenic shock
    d. metabolic shock

45. The underlying cause of hypoperfusion that occurs from cardiogenic shock involves:
    a. loss of fluid into body tissues
    b. relaxation and dilation of blood vessels throughout the body
    c. an inability of the lungs to exchange oxygen and carbon dioxide
    d. pump failure

46. Neurogenic shock can occur when:
    a. the heart muscle becomes too weak to function properly
    b. the spinal cord is damaged, resulting in an interruption of nerve impulses to the blood vessels
    c. a patient is exposed to severe emotional stress
    d. a patient experiences a severe allergic reaction

■ **Additional Points for Discussion** ■

1. What are some ways to place the PASG on a patient?

2. What are your local protocols for use, inflation, and deflation of the PASG?

3. What procedure does your department employ for cleaning and disinfecting the PASG after use?

4. Which hospitals in your area are designated trauma centers?

5. What are the local policies regarding when a patient should be transported to a trauma center?

ANSWERS TO CHAPTER 10 REVIEW QUESTIONS

1. **b.** Shock is defined as inadequate perfusion of the body's cells and tissues with oxygen and nutrients, as well as inadequate removal of metabolic waste products.

2. **a.** Hemorrhagic shock is hypoperfusion caused by blood loss.

3. **d.** A drop in blood pressure is a late sign of shock. Infants and children often maintain a good blood pressure until they are very close to death. An increase in pulse rate is a better indicator of shock in the early stages. The EMT must be alert to recognize shock well before the blood pressure drop occurs.

4. **d.** Capillary refill time should be checked only on infants and children younger than 6 years.

5. **a.** Normal capillary refill time in infants and children is less than 2 seconds.

6. **c.** Restlessness and anxiety, or a change in mental status caused by a decreased delivery of oxygen to the brain tissues, may be the first indicator of shock. Shock patients also develop an increased pulse rate, moist skin, and dilated pupils.

7. **b.** For perfusion to be maintained, there must be an intact pump (the heart), adequate fluid in the system (the blood), and intact pipes (the blood vessels).

8. **b.** Airway and breathing are the first priority in managing shock. Major bleeding should be controlled, and oxygen should be administered as soon as possible. Place the patient in the shock position and keep the patient warm, but do not overheat the patient.

9. **c.** The shock position involves elevating only the patient's lower extremities 8" to 12" if no spinal injury is suspected. Slanting the patient's entire body (such as in the Trendelenburg position) should be avoided if possible, because this causes the abdominal organs to put pressure on the diaphragm, thereby hindering breathing.

10. **a.** The shock patient's vital signs should be checked every 5 minutes. Although this is not always practical in the field, it should be attempted.

11. **d.** When managing a patient with obvious external blood loss, the EMT should wear appropriate personal protective equipment as dictated by the circumstances. For example, if minimal bleeding without the risk of splash is encountered, gloves may be all that are needed. However, in the event of severe bleeding, the risk of splashing or spurting is much greater, and eye protection, gown, and mask should be used. Use of personal protective equipment should never be based on the patient's admission of having a communicable disease. All patients must be assumed to pose a risk to the EMT.

12. **c.** The loss of 1 L of blood in an adult patient can cause hypovolemic shock. In children, a loss of 500 cc of blood is serious, as is a loss of 100 to 200 cc of blood in infants.

13. **c.** Venous bleeding can be recognized as dark-red blood that flows steadily. This type of bleeding is often easily controlled with direct pressure.

14. **a.** Arterial bleeding is bright red, and the blood spurts with each heartbeat. This type of bleeding may not be easily controlled and can be rapidly fatal.

15. **b.** Bleeding from the capillaries is characterized by a slow, oozing flow of dark-red blood. Pressure points are not used to control capillary bleeding.

16. **a.** Application of direct pressure is the first step to control bleeding. The pressure may be concentrated (such as when a fingertip is used to press on the bleeding point) or diffuse (such as when pressure is applied over a larger area of injury). Diffuse pressure occludes the arteries and veins that supply blood to the injured area.

17. **d.** A gauze bandage, the hand, or an air splint may be used to apply direct pressure to a wound. A narrow cravat should not be used because it applies too much pressure to a narrow area and may impair circulation or damage underlying blood vessels and nerves.

18. **d.** Elevation of an extremity may supplement direct pressure for bleeding control. Ice should never be placed directly on a wound.

19. **c.** The brachial artery, located in the upper arm, is the pressure point of choice for controlling bleeding from a forearm injury.

20. **d.** The femoral artery, located in the groin, is the best pressure point to use to control bleeding from a leg injury.

21. **b.** Tourniquets should be used only as a last resort, after trying all other bleeding-control techniques. They are not automatically necessary in cases of amputation or crush injury.

22. **a.** When a bandage is used as a tourniquet, it should be wrapped twice around an extremity before being tightened. It should be 4 inches wide and six to eight layers deep. The tourniquet is applied proximal to the wound, but as distal on the extremity as possible. It should never be loosened once it is applied, as this may flood the body with acidotic blood.

23. **b.** Tourniquets must be applied tightly enough to occlude arterial blood flow. If only venous blood flow is occluded, bleeding may become worse because the bleeding site is still supplied with blood, but return of venous blood is restricted.

24. **a.** After applying a tourniquet, document its use and the time it was applied on the EMS report. Some sources advocate writing the letters "TK" and the time the tourniquet was applied on the patient's forehead.

25. **d.** Blood pressure cuffs may gradually lose pressure. They are wide enough to be used as tourniquets; however, if used as such they must be constantly monitored for pressure loss. Hemostats may be used to clamp the cuff tubes, potentially reducing pressure loss.

26. **c.** *Epistaxis* is another term for nosebleed. Epinephrine (also known as adrenalin) is a hormone produced by the adrenal glands. Epiphyseal means pertaining to long bones, and epidural means "upon the dura."

27. **b.** To manage a nosebleed when there is no associated spinal injury, the EMT should have the patient lean forward if possible. This helps prevent blood from going down the patient's throat. The EMT may also pinch the fleshy portion of the patient's nostrils together.

28. **c.** When managing a patient with a head injury accompanied by a nosebleed, do not attempt to stop the bleeding, because this can increase pressure in the head. Do not tip the head, because head injuries may be accompanied by neck injuries, which should be stabilized by appropriate means.

29. **d.** Bleeding in the stomach should be suspected if emesis looks like coffee grounds. This appearance is caused by the partial digestion of the blood.

30. **c.** Tarry-looking stool is an indication of internal bleeding in the upper intestines. Bright-red blood may be noted if bleeding is from the lower intestines.

31. **b.** Signs of internal bleeding include bright blood in stool or vomitus; an enlarging, tender, rigid abdomen; and signs of hypovolemic shock. The patient may complain of extreme thirst.

32. **c.** An EMT who suspects that the patient has internal bleeding must be alert for the development of nausea and/or vomiting.

33. **a.** A pelvic injury with signs of abdominal bleeding is an indication for the use of the PASG. The PASG should not be used if the patient has chest injuries or an isolated head injury.

34. **c.** The PASG should not be applied if chest auscultation reveals sounds indicating fluid in the lungs.

35. **a.** The top of the PASG should lie below the last pair of ribs.

36. **c.** The PASG should be inflated until the hook-and-loop tape starts to crackle or the pop-off valves release. Gauges tend to be inaccurate and are not often used. If gauges are used, a pressure of 60 mm Hg is recommended. Always follow your local protocols.

37. **d.** Deflation of the PASG should not be done in the field. It should be accomplished by trained personnel in a clinical setting. Generally, deflations should be stopped after each 5 mm Hg drop in the patient's blood pressure. The EMT should be familiar with deflation procedures in the event that instruction needs to be given to hospital personnel who are less familiar with the device. Always follow your local protocols for deflation.

❋ ENRICHMENT QUESTIONS

38. **a.** Digital pressure should not be used alone. The EMT should continue to apply direct pressure to the wound, as the bleeding area may be supplied by more than one artery. Digital pressure should be applied on the pressure point as close to the wound as possible.

39. Match each bone injury with its associated blood loss.
femur
humerus
pelvis
rib
tibia

___rib___	125 cc (¼ unit)
___humerus___	250 cc (½ unit)
___tibia___	500 to 750 cc (1 to 1½ units)
___femur___	1,000 cc (2 units)
___pelvis___	1,000 to 10,000 cc (2 to 20 units)

40. **c.** Bilateral femur fractures may be accompanied by moderate-to-severe shock due to severe bleeding into the tissues surrounding the fractured area of bone.

41. **d.** In trauma care, the "golden hour" begins when the injury occurs.

42. **d.** The low blood pressure and accompanying lack of perfusion associated with septic and neurogenic shock are the result of widespread vasodilation. In the case of septic shock, the vasodilation is caused by toxins released into the bloodstream. With neurogenic shock, nervous system dysfunction (such as when spinal cord damage occurs) causes blood vessels to relax and dilate.

43. **a.** Septic shock occurs as a result of infection in the body system. Hypoperfusion occurs because the blood vessels lose their ability to constrict.

44. **c.** Psychogenic shock is caused by an emotional response to a traumatic situation. This is the same as fainting. Generally, patients recover quickly from psychogenic shock and vital signs are likely to be normal upon arrival of EMS.

45. **d.** Cardiogenic shock is basically a form of pump failure. There is enough blood in the system and the "pipes," the blood vessels, are intact. However, the heart is too weak to keep up with the body's demand for oxygen and nutrient-rich blood.

46. **b.** The hypoperfusion experienced by patients in neurogenic shock is due to an interruption of nerve impulses to the muscles and arteries, which results in dilation of the blood vessels. The dilation increases the volume of the circulatory system beyond the point where it can be filled by the body's normal volume of blood. Neurogenic shock is most often associated with spinal cord injuries.

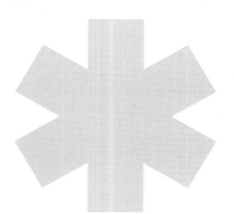

11

Soft-Tissue Injuries

CHAPTER 11 REVIEW QUESTIONS

1. An important aspect of dealing with open soft-tissue injuries is:
   a. that soft-tissue injuries are generally life-threatening
   b. to pay particular attention to avoiding contact with body substances
   c. that bleeding control takes priority over all other care
   d. that the injuries are generally worse than they appear

2. An example of a closed soft-tissue injury would be:
   a. an incision
   b. a hematoma
   c. a compound fracture
   d. an abrasion

3. When bruising is noted over the area of a vital organ:
   a. a superficial injury should be suspected
   b. direct pressure should be applied to the area
   c. damage to the underlying organ and internal bleeding should be suspected
   d. it is of concern only if it is noted on the abdomen and not the chest

4. Match the types of open soft-tissue injuries below with their descriptions.
   abrasion
   amputation
   avulsion
   laceration
   puncture

   _____ A break in the skin caused by forceful impact with a sharp object. The wound edges may be regular (linear) or irregular (stellate).

   _____ Caused by a simple scraping or scratching of the outer layer of the skin. Examples include "rug burns" or "friction burns."

   _____ A portion of tissue or skin that is torn loose and left hanging as a flap or is completely pulled from the body.

   _____ A small opening or perforation of the skin typically caused by pointed sharp objects.

   _____ The removal of an appendage (such as an arm) from the body.

5. A consideration when managing abrasions is that:
   a. bleeding may be severe
   b. they may become contaminated by foreign matter
   c. pain is usually minimal
   d. sterile dressings are not needed because the wound is not deep

6. Bleeding from a laceration:
   a. is always easy to control
   b. usually cannot be controlled using direct pressure
   c. may be severe and difficult to control
   d. primarily from the capillaries

7. A gunshot wound with no exit point is classified as a:
   a. laceration
   b. puncture wound
   c. perforating wound
   d. sterile wound

8. Another term for a bruise is:
   a. abrasion
   b. urticaria
   c. hematocrit
   d. contusion

9. A lump at a wound site caused by blood collecting within damaged tissue is a:
   a. hematoma
   b. varicose vein
   c. fistula
   d. melanoma

10. One of the goals of managing open wounds is to:
    a. thoroughly clean the wound before dressing it
    b. remove any clots that have formed prior to the arrival of EMS
    c. immediately apply a bandage
    d. prevent further contamination of the wound

11. A dressing should do all of the following *except*:
    a. hold a bandage in place
    b. help control bleeding
    c. prevent further contamination and infection
    d. protect the wound from further injury or damage

12. When bandaging an extremity:
    a. place knots over the wound
    b. cover all fingertips and toes to prevent further injury
    c. secure any loose bandage ends
    d. wrap the bandage tightly enough to occlude venous flow

13. When managing an impaled object:
    a. control bleeding by applying pressure on the object
    b. stabilize the object with a bulky dressing
    c. remove the object and apply direct pressure to the wound to control bleeding
    d. never remove the object

14. Examine the patient for an exit wound whenever:
    a. a penetration or puncture injury is encountered
    b. an avulsion has occurred
    c. a partial amputation has occurred
    d. a stellate laceration is discovered

15. Early management of an open chest injury includes:
    a. covering the wound with saline-soaked gauze pads
    b. supporting the injured area with sandbags
    c. sealing the wound with an occlusive dressing
    d. placing the patient on a backboard

16. If no spinal injuries are present,
    a patient with an open chest injury
    should be placed:
    a. supine with the legs elevated
    b. in a position of comfort, usually sitting
    c. in a prone position
    d. on the right side with the head lower
       than the legs

17. A critical issue when managing open chest
    injuries is:
    a. early application of a cervical collar
    b. rapid access to an automated
       external defibrillator
    c. access to a flow-restricted, oxygen-
       powered ventilation device
    d. early administration of
       high-flow oxygen

18. Management of an evisceration includes:
    a. replacing the organ within
       the abdomen
    b. applying a moist, sterile dressing to
       the area and covering it with an
       occlusive dressing
    c. applying direct pressure to the
       evisceration to control bleeding
    d. applying the pneumatic anti-shock
       garment (PASG) and inflating the leg
       and abdominal chambers

19. The position of choice for a patient with
    an evisceration and no accompanying
    spinal or leg injuries is on the:
    a. back with the hips and knees flexed
    b. back with the hips and knees straight
    c. left side
    d. right side

20. An impaled object may need to be
    removed if it:
    a. interferes with the airway
    b. is lodged in the ear
    c. is too small to be x-rayed
    d. is lodged in the nose

21. To package an amputated part for
    transportation to the hospital:
    a. pack it in ice
    b. immerse the part in sterile water
    c. wrap it in a sterile dressing and keep
       it cool
    d. wrap it in a wet, sterile dressing and
       keep it warm

22. When managing a partial avulsion
    or amputation:
    a. leave the part in the position found
    b. complete the amputation with
       sterile scissors
    c. apply direct pressure to the skin flap
       to control bleeding
    d. gently straighten and align any
       skin bridges

23. A serious complication associated with an
    open neck injury is:
    a. air embolism
    b. tracheal deviation
    c. increased blood pressure
    d. neck vein distention

24. Management of an open neck injury
    may include:
    a. placing the patient in a sitting position
    b. applying digital pressure to a
       brachial artery
    c. covering the wound with a sterile
       occlusive dressing
    d. applying cold packs to the injury site

25. When managing a patient with an injury
    to the soft tissue of the neck, always
    suspect accompanying:
    a. rib injuries
    b. jaw injuries
    c. cervical spine injury
    d. chest injuries

26. When managing a penetrating injury to the eye:
    a. cover the uninjured eye also
    b. leave the uninjured eye uncovered
    c. apply dry gauze pads to the eye
    d. use a compression dressing

27. When managing a patient with an impaled object in the eye:
    a. remove the object if it interferes with placement of a metal eye shield
    b. remove the object if transport time to the hospital is greater than 20 minutes
    c. remove the object and apply pressure to the wound
    d. never remove the object

28. When flushing a patient's eyes, the EMT should:
    a. flush from the outside corner to the inside corner
    b. slowly drip the water into the eye
    c. flush from the inside corner to the outside corner
    d. instruct the patient to close his or her eyes during the irrigation process

29. The major concern when managing a patient with a mouth injury is:
    a. airway compromise
    b. permanent disfigurement
    c. hypoperfusion
    d. swelling of brain tissue

30. Burn injuries are typically classified as any of the following *except*:
    a. chemical
    b. steam
    c. electrical
    d. thermal

31. A burn characterized by reddening, blister formation, and intense pain is a:
    a. full-thickness burn
    b. superficial burn
    c. partial-thickness burn
    d. medium-thickness burn

Questions 32 through 34 refer to the Rule of Nines.

32. Using the list of body-surface-area percentages below, label each part of the *adult* in Figure 11-1. (Some percentages may be used more than once.)
    1%
    9%
    18%

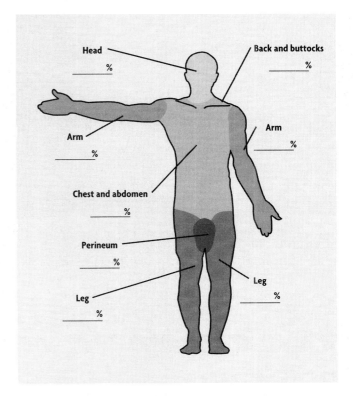

Figure 11-1 Adult.

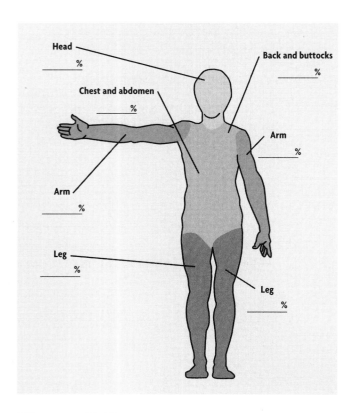

Figure 11-2 Child.

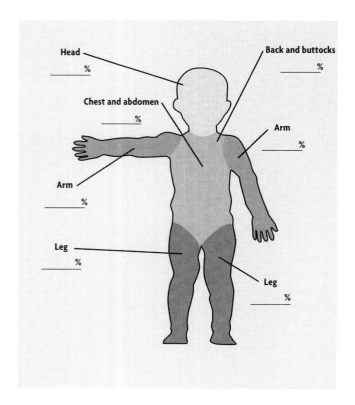

Figure 11-3 Infant.

33. Using the list of body-surface-area percentages below, label each part of the *child* in Figure 11-2. (Some percentages may be used more than once.)
9%
14%
16%
18%

34. Using the list of body-surface-area percentages below, label each part of the *infant* in Figure 11-3. (Some percentages may be used more than once.)
9%
14%
18%

For questions 35 through 37, use the Rule of Nines to calculate the approximate percentage of burns.

35. A 48-year-old man was injured in a gas heater explosion. He has burns covering his entire right arm, entire back, and the back of his head. You estimate the burns to cover a body surface area of about:
a. 18%
b. 27%
c. 31%
d. 40%

36. A 5-year-old girl pulled a pot of boiling water off the stove while helping her mother make supper. She has burns on the chest, abdomen, and front of both legs. You estimate the burns to cover a body surface area of about:
a. 22%
b. 34%
c. 48%
d. 56%

37. An 8-month-old baby has been rescued from a burning house by firefighters. Upon examination, you find that the infant has partial-thickness burns on the buttocks and back of both legs. You estimate the burns to cover a body surface area of about:
    a. 9%
    b. 14%
    c. 23%
    d. 30%

38. Superficial burns involve:
    a. only the dermis
    b. only the epidermis
    c. the epidermis and dermis
    d. all the layers of the skin

39. Respiratory tract burns should be suspected if a patient:
    a. has singed or sooty nasal hairs, nostrils, or lips
    b. has a hoarse voice
    c. was in a closed room during a fire
    d. all of the above

40. Patients with suspected inhalation injuries:
    a. should not be given oxygen to avoid drying of the mucus membranes
    b. will display signs of respiratory distress within 1 hour of the injury
    c. should always be transported to the hospital
    d. normally have a cherry-red skin color

41. The palm of a patient's hand may be used as a guide when estimating burn percentages of small areas because it represents an area of approximately:
    a. 0.5% of body surface
    b. 1% of body surface
    c. 2% of body surface
    d. 3% of body surface

42. Use the list below to categorize the following burns.
    minor
    moderate
    critical

    _____ A timer on a tanning bed malfunctions. Superficial burns cover 85% of the patient.

    _____ A weekend mechanic removes the cap from a hot radiator. He manages to protect his face but has partial-thickness burns covering 10% of the front of his chest and abdomen.

    _____ A spark ignites a welder's shirt. Workmates quickly extinguish the fire, but not before it has caused full- and partial-thickness burns to both arms and the chest. 18% of surface area sustained partial-thickness burns and 5% sustained full-thickness burns.

    _____ A woman cooking supper spills a pot of boiling water on her legs. Partial-thickness burns cover 18% to 20% of body surface area.

    _____ A roofer wearing shorts and no shirt has hot tar dropped on his body. Approximately 20% to 24% of the body surface has partial-thickness burns; one arm is completely encompassed.

43. For adults, moderate burns include:
    a. full-thickness burns covering less than 10% of the body and involving hands, feet, face, or groin
    b. superficial burns covering more than 30% of the body
    c. partial-thickness burns involving 15% to 30% of the body
    d. partial-thickness burns covering more than 40% of the body

44. The age of a burn victim is of special concern to the EMT if the patient:
    a. is between 20 and 45 years of age
    b. is younger than 5 years or older than 55 years
    c. is younger than 10 years or older than 50 years
    d. has a history of febrile seizures

45. A partial-thickness burn in a child is considered moderate if it covers:
    a. 5% to 10% of the body
    b. 10% to 20% of the body
    c. 20% to 30% of the body
    d. 30% to 40% of the body

46. Moderate pain with associated redness but no blistering is characteristic of a:
    a. superficial burn
    b. partial-thickness burn
    c. medium-thickness burn
    d. full-thickness burn

47. A burn associated with a painful, swollen, deformed extremity would be considered:
    a. minor
    b. moderate, provided that it involves only a lower extremity
    c. moderate, regardless of the extremity involved
    d. critical

48. The first step in managing a burn patient is to:
    a. estimate the percentage of burns
    b. open the airway and assess breathing
    c. stop the burning process
    d. apply sterile burn dressings

49. A burn characterized by leathery, dry skin that may appear white or charred, and may be accompanied by little or no pain is a:
    a. superficial burn
    b. partial-thickness burn
    c. medium-thickness burn
    d. full-thickness burn

50. When caring for burns to the hands or feet:
    a. apply burn cream on each individual digit
    b. place nothing between the fingers or toes
    c. separate each digit with sterile gauze
    d. advanced medical care is needed only if full-thickness burns are present

51. Burn management should include:
    a. applying ice directly to the burn
    b. removing jewelry and smoldering clothing
    c. removing charred clothing stuck to a burn
    d. removing hot tar from a burn

52. Ointments or greases should:
    a. be used on burns only if they are sterile
    b. never be used on burns by EMTs
    c. be applied immediately after the burning process has stopped
    d. be applied only to extremity burns

53. When managing a patient with burns caused by a chemical powder:
    a. cover the chemical with a sterile, moist dressing
    b. brush off as much powder as possible
    c. wash the chemical off slowly
    d. cover the chemical with a sterile, dry dressing

54. Irrigate liquid chemical burns to the body:
    a. only with sterile solutions
    b. with a neutralizing solution
    c. for no longer than 15 minutes
    d. with copious amounts of water

55. Chemical burns to the eyes should be irrigated:
    a. with a neutralizing solution
    b. only if the procedure does not interfere with transport
    c. until the patient reaches the hospital
    d. for no longer than 10 minutes

56. When caring for a patient who has suffered an electrical burn, the EMT must:
    a. ground the patient first to discharge any electricity remaining in the patient
    b. check for entrance and exit wounds
    c. pull the patient off energized wires
    d. ascertain the exact voltage that caused the burn

57. Electrical burns differ from other burns in that:
    a. there is no injury from heat
    b. they heal faster than ordinary burns
    c. damage is always limited to the dermis and epidermis
    d. tissue damage may be deeper and more severe than it appears

58. A major problem associated with lightning or electrical burns is:
    a. respiratory and cardiac arrest
    b. abdominal injury
    c. head bleed
    d. tension pneumothorax

ENRICHMENT QUESTIONS

59. If blood soaks through dressings:
    a. apply fresh dressings over the blood-soaked dressings and continue applying pressure
    b. remove all the blood-soaked dressings and apply fresh ones
    c. apply a tourniquet
    d. lower an extremity below the level of the heart

60. If, after an open chest injury is sealed, the patient becomes cyanotic and dyspnea increases:
    a. place a second, larger occlusive dressing over the first
    b. release the dressing to allow air to escape
    c. turn the victim onto the side opposite the wound
    d. decrease the oxygen flow to the patient to avoid hyperventilation

61. If a patient is found with an object impaled through the cheek:
    a. do not remove the object
    b. remove the object by carefully pulling it out in the direction opposite from which it entered the cheek
    c. remove the object with a twisting motion
    d. remove the object by carefully pulling it out in the same direction it entered the cheek

62. Injuries to the neck or throat:
    a. are never serious
    b. are serious only if they involve open wounds
    c. are classified as open or sharp
    d. should always be considered serious

63. Management of a burned eye or eyelid includes:
    a. leaving the eyes uncovered
    b. covering both eyes with dry, sterile dressings
    c. covering both eyes with moist dressings
    d. covering both eyes with occlusive dressings

64. Before applying a metal eyeshield:
    a. pad the edges of the eyeshield
    b. flush the patient's eye
    c. place an occlusive dressing over the eye
    d. cover the holes with tape

65. Lacerations of the eyeball can be managed by:
    a. applying direct pressure to the eye
    b. covering the eye with a metal eyeshield or protective cup
    c. covering the eye with a gauze pad
    d. irrigating the eye with sterile water

66. An important consideration when managing burns is that:
    a. burn patients easily lose body heat
    b. all burn patients should go to the nearest hospital
    c. burn patients are often overheated
    d. there is no risk of shock unless other injuries are present

67. The unusual, opposite motion of a flail segment seen during respirations is known as:
    a. paroxysmal movement
    b. paradoxical movement
    c. oppositional movement
    d. inordinate movement

68. Management of a patient with a flail chest would include:
    a. applying the PASG
    b. transporting the patient without using the lights and siren
    c. stabilizing the flail segment and assisting the patient's ventilations
    d. avoiding any contact with the flail segment

69. When air escapes into the soft tissue of the chest wall or neck, the condition is known as:
    a. rhonchi
    b. subcutaneous emphysema
    c. ischemia
    d. parenchyma

70. When tracheal deviation develops from a tension pneumothorax:
    a. the trachea deviates away from the injured side
    b. tracheal displacement always occurs immediately
    c. the trachea deviates toward the injured side
    d. the deviation is easily detectable

71. The neck veins of a patient with a tension pneumothorax will most likely be:
    a. normal
    b. flat
    c. unaffected
    d. distended

72. Pulmonary contusions are almost always associated with:
    a. stab wounds
    b. pneumothorax
    c. blunt injuries
    d. unconsciousness

73. A critical injury associated with rapid deceleration, such as occurs when a car suddenly stops after hitting an immoveable object, is:
    a. spontaneous pneumothorax
    b. myocardial infarction
    c. aortic tear
    d. pulsus paradoxus

74. A patient who has suffered a recent injury or blow to the left upper quadrant of the abdomen and who is experiencing pain in the left shoulder should be suspected of having a:
    a. ruptured spleen
    b. retroperitoneal bleed
    c. ruptured appendix
    d. cardiac tamponade

75. At a vehicle crash scene, abdominal injuries should especially be suspected if:
    a. the steering wheel is bent
    b. the dashboard is broken
    c. the front windshield is cracked
    d. a passenger is wearing a lap belt but not a shoulder belt

76. When managing a male patient with a genital injury:
    a. use a moist sterile dressing for open wounds
    b. avoid direct pressure when treating lacerations
    c. do not expose the area; leave any physical examination for hospital personnel
    d. avoid applying cold packs to the injury

77. You are assessing a female patient who is bleeding from the external genitalia. Management of this patient includes:
    a. packing the vagina with dressings to control bleeding
    b. advising the patient to see her gynecologist as soon as possible
    c. advising the patient that transportation by ambulance is necessary only if an open injury is involved
    d. placing nothing in the vagina

78. Management of an extruded eyeball would include:
    a. replacing the eyeball in the socket to prevent drying out of the tissue
    b. covering the eyeball with a dry, sterile dressing
    c. covering the eyeball with a moist dressing
    d. covering the eyeball with a petrolatum-coated dressing

79. In general, when a patient is wearing contact lenses:
    a. do not remove them
    b. always remove them
    c. remove them only if there is trauma to the eye
    d. do not remove them if there has been a chemical burn to the eye

80. Blunt trauma or a blow to the eye may result in a:
    a. basilar skull fracture
    b. temporal fracture
    c. mandibular fracture
    d. blow-out fracture

81. Injuries to the larynx or trachea may produce:
    a. rhonchi
    b. yellow sputum
    c. hoarseness
    d. vomiting

82. Wet dressings may be applied to burn areas covering:
    a. no more than 5% of the body surface area
    b. 9% or less of the body surface area
    c. up to 21% of the body surface area
    d. 33% or less of the body surface area

83. A patient with serious burns who presents with rapid onset of signs of hypoperfusion likely has:
    a. a spinal injury that caused neurogenic shock
    b. lost a large quantity of fluid because of seepage from the burns
    c. another serious injury causing the hypoperfusion
    d. hypoglycemia as a result of being burned

84. The maximum time a minor burn should be immersed in cool water is:
    a. 5 minutes
    b. 10 minutes
    c. 15 minutes
    d. 20 minutes

85. Light burns to the eyes caused by ultraviolet rays from sun lamps or arc welding units may be treated by:
    a. placing sterile, moistened pads over both eyes
    b. placing dry, sterile pads over both eyes
    c. placing paper cups over both eyes
    d. applying warm compresses to the eyes

■ Additional Points for Discussion ■

1. What are some types of commercially produced occlusive dressings?

2. If a commercially produced occlusive dressing is not available, what other items carried on the ambulance may be adapted?

3. What are your procedures for notifying local authorities of an animal attack or bite?

4. Where is the nearest rabies control center for your area?

5. Which hospital(s) in your area have the capability of reattaching an amputated limb?

6. What are your local protocols regarding removal of contact lenses?

7. How would you remove the following?

    • Hard contact lens:

    • Soft contact lens:

8. To which hospital(s) in your area would you transport a patient with severe burns?

9. Do your local protocols allow the use of wet dressings?

    • If so, in what cases?

    • What is the maximum amount of body surface that may be covered by wet dressings?

10. To which hospital(s) would you transport a patient with a chemical burn or contamination?

11. What precautions can be taken before transporting to avoid unnecessary contamination of the ambulance and equipment?

ANSWERS TO CHAPTER 11 REVIEW QUESTIONS

1. **b.** When dealing with open soft-tissue injuries, the EMT should pay particular attention to avoiding contact with body substances. Such precautions include wearing gloves and other personal protective equipment, as well as washing the hands as soon as possible after managing the patient. A waterless hand cleaner should be used if running water is not available. Soft-tissue injuries are generally not life-threatening and tend to look much worse than they really are. Airway control still takes priority over bleeding control.

2. **b.** A hematoma is an example of a closed soft-tissue injury. A contusion is another example.

3. **c.** When bruising is noted over the area of a vital organ, suspect damage to the underlying organ and possible internal bleeding. Direct pressure does not control internal bleeding. Although the ribs provide some protection, a blow of enough force to bruise the chest wall can also bruise the underlying lung or heart tissue. Although this may not cause internal bleeding as severe as that associated with abdominal organs, the results can be equally devastating.

4. Match the types of open soft-tissue injuries below with their descriptions.
   abrasion
   amputation
   avulsion
   laceration
   puncture

   ___laceration___   A break in the skin caused by forceful impact with a sharp object. The wound edges may be regular (linear) or irregular (stellate).

   ___abrasion___   Caused by a simple scraping or scratching of the outer layer of the skin. Examples include "rug burns" or "friction burns."

   ___avulsion___   A portion of tissue or skin that is torn loose and left hanging as a flap or is completely pulled from the body.

   ___puncture___   A small opening or perforation of the skin typically caused by pointed sharp objects.

   ___amputation___   The removal of an appendage (such as an arm) from the body.

5. **b.** Abrasions are often contaminated by foreign matter since they are associated with friction between the skin and another object, such as ground or pavement. As a result, risk of infection is increased. Bleeding is usually minor and from the capillary beds. Abrasions may be very painful due to the large surface area involved.

6. **c.** Bleeding from a laceration may be severe and difficult to control depending on location and depth. However, in most cases the bleeding can be controlled using direct pressure.

7. **b.** Stab wounds and gunshot wounds with no exit point are classified as puncture wounds. For a gunshot wound to be considered a "perforating wound," it must travel through the body and cause entrance and exit wounds. The notion that gunshot wounds are sterile as a result of the heat of the bullet is false—contamination can occur with bits of clothing and dirt carried deep into the wound.

8. **d.** A contusion is a bruise and can be managed with cold application. Urticaria are itchy wheals or hives, and a hematocrit measures the volume of red blood cells in a specimen.

9. **a.** A hematoma is a lump caused by blood collecting within damaged tissue. Varicose veins are distended veins, a fistula is an abnormal passage, and a melanoma is a tumor or growth.

10. **d.** Preventing further contamination of the wound is a goal of wound management. Other goals include bleeding control and immobilizing the injured part. Thorough cleaning should not be attempted by the EMT, and clots should not be removed. Although open wounds may be graphic, they should not sidetrack the EMT from checking for more serious, life-threatening injuries.

11. **a.** Dressings help control bleeding, prevent further contamination and infection, and protect the wound from further injury or damage. Dressings are held in place by bandages.

12. **c.** Loose bandage ends should be secured so they do not catch on anything. Do not place knots over wounds, over fractures, on the skin, or on the patient's back. Bandages should not be so tight that they restrict circulation. Do not cover fingertips or toes as this will make it difficult to check for signs of impaired circulation.

13. **b.** Impaled objects should be stabilized with bulky dressings. Do not apply pressure to the object. Although the object is usually left in place, there are situations when the object must be removed (follow local protocols). Long objects may be carefully shortened to facilitate transport.

14. **a.** Whenever a penetrating or puncture injury is encountered, the EMT should check for an exit wound. A stellate laceration has irregular edges.

15. **c.** Early management of an open chest injury includes sealing the wound with an occlusive dressing. This should be accomplished at the same time as the airway step.

16. **b.** If no spinal injuries are suspected, a patient with an open chest injury should be placed in a position of comfort that does not interfere with breathing.

17. **d.** Early administration of high-flow oxygen is critical when managing open chest injuries.

18. **b.** Eviscerations should be covered with moist, sterile dressings that are then covered with an occlusive dressing. The organs should not be replaced, and direct pressure should not be applied to the area. The abdominal compartment of the PASG should not be inflated over an evisceration.

19. **a.** If there are no accompanying spinal or leg injuries, transport an evisceration patient on his or her back with the hips and knees flexed.

20. **a.** An impaled object may need to be removed if it interferes with the airway or with chest compressions or patient transportation. Objects lodged in the ear or nose should not be removed.

21. **c.** An amputated part should be wrapped in a sterile dressing and kept cool. It should not be immersed or soaked in water or allowed to freeze. Always follow local protocols.

22. **d.** Any skin bridges should be gently straightened and aligned to maintain circulation in the partially avulsed or amputated part. Skin bridges may also be used to cover the stump if surgical amputation is necessary. The EMT should never complete an amputation or apply pressure to the skin bridge.

23. **a.** Air embolism may occur when a large neck vein is lacerated.

24. **c.** A neck vein laceration should be covered with an occlusive dressing to reduce chances of air embolism. The patient should not stand or sit up because this increases the chances of air embolism.

25. **c.** The EMT should suspect cervical spine injury when an injury to the soft tissue of the neck is encountered.

26. **a.** When managing a penetrating injury to the eye, cover both eyes. If the uninjured eye is not covered, the injured eye will move in tandem with the uninjured eye. This is known as sympathetic movement. Do not cover an exposed part of the eyeball with dry gauze; this can be irritating and the gauze will absorb eye fluids.

27. **d.** Objects impaled in the eye should not be removed. Stabilize the object, if possible, and cover it with a cone to protect the protruding object from being accidentally displaced. Since both eyes move together, cover the uninjured eye to minimize the chances of eye movement.

28. **c.** Eyes should be flushed from the corner closest to the nose to the outside corner to avoid contaminating the uninjured eye with the runoff. Flushing of both eyes can be accomplished using a nasal cannula attached to intravenous tubing if available.

29. **a.** The EMT must always monitor a patient with a mouth injury for airway compromise. Loose teeth and blood can present problems but may be managed with aggressive suctioning.

30. **b.** Burns may be classified as thermal, chemical, or electrical. Some sources also add radiation burns as a fourth category. A steam burn is a thermal burn.

31. **c.** Partial-thickness burns are characterized by reddening, blister formation, and intense pain.

32. Using the list of body-surface-area percentages below, label each part of the *adult* in Figure 11-1. (Some percentages may be used more than once.)
1%
9%
18%

33. Using the list of body-surface-area percentages below, label each part of the *child* in Figure 11-2. (Some percentages may be used more than once.)
9%
14%
16%
18%

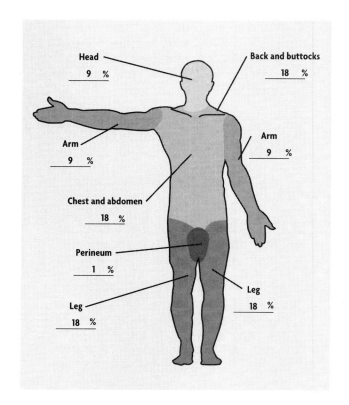

Figure 11-1 Adult.

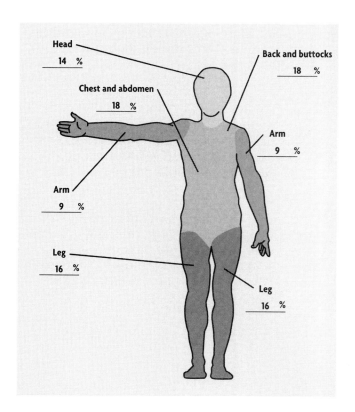

Figure 11-2 Child.

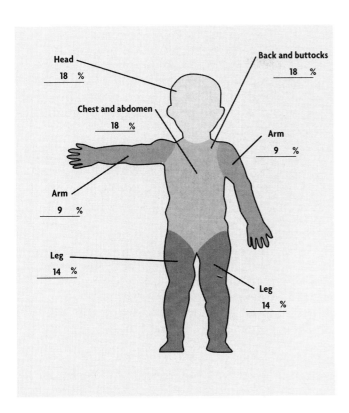

Figure 11-3 Infant.

34. Using the list of body-surface-area percentages below, label each part of the *infant* in Figure 11-3. (Some percentages may be used more than once.)
9%
14%
18%

35. **c.** The burns cover approximately 31% of body surface area (right arm = 9%, entire back = 18%, back of head = 4%).

36. **b.** Approximately 34% of body surface area is involved (chest and abdomen = 18%, fronts of both legs = 16%).

37. **c.** The infant has burns covering approximately 23% of its body (buttocks = 9%, backs of legs = 14%).

38. **b.** A superficial burn involves only the epidermis. Partial-thickness burns involve the epidermis and part of the dermis. Full-thickness burns involve the full thickness of the skin and may involve underlying muscles, bones, or other structures.

39. **d.** All of the above. Singed or sooty nasal hairs, nostrils, or lips or a hoarse voice are signs of possible respiratory tract burns. Also, respiratory tract burns should be suspected if a patient was in a closed room or confined area that was on fire.

40. **c.** Always transport patients with suspected inhalation injuries to the hospital. The structures of the respiratory tract may swell to a point that the airway becomes occluded.

41. **b.** Generally, the palm of the patient's hand equals approximately 1% of body surface area. This can be helpful when estimating burn percentages of small areas.

42. Use the list below to categorize the following burns.
minor
moderate
critical

_____moderate_____ A timer on a tanning bed malfunctions. Superficial burns cover 85% of the patient.

_____minor_____ A weekend mechanic removes the cap from a hot radiator. He manages to protect his face but has partial-thickness burns covering 10% of the front of his chest and abdomen.

_____critical_____ A spark ignites a welder's shirt. Workmates quickly extinguish the fire, but not before it has caused full- and partial-thickness burns to both arms and the chest. 18% of surface area sustained partial-thickness burns and 5% sustained full-thickness burns.

_____moderate_____ A woman cooking supper spills a pot of boiling water on her legs. Partial-thickness burns cover 18% to 20% of body surface area.

_____critical_____ A roofer wearing shorts and no shirt has hot tar dropped on his body. Approximately 20% to 24% of the body surface has partial-thickness burns; one arm is completely encompassed.

43. c. For adults, moderate burns include superficial burns covering more than 50% to 75% of the body, partial-thickness burns covering 15% to 30% of the body, or full-thickness burns (not involving face, hands, feet, or genitals) covering 2% to 10% of the body.

44. b. The age of a burn patient is of special concern if the patient is younger than 5 years or older than 55 years.

45. b. In a child, any partial-thickness burn covering 10% to 20% of the body is considered moderate. Any full-thickness or partial-thickness burn covering more than 20% of the body is considered critical.

46. a. Superficial burns are characterized by redness, moderate pain, and no blister formation.

47. d. Burns associated with a painful, swollen, deformed extremity or that involve the respiratory tract are considered critical. They are considered a high-priority injury.

48. c. The burning process must be stopped first or the injury process will continue. An open airway and artificial ventilations will do little good if a patient's tissues are still burning.

49. d. Full-thickness burns are accompanied by little or no pain due to destruction of nerve endings. The skin may be white or charred, and dry and leathery.

50. **c.** When burns of the hands or feet are being dressed, each finger or toe should be separated with a sterile dressing to keep them from sticking together.

51. **b.** Jewelry and smoldering clothing should be removed from the burn area. Clothing that is sticking to the burn should be cooled and left in place to avoid removing any burned skin. Attempting to remove tar may also cause further tissue injury.

52. **b.** Never use ointments or grease on burns, even if sterile, because they will trap heat in the tissues.

53. **b.** Powdered chemicals should be brushed off as much as possible, after which the remaining residue may be washed off with copious amounts of water. A special problem associated with some chemicals is that they react with water.

54. **d.** Liquid chemical burns should be flushed with copious amounts of water. A small amount or trickle may do more harm than good in some cases. The water does not have to be sterile. Neutralizing solutions should be avoided, because these often produce heat as the neutralizing takes place. Continue to flush during transportation to the hospital.

55. **c.** Chemical burns to the eyes should be flushed until the patient reaches the hospital. A sterile solution should be used if possible. Eyes should be flushed from the corner closest to the nose to the outside corner to avoid contaminating the uninjured eye with the runoff. Flushing of both eyes can be accomplished using a nasal cannula attached to intravenous tubing if available.

56. **b.** Once it is safe to do so, patients who have contacted electrical wires or equipment must be checked for entrance and exit wounds. Electricity does not remain in the patient after the patient is removed from the source. If a patient is still in contact with the electrical source, do not touch the patient. Attempt to turn the power off.

57. **d.** Tissue damage caused by electrical burns may be much deeper and more severe than it appears. Electricity readily travels along nerves, blood vessels, and muscles, and is capable of causing severe damage throughout its course of travel.

58. **a.** Lightning and electrical shocks may cause respiratory and cardiac arrest. Although it is not high voltage, 110-volt house current causes most electrocutions because wires and equipment using this current are accessible to most people.

✳ ENRICHMENT QUESTIONS

59. **a.** If blood soaks through a dressing, the dressing should not be removed, because this may dislodge a partially formed clot. Additional dressings should be placed over the soaked dressing. However, if too many layers are applied, pressure may be lost and bleeding control rendered inadequate. The EMT may consider removing all but the few layers of dressings closest to the wound. Fresh dressings can be applied over these.

60. **b.** If, after an open chest injury is sealed, the patient becomes cyanotic and dyspnea increases, pressure has probably built up in the chest cavity. The EMT should release the dressing to allow air to escape.

61. **d.** Objects that perforate the cheek wall should usually be removed if they interfere with the airway or may become dislodged and obstruct the airway. Remove the object by carefully pulling it out in the same direction it entered the cheek. If the object cannot easily be removed, stabilize it and leave it in place.

62. **d.** Injuries to the neck or throat should always be considered serious due to the large number of structures located in such a small area. Neck injuries are classified as blunt or penetrating in nature.

63. **c.** When burns to the eyes or eyelids are encountered, cover both eyes with moist dressings.

64. **a.** The edges of a metal eyeshield should be padded before it is applied.

65. **b.** A lacerated eye should be covered with a metal eyeshield or protective cup. Never apply pressure to a lacerated eye because this can cause a loss of fluid from inside the eye.

66. **a.** Burn patients lose body heat easily (and quickly) since the skin no longer can function as a heat regulator. The EMT must be alert for this and keep the patient in a warm environment.

67. **b.** Paradoxical movement is the unusual, opposite motion of a flail segment seen during respirations.

68. **c.** Management of a flail chest includes stabilizing the flail segment and assisting the patient's ventilations. This should be accomplished gently. A pillow can be used to stabilize the segment. Use of the PASG should be avoided in these patients since they are at high risk of developing pulmonary edema.

69. **b.** Subcutaneous emphysema is a collection of air in the soft tissue. This often is associated with some type of disruption of the tracheobronchial tree and is a serious finding. Rhonchi refers to an abnormal lung sound, parenchyma is the substance of a gland or solid organ, and ischemia involves inadequate blood flow to a tissue.

70. **a.** In a tension pneumothorax, the trachea will deviate away from the injured side and toward the uninjured side. Death is due to a kinking of the superior vena cava caused by deviation of the mediastinum. It should be remembered, however, that tracheal deviation is a late sign of tension pneumothorax and may be difficult to detect.

71. **d.** Jugular vein distention is a sign of tension pneumothorax. The distention is caused by the increase in intrathoracic pressure. If the patient is also hypovolemic, distention may not be as noticeable.

72. **c.** Pulmonary contusions are commonly associated with blunt injuries. The underlying area of lung bruising will be directly proportional to the area of injury. EMTs who start IVs must be especially careful not to cause fluid overload in patients with lung contusions. Aggressive CPR may also cause pulmonary contusion.

73. **c.** Rapid deceleration may cause aortic tear or disruption, which results in rapid and serious blood loss. This is the most common cause of sudden death related to rapid deceleration often associated with high-speed vehicle crashes.

74. **a.** A ruptured spleen should be suspected in a patient who has suffered a recent injury or blow to the left upper quadrant of the abdomen and who is experiencing pain in the left shoulder. The pain in the left shoulder is referred pain, caused by aggravation of the phrenic nerve.

75. **d.** If a passenger in a vehicle was wearing a lap belt but no shoulder belt, suspect abdominal injuries. Also, even in situations when the patient is wearing a shoulder belt, if the lap belt is worn too loose, the patient can "submarine" under the lap belt and sustain abdominal injuries.

76. **a.** A moist sterile dressing should be applied to open wounds of the male genitalia. Direct pressure may be used to control bleeding, and cold packs may be applied to blunt injuries. If a genital injury is suspected, the EMT should expose the area and do a routine examination to be sure no tissue has been avulsed.

77. **d.** The EMT should never place anything in the patient's vagina. Any female patient with a blunt injury to the genitalia should be evaluated in the hospital, as the EMT cannot tell if the internal reproductive organs have also been injured or damaged.

78. **c.** Extruded eyeballs should be covered with moist sterile dressings. Do not attempt to replace the eyeball or cover it with dry or petrolatum-coated dressings.

79. **a.** Generally, contact lenses should not be removed in the field. An exception is when a chemical burn to the eye occurs, because the lenses may trap some of the chemical underneath them. Never remove contact lenses if there is trauma to the eye itself.

80. **d.** Blunt trauma to the eye may result in a blow-out fracture to the floor of the orbit.

81. **c.** A patient with an injury to the larynx or trachea may present with hoarseness. Monitor the patient closely as he or she may develop an occluded airway.

82. **b.** Generally, wet dressings should only be applied only to total burn areas of 9% or less. If a greater area is covered with wet dressings, the patient may become hypothermic. Always follow local protocols regarding use of wet dressings.

83. **c.** Burns, even those that cover a rather large area of the body, do not cause rapid hypovolemia and rapid hypoperfusion. Since burns look serious, they can often cause an EMT to overlook other less obvious but more severe injuries. A thorough patient examination and assessment will minimize the possibility of missing other injuries.

84. **b.** Minor burns should not be immersed in cool water for longer than 10 minutes.

85. **a.** Sterile, moistened pads may be placed over the eyes of a patient who has experienced burns from ultraviolet rays. Cold application may also reduce the pain.

12

Musculoskeletal Care

D.O.T. Curriculum Objectives Covered in This Chapter:

Lesson 5-3

CHAPTER 12 REVIEW QUESTIONS

1. Two basic groups into which all musculoskeletal injuries may be classified are:
   a. open and closed
   b. deformed and simple
   c. open and compound
   d. simple and angulated

2. The mechanism of injury that causes a musculoskeletal injury may be classified as:
   a. primary or secondary
   b. simple or complex
   c. direct or indirect
   d. lateral or medial

3. Signs and symptoms of an underlying bone or joint injury may include:
   a. pain and deformity
   b. swelling and discoloration
   c. loss of use of an extremity
   d. all of the above

4. The sound or sensation noted when broken bones rub together is known as:
   a. rales
   b. crepitus
   c. rhonchi
   d. bruit

5. When a patient presents with multiple musculoskeletal injuries and hypoperfusion:
   a. splint all injuries prior to moving the patient to prevent further blood loss
   b. splint only open musculoskeletal injuries prior to moving the patient
   c. perform full-body immobilization with a backboard and immediately transport
   d. place the patient in a position of comfort

6. Evaluate motor, sensory, and circulatory status of an injured extremity:
   a. before and after splinting
   b. only if there is numbness or loss of sensation below the injury site
   c. only if a deformity is present
   d. only before splinting

7. When properly applied, a splint can:
   a. increase damage to muscle, nerves, and blood vessels
   b. diminish pain
   c. cause a closed injury to become an open injury
   d. all of the above

8. When applied to an injured extremity, the splint should:
   a. immobilize 4 inches above and below the injury
   b. immobilize one joint above and one joint below the injury
   c. be the same length as the bone
   d. be at least half the length of the limb

9. To help reduce the swelling that often accompanies musculoskeletal injuries:
   a. massage the injured area
   b. rub ice on the injured area
   c. place the patient in Trendelenburg position
   d. apply a cold pack to the injured area

10. Reducing blood flow to an injured extremity is best accomplished by:
    a. elevating the extremity
    b. lowering the extremity
    c. applying constricting bands
    d. applying pressure to arterial pressure points

11. If a patient has a severely deformed bone injury and no distal pulses, the limb should:
    a. always be splinted in the position found
    b. be realigned while pushing on the limb
    c. be realigned using gentle traction
    d. be splinted using a traction splint

12. If an open musculoskeletal injury with a protruding bone is encountered:
    a. do not try to replace the bone
    b. avoid splinting the limb
    c. use gentle traction to replace the bone
    d. use a traction splint

13. In general, joint injuries should be:
    a. realigned prior to splinting
    b. managed with a traction splint
    c. transported without splinting to reduce scene time
    d. splinted in the position found

14. When applying a splint to a joint injury:
    a. straighten the joint to its normal position
    b. wrap the joint with an elastic bandage prior to splinting
    c. immobilize the bones above and below the joint
    d. leave shoes and clothing in place to avoid unnecessary manipulation of the limb

15. Serious blood loss may often accompany:
    a. a clavicle injury
    b. an elbow injury
    c. a tibia injury
    d. a femur injury

16. A wire ladder splint is an example of a:
    a. soft splint
    b. rigid splint
    c. lateral splint
    d. traction splint

17. A vacuum splint is an example of:
    a. a pneumatic splint
    b. an air splint
    c. a rigid splint
    d. a compound splint

18. A type of splint that can be used to apply pressure to a bleeding area as well as immobilize an injury is:
    a. a sling and swathe
    b. an air splint
    c. a rigid splint
    d. a traction splint

19. Using the list below, match the most commonly used type of splint to each injury. (More than one type of splint may be appropriate. Include all that apply.)
    pillow
    rigid
    sling and swathe
    traction
    vacuum

    _____ mid-femur injury

    _____ ankle injury

    _____ forearm injury

    _____ shoulder injury

    _____ knee injury

20. Before a board splint is used, it should be:
    a. padded
    b. lubricated
    c. powdered
    d. wrapped with plastic or aluminum foil

21. Hand injuries should be splinted:
    a. with the fist clenched
    b. with the fingers outstretched and spread
    c. in the position of function
    d. with the fingers outstretched and together

22. When using a bipolar traction splint to manage a patient with a mid-femur injury, one EMT should begin applying traction:
    a. immediately using manual traction
    b. after sliding the splint under the leg
    c. only if directed to do so by medical direction
    d. after securing the leg to the splint

23. Before applying the traction splint, the patient's shoe is normally:
    a. left in place
    b. removed
    c. unlaced and left in place
    d. taped to the ankle hitch

24. Application of a bipolar traction splint requires:
    a. one EMT
    b. two EMTs
    c. three EMTs
    d. four EMTs

25. When moving a patient with a suspected pelvic injury, do not:
    a. tighten the backboard straps
    b. use a scoop stretcher
    c. place the patient on his or her back
    d. log-roll the patient

26. A complication that may result from applying splints and bandages too tightly is:
    a. angulated joints
    b. a compound deformity
    c. reduced distal circulation
    d. compensatory syndrome

27. A sling and swathe would be most appropriate type of splint to use for an injury to the:
    a. sternum
    b. hand
    c. shoulder
    d. tibia

28. Of the following, the bone that would require the greatest force to break is the:
    a. femur
    b. humerus
    c. tibia
    d. clavicle

29. The EMT's primary concern when managing a patient with a suspected pelvic fracture should be the:
    a. likelihood that the nerves controlling the legs were damaged
    b. increased likelihood of accompanying lower leg injuries
    c. high potential for severe blood loss and accompanying hypoperfusion
    d. possibility of injuries to the patient's reproductive organs

❋ ENRICHMENT QUESTIONS

30. Pelvic injuries are best immobilized using:
    a. a traction splint
    b. padded board splints
    c. a Thomas half-ring
    d. the pneumatic anti-shock garment (PASG) and a backboard

31. The most reliable sign of an underlying fracture is:
    a. swelling
    b. ecchymosis
    c. a contusion
    d. point tenderness

32. Hip fractures are often accompanied by:
    a. lengthening of the injured leg
    b. an outward rotation of the foot
    c. knee dislocations
    d. associated ankle fractures

33. A frequent complication accompanying a posterior dislocation of the hip is:
    a. an outward rotation of the thigh
    b. loss of all distal pulses
    c. sciatic nerve injury
    d. extension of the limb

34. When managing a patient with a femur fracture who also has significant hypotension, the EMT:
    a. can use the PASG only if a traction splint is not used
    b. should place the PASG over a traction splint
    c. can place a traction splint over the PASG
    d. should use a traction splint only if the leg sections of the PASG are removable

35. A patient with a humerus fracture who is experiencing an inability to raise the wrist should be suspected of having:
    a. a radial nerve injury
    b. an accompanying cervical fracture
    c. an accompanying radius or ulna fracture
    d. a dislocated elbow

36. When managing a knee dislocation:
    a. do not check distal pulses until after the leg is splinted
    b. distal pulses should be checked early in the patient examination
    c. always straighten the knee before splinting
    d. immobilize the knee with a traction splint

■ **Additional Points for Discussion** ■

1. Review the various types of splints carried on your ambulances and their proper application.

2. What type(s) of traction splint does your department carry?

3. Review the proper application of the splint(s).

ANSWERS TO CHAPTER 12 REVIEW QUESTIONS

1. **a.** Musculoskeletal injuries may be classified as open or closed. Open injuries break the skin and closed injuries do not.

2. **c.** The mechanism of injury associated with musculoskeletal injuries may be classified as direct or indirect. With a direct injury, a force is directly applied to an area of the body, causing an injury at that location. With an indirect injury, the force is exerted in one area but the injury occurs in a different location on the bone or at a joint.

3. **d.** All of the above. Signs and symptoms of an underlying bone or joint injury include pain, deformity, swelling, discoloration, loss of use or joints locked, tenderness, grating, and exposed bone fragments or ends.

4. **b.** The sound or sensation noted when broken bones rub together is known as crepitus. It is also called grating. Rales and rhonchi are abnormal breath sounds. A bruit is an abnormal sound or murmur heard when auscultating a blood vessel or the heart.

5. **c.** Perform a rapid extrication and transport immediately — the backboard can function as a full-body splint. When a patient presents with multiple musculoskeletal injuries accompanied by hypoperfusion, time should not be wasted splinting every injury prior to moving.

6. **a.** Evaluate the motor, sensory, and circulatory status of an injured limb before and after splinting.

7. **b.** When properly applied, a splint can diminish pain. Splinting also reduces damage to muscles, nerves, and blood vessels and can prevent a closed injury from becoming an open injury.

8. **b.** Splints should immobilize one joint above and one joint below the injury.

9. **d.** A cold pack may be applied to the injured area to help reduce swelling. Do not rub ice directly on the area, because this can cause cold injury to the tissue.

10. **a.** Elevating an injured extremity reduces blood flow to the injured area.

11. **c.** Angulated or deformed bone injuries without distal pulses should be realigned using gentle traction pulled along the long axis of the bone.

12. **a.** Do not try to replace a protruding bone. Apply a sterile dressing over the bone end or open wound.

13. **d.** Generally, joint injuries should be splinted in the position found. If circulation is impaired, contact medical direction for advice.

14. **c.** When applying a splint to a joint injury, the splint should immobilize the bones above and below the joint. Distal pulses should always be checked, and the EMT should be alert for signs of circulatory impairment and bruising. This requires removing shoes and clothing from the injury site.

15. **d.** A femur injury may be accompanied by serious blood loss into the surrounding tissues. The situation is even more serious if both femurs are injured.

16. **b.** A wire ladder splint is an example of a rigid splint. Its shape can be formed to the injury. Other examples of rigid splints include padded board splints as well as plastic, metal, or cardboard splints.

17. **a.** Vacuum splints and air splints are both examples of pneumatic splints.

18. **b.** Air splints may be used to apply pressure to a bleeding area as well as to immobilize an injury.

19. Using the list below, match the most commonly used type of splint to each injury. (More than one type of splint may be appropriate. Include all that apply.)
pillow
rigid
sling and swathe
traction
vacuum

_____traction_____	mid-femur injury
_____pillow_____	ankle injury
vacuum, rigid, _sling and swathe_	forearm injury
sling and swathe	shoulder injury
vacuum, rigid	knee injury

20. **a.** Board splints should be padded before they are used.

21. **c.** Hand and foot injuries should be splinted in the position of function.

22. **a.** When traction to an injured femur is indicated, manual traction should be applied immediately if there are no life-threatening injuries present. Do not wait for the traction splint before applying manual traction. Do not use a traction splint if the injury is close to the knee or if there is an accompanying injury to the pelvis, hip, knee, lower leg, or ankle. Traction splints should not be used if the patient has a partial amputation with bone separation.

23. **b.** A patient's shoe should be removed before applying the traction splint. This allows the EMT to check distal pulses and continue to monitor circulatory status after the splint is applied.

24. **b.** Two EMTs are required to apply a bipolar traction splint (e.g., a Hare traction splint). Although only one EMT is needed to apply a unipolar traction splint (e.g., a Sager splint), it is still preferable to have two EMTs involved. This allows one EMT to manually stabilize the leg while the other applies the splint.

25. **d.** Patients with suspected pelvic injuries should not be log-rolled. The scoop stretcher or a backboard can be used, and straps should always be used to secure the patient. Pelvic injuries are associated with serious blood loss and shock.

26. **c.** Reduced distal circulation may result from applying splints and bandages too tightly. If this condition is suspected, loosen splints and bandages and reassess.

27. **c.** A sling and swathe would be most appropriate type of splint to use for an injury to the shoulder.

28. **a.** The femur is the largest bone of the body and requires the greatest force to break.

29. **c.** The EMT's primary concern when managing a patient with a suspected pelvic fracture is that these injuries have a high potential for severe blood loss and resulting hypoperfusion. This bleeding cannot be adequately controlled in the field. These patients need rapid transport to a hospital capable of dealing with such a potentially devastating injury. Use of the PASG should be considered based on local protocols.

❋ **ENRICHMENT QUESTIONS**

30. **d.** Pelvic injuries are best immobilized using a PASG and a backboard.

31. **d.** Point tenderness is the most reliable sign of an underlying fracture. Contusion is another term for bruise, and ecchymosis refers to soft-tissue discoloration associated with a closed wound.

32. **b.** Hip fractures are commonly accompanied by an outward rotation and shortening of the injured leg.

33. **c.** Posterior dislocations of the hip may be accompanied by sciatic nerve injury. The patient will have decreased sensation in the leg and foot, and weakness of the foot muscles with accompanying foot drop. The hip joint will be flexed with an inward rotation of the thigh.

34. **c.** If a patient has a femur fracture and is also displaying signs and symptoms of significant hypovolemia, the PASG may be used in conjunction with the Sager traction splint. After placing the patient in the PASG, the traction splint can be applied over the garment. Always follow local protocols regarding the use of the PASG.

35. **a.** A radial nerve injury should be suspected if a patient with a humerus fracture is unable to raise the wrist.

36. **b.** Knee dislocations have a high incidence of permanent damage. Distal pulses must be checked early in the patient examination, and the knee should normally not be straightened.

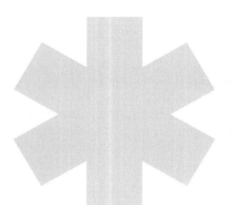

13

Head and Spinal Injuries

D.O.T. Curriculum Objectives Covered in This Chapter:

Lesson 5-4

CHAPTER 13 REVIEW QUESTIONS

1. Until proven otherwise, all unconscious trauma patients should be suspected of having:
   a. hyperglycemia
   b. DNR orders
   c. high blood pressure
   d. a spinal injury

2. A mechanism of injury at the scene of a vehicle collision that indicates a patient may have suffered a traumatic head injury is a:
   a. bent steering column
   b. cracked or deformed windshield
   c. cracked dashboard
   d. broken gearshift lever

3. Indications for applying a cervical collar include:
   a. the patient's medical history
   b. the patient's signs and symptoms
   c. the mechanism of injury
   d. all of the above

4. Cervical spine stabilization should be accomplished while performing the:
   a. ongoing assessment
   b. focused history
   c. initial assessment
   d. detailed assessment

5. If an injury to the head or spinal cord is suspected:
   a. ask the patient if it hurts to move his or her head to check for neck pain
   b. check for sensory and motor function in all four extremities
   c. have the patient stand and ask if he or she feels dizzy
   d. check reflexes and capillary refill in all four extremities

6. Adequate cervical spine immobilization may be obtained by:
   a. applying a rigid cervical collar to the patient and sitting the patient in the captain's chair in the ambulance
   b. using a soft cervical collar, scoop stretcher, and cervical immobilization device
   c. using a rigid cervical collar and a long backboard
   d. any of the above means

7. When applying a cervical collar, remember:
   a. to continue to provide manual stabilization until the patient's head can be secured to a backboard
   b. to use whatever size collar is most comfortable for the patient
   c. that all cervical collars are sized the same way
   d. all of the above

8. Rapid extrication is indicated when:
   a. there are other patients with minor injuries in the vehicle who also need extrication
   b. the patient's condition is unstable
   c. the EMT prefers not to use other methods for moving the patient
   d. only two EMTs are available to move the patient

9. Log-rolling a patient should be directed by the:
   a. EMT at the patient's waist
   b. EMT at the patient's shoulders
   c. EMT controlling the patient's head
   d. senior EMS officer

10. If only two EMTs are available to perform a log-roll, one EMT should be positioned:
    a. at the patient's head and the other at the patient's torso
    b. at the patient's shoulders and the other at the patient's hips
    c. at the patient's head and the other at the patient's legs
    d. at the patient's torso and the other slides the board under the patient

11. During the log-roll:
    a. check sensory and motor function in all extremities
    b. apply a cervical collar to the patient
    c. reassess patient vital signs
    d. assess the patient's back

12. If a standing patient complains of neck and back pain but is able to walk:
    a. there probably is no spinal injury
    b. place the backboard on the cot next to the patient and have the patient lie down on the backboard
    c. apply a short backboard and walk the patient to the ambulance
    d. immobilize the patient to a backboard while the patient is standing

13. Secure the patient's head to a long backboard:
    a. before applying any backboard straps
    b. after securing the patient's torso to the board
    c. before securing the patient's torso to the board
    d. after securing the patient's legs to the board

14. If there are void spaces between the long backboard and the patient's head and torso:
    a. gently manipulate the patient to conform to the long backboard
    b. remove the patient from the long backboard and use the cot mattress for support
    c. pad between the patient and the long backboard
    d. ignore the void spaces because manipulating the patient may cause further spinal injury

15. After a patient is removed from a vehicle using a rigid short board or a vest-type extrication device, the patient should be:
    a. placed flat on an ambulance cot without a backboard
    b. removed from the device and then placed on a long backboard
    c. left in the device and placed on an ambulance cot in a sitting position
    d. left in the extrication device and secured to a long backboard

16. When managing infants and children with spinal injuries:
    a. place padding from the shoulders to the heels if necessary to provide proper immobilization
    b. do not use a long backboard for immobilization
    c. do not immobilize the patient if it causes excessive restlessness and agitation
    d. do not secure the patient's head to the backboard

17. Bleeding from scalp injuries:
    a. always indicates a more severe underlying head injury
    b. is very easy to control
    c. normally is arterial in nature
    d. often looks worse than it is

18. The best indicator that a patient has a brain injury is:
    a. altered mental status
    b. increasing pulse
    c. decreased breathing rate
    d. constricted pupils

19. Injury or damage to brain tissue may cause:
    a. a decreased need for oxygen
    b. an increase in pressure inside the skull
    c. a gradual constriction of both pupils
    d. a temporary decrease in brain size

20. A significant sign of skull injury is:
    a. distended neck veins
    b. regular breathing patterns
    c. pale skin
    d. bruising around the eyes or behind the ears

21. When a patient with a traumatic head injury accompanied by a low blood pressure and rapid pulse rate is encountered:
    a. position the patient on the right side with the head lower than the feet
    b. place the patient in a sitting position
    c. suspect other injuries or bleeding
    d. suspect a diabetic emergency

22. Check the level of consciousness of an unstable patient with a head injury:
    a. every 5 minutes
    b. only if changes in mental status are noted
    c. every 15 minutes
    d. only if the vital signs change

23. If a patient with a head injury is bleeding from the nose or ears, be alert for the presence of:
    a. lymph
    b. mucus
    c. cerebrospinal fluid
    d. saline fluid

24. To control bleeding from an open or depressed skull injury:
    a. use a loose, bulky dressing
    b. apply firm pressure to the injury site
    c. apply digital pressure to the carotid arteries
    d. pack the wound with gauze

25. When managing patients with a head injury:
    a. also suspect a neck injury
    b. have the patient move his or her head to check for neck pain
    c. there is no need for concern unless the pupils are unequal
    d. apply a cervical collar and transport the patient sitting upright

26. A patient with a head injury may quickly develop:
    a. an increased level of consciousness
    b. chest pain
    c. nausea and vomiting
    d. hyperglycemia

27. Nontraumatic brain injuries may be a result of:
    a. breathing problems
    b. hemorrhaging or clots
    c. hyperventilation
    d. liver dysfunction

28. A semi-responsive patient with a medical or nontraumatic brain injury should usually be positioned:
    a. on the right side with the head lower than the feet
    b. prone
    c. in the shock position
    d. on the left side

29. Carefully remove a motorcycle or football helmet from a patient if the helmet:
    a. fits the patient's head well
    b. does not have a chin strap
    c. interferes with the airway
    d. does not have a visor

30. The most critical factor when removing a helmet is:
    a. monitoring the pulse for changes
    b. maintaining good cervical spine control
    c. not obstructing the airway
    d. minimizing damage to the helmet

31. Proper removal of a helmet requires at least:
    a. one EMT
    b. two EMTs
    c. three EMTs
    d. four EMTs

✻ ENRICHMENT QUESTIONS

32. If a patient who is secured to a long backboard may vomit:
    a. turn the patient's head to one side
    b. roll the secured patient and board to one side as a unit
    c. release the straps and sit the patient up
    d. leave the patient in a supine position and attempt to suction

33. Managing scalp injuries should include all of the following *except*:
    a. controlling bleeding
    b. applying a sterile dressing over the wound
    c. cleaning and irrigating the wound
    d. leaving dirt or glass fragments in place

34. Concerning unequal pupils, remember that:
    a. unequal pupils are an early sign of head injury
    b. medications will not affect pupils
    c. unequal pupils always indicate a severe head injury
    d. some individuals normally have unequal pupils

35. The blood pressure of a patient with a severe head injury and increased intracranial pressure will:
    a. decrease
    b. increase
    c. remain the same
    d. increase or decrease directly proportional to the pulse

36. A patient who is an alcoholic is more prone to develop:
    a. a spontaneous pneumothorax
    b. hemophilia
    c. a kidney stone
    d. intracranial bleeding

■ **Additional Points for Discussion** ■

1. Review the local protocols regarding the appropriate circumstances for the removal of motorcycle or football helmets.

2. Review the suggested local procedure for removing a helmet from a patient's head.

3. Review the types and proper use of the following spinal immobilization equipment used by your department.

   • Cervical collars:

   • Extrication devices:

   • Head blocks and cervical immobilization devices:

4. What locations (such as buildings or industrial complexes) in your territory may require special packaging and removal techniques for patients?

ANSWERS TO CHAPTER 13 REVIEW QUESTIONS

1. **d.** Suspect a spinal injury when managing an injured, unconscious patient. Although physical signs of spinal injury may not be present, be alert for such injury.

2. **b.** Suspect traumatic head injury if a cracked or deformed windshield is noted. A "spiderweb" pattern is typically seen where the patient's head struck the windshield.

3. **d.** All of the above. A cervical collar should be used based on the history, patient signs and symptoms, or mechanism of action.

4. **c.** Cervical spine stabilization should be accomplished while performing the initial assessment.

5. **b.** A patient with a suspected injury of the head or spinal cord should have sensory and motor function checked in all four extremities. The patient should not be asked to stand, and the neck should not be moved.

6. **c.** A rigid cervical collar and long backboard (or scoop stretcher) must be used to adequately immobilize the cervical spine in the field. In addition, a cervical immobilization device (such as head blocks) should be used if available. Soft cervical collars are not acceptable immobilization devices in the field.

7. **a.** Even after a cervical collar is applied, maintain manual stabilization until the patient can be secured to a backboard. There are a variety of sizes of collars available from many manufacturers. The proper size cervical collar should be used. Follow manufacturer's instructions on choosing the proper size collar for each patient.

8. **b.** Rapid extrication is indicated when the patient is unstable and needs to be immediately moved and transported, or when the scene is unsafe. It may also be used if a less seriously injured patient is blocking access to a more seriously injured patient. Rapid extrication should not be performed simply because the EMT prefers to move the patient by this method. The number of EMTs present should not be a factor. Other rescue personnel or bystanders may be used to assist extrication regardless of whether it is done rapidly.

9. **c.** The EMT controlling the head directs the log-rolling operation.

10. **a.** If only two EMTs are available to perform a log-roll, one EMT controls the patient's head and neck and the other should be positioned at the patient's torso to control the shoulders and hips.

11. **d.** The patient's entire posterior, or back, should be assessed when the patient is rolled. A cervical collar should already be in place. Sensory and motor function as well as vital signs can be reassessed after the patient is secured to the board.

12. **d.** A standing patient who is complaining of neck and back pain should be secured to a backboard while still standing. A patient's ability to walk does not indicate that a spinal injury does not exist.

13. **b.** Secure the patient's head to the long backboard after the torso has been secured to the board. Secure the legs to the board after the torso and head are immobilized.

14. **c.** Pads should be placed to fill voids between the long backboard and the patient's head and torso to prevent any movement. This should be done carefully and in a manner that does not move the patient unnecessarily.

15. **d.** After a patient is removed from a vehicle using a rigid short board or vest-type extrication device, secure the patient to a long backboard while he or she is still in the device.

16. **a.** When immobilizing infants and children, place padding from the shoulders to the heels to fill voids under the patient because a child's head is normally larger in proportion to the size of the body than an adult's. The patient should still be secured to the board. A variety of devices may be used, such as long backboard, short backboard, commercial immobilization device, or padded board splint. Use the device that is the most appropriate for the size of the child. Do not neglect proper immobilization simply because it agitates the patient.

17. **d.** Bleeding from scalp injuries always looks worse than it is and is not always accompanied by a more severe underlying head injury. The bleeding usually comes from the capillaries but may be difficult to stop because of the number of vessels involved.

18. **a.** Altered or decreasing mental status should alert the EMT to the possible presence of a head injury.

19. **b.** Brain damage or injury may cause an increase in pressure inside the skull.

20. **d.** Bruising around the patient's eyes or behind the patient's ears is a significant sign of skull injury.

21. **c.** A patient with a head injury who presents with a low blood pressure and a rapid pulse rate probably has other injuries or bleeding. Isolated head injuries do not usually produce low blood pressure in the early stages.

22. **a.** Check the level of consciousness of an unstable patient with a head injury every 5 minutes. Any changes, whether good or bad, should be noted.

23. **c.** Be alert for the presence of cerebrospinal fluid mixed with blood that is discharged from the nose or ears.

24. **a.** Use a loose, bulky dressing to control bleeding from an open or depressed skull injury. Do not pack the wound or apply pressure to the injury site.

25. **a.** Always suspect a neck injury when treating a patient with a head injury.

26. **c.** Increasing pressure inside the head can cause nausea and vomiting. The patient's level of consciousness will decrease.

27. **b.** Hemorrhaging or clots within the head can cause nontraumatic brain injury.

28. **d.** Position a semi-responsive patient with a medical or nontraumatic brain injury on the left side to help keep the airway clear.

29. **c.** Generally, if a helmet interferes with airway control or is so loose that cervical spine immobilization cannot be accomplished, it should be removed. Local protocols concerning removal of helmets should be followed.

30. **b.** The most critical factor when removing a helmet is maintaining good cervical spine control, which can be difficult. Practice is necessary to develop this skill.

31. **b.** Proper removal of a helmet requires at least two EMTs.

❋ **ENRICHMENT QUESTIONS**

32. **b.** If a patient who is properly secured to a long backboard begins to vomit, roll the board and the patient to one side as a unit. Patients should not sit up, and their heads should not be turned to the side.

33. **c.** Scalp wounds should not be cleaned or irrigated, as this may force foreign matter into the brain tissue if an underlying open skull fracture is present. A loose, bulky sterile dressing can be applied to control bleeding.

34. **d.** Remember that some individuals have normally unequal pupils. When related to head injuries, unequal pupils usually occur late, not early, in the incident, as pressure on the optic nerve increases. Although unequal pupils are a bad sign in an unresponsive patient with a head injury, unequal pupils alone do not always signify head injury. Medications can also affect pupil size and reactivity.

35. **b.** As the intracranial pressure increases, the blood pressure increases. This is to overcome the resistance to blood flow created by the swelling of brain tissue. At the same time, the pulse rate will normally decrease.

36. **d.** Alcoholics are prone to the development of intracranial bleeding. This is due to impaired clotting mechanisms caused by liver damage and because of frequent falls. A patient with intracranial bleeding may appear drunk, so the EMT must be careful not to mistake a serious case of intracranial bleeding for simple intoxication.

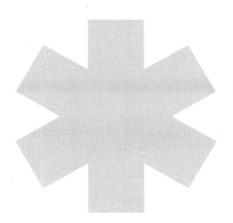

14

Infants and Children

D.O.T. Curriculum Objectives Covered in This Chapter:

Lesson 6-1

CHAPTER 14 REVIEW QUESTIONS

1. Managing infants and children is different from treating adults because younger patients:
   a. are more trusting and less fearful
   b. like to ride in ambulances
   c. tend to be more fearful and may have difficulty communicating
   d. have less difficulty communicating

2. When an infant or child with a non–life-threatening problem is encountered:
   a. take a little more time to perform the examination
   b. treat the infant or child like a small adult
   c. it is not necessary to perform an assessment
   d. perform the examination the same way it would be performed on an adult

3. If a procedure must be performed that may cause pain:
   a. restrain the child before proceeding
   b. tell the child it will not hurt
   c. tell the child in advance it will hurt
   d. have the parents leave the room

4. When caring for a sick or injured child:
   a. never allow parents to be present
   b. allow parents to be present only if absolutely necessary
   c. allow only one parent to be present at any time
   d. make judicious use of the parents for assistance

5. The first priority when assessing an infant or child is evaluating:
   a. airway and breathing
   b. pulse and blood pressure
   c. amount of movement
   d. response to external stimuli

6. An important consideration when managing a sick or injured infant or child is:
   a. the EMT's general impression of the child
   b. whether the child has a good blood pressure reading
   c. when the child last took a nap
   d. that both parents are present before care is begun

7. When performing a detailed physical exam on a newborn or infant, first examine the:
   a. head
   b. neck
   c. abdomen
   d. heart and lungs

8. When performing a detailed physical exam on a toddler:
   a. start with vital signs
   b. use a trunk-to-head approach
   c. examine only exposed areas
   d. use a head-to-toe approach

9. The number one cause of death among infants and children is:
   a. traumatic injury
   b. poisoning
   c. drowning
   d. child abuse

10. When opening the airway of an infant or child:
    a. tilt the head forward
    b. keep the neck totally neutral
    c. tilt the head as far back as possible
    d. do not hyperextend the neck

11. If a child is breathing rapidly and exhibits signs of increased breathing effort:
    a. respiratory fatigue or general fatigue may rapidly develop
    b. the child is likely reacting normally to a stressful situation
    c. immediately assist the child to use a prescribed inhaler
    d. use caution administering oxygen, as it can cause respiratory arrest

12. To insert an oral airway in a child:
    a. insert the airway right-side up without using the rotating maneuver that would be used for an adult
    b. the EMT must receive an order from medical direction
    c. insert the airway upside-down and rotate it once in the proper position
    d. visualize the oropharynx first with a laryngoscope

13. When using a rigid suction catheter to suction an infant or a young child, a key concern is that suctioning may cause:
    a. an increase of the blood pressure
    b. an increase in oxygen levels in the blood
    c. a decrease of carbon dioxide levels in the blood
    d. a slowing of the heart rate

14. For newborns with breathing problems:
    a. the use of oxygen is optional
    b. oxygen should be used only if CPR is necessary
    c. the use of oxygen should be avoided, as it can cause blindness
    d. oxygen should be carefully administered

15. If a seriously ill or injured infant or child will not tolerate an oxygen mask:
    a. restrain the child and force him or her to wear the mask
    b. use a blow-by technique to enrich the surrounding air
    c. wait for the child to calm down, then administer oxygen
    d. refrain from using oxygen because the stress can worsen the medical problem

16. The best way to determine the breathing rate of a newborn or infant is to:
    a. watch the chest rise from a distance
    b. listen with a stethoscope
    c. place one hand on the patient's chest
    d. place one hand on the patient's abdomen

17. Regarding respiratory distress in infants and children, all of the following statements are correct *except*:
    a. nasal flaring in children is a sign of increased respiratory effort
    b. infants and children have a relatively large respiratory reserve
    c. "see-saw" breathing is more commonly seen in infants than adults
    d. infants and children often use accessory muscles to enhance respiratory effort

18. The best place to look for cyanosis in an infant or child is the:
    a. oral mucosa
    b. abdomen
    c. hands
    d. feet

19. The pulse of infants and children is normally:
    a. slower than that of an adult
    b. faster than that of an adult
    c. the same as that of an adult
    d. weak and thready

20. Blood pressure should be assessed:
    a. only on children younger than 6 years
    b. on all infants and children
    c. only on children older than 3 years
    d. only on children who have sustained trauma

21. A sign of an upper airway obstruction is:
    a. stridor on inspiration
    b. wheezing on expiration
    c. rhonchi
    d. rales

22. Lower airway disease should be suspected if the EMT notes:
    a. stridor on inspiration
    b. wheezing on expiration
    c. a slow breathing rate
    d. a sore throat and drooling

23. The point at which an infant or child is considered to be in respiratory arrest is when the breathing rate drops below:
    a. 8 breaths per minute
    b. 10 breaths per minute
    c. 12 breaths per minute
    d. 14 breaths per minute

24. Oxygen should be given to infants and children:
    a. only if trauma is present
    b. only if the child will tolerate it
    c. anytime a breathing emergency is present
    d. whenever a child has a breathing rate over 16

25. Febrile seizures:
    a. seldom need evaluation at a hospital
    b. occur in most infants with fevers
    c. signify serious brain disorders
    d. occur because of a rapid rise in temperature

26. If a child with a history of seizures has just had a seizure, an important question is whether the:
    a. seizure is following a normal seizure pattern
    b. child is taking antiemetic medications
    c. child is nauseated and vomiting
    d. all of the above

27. When a child accidentally ingests poison:
    a. administer glucose if he is semi-responsive
    b. there is no need for transport if the child does not appear to be in distress
    c. make the patient vomit
    d. contact medical direction about administering activated charcoal

28. A fever is of particular concern if the child also:
    a. complains of an earache
    b. has a rash
    c. feels achy
    d. cries when being examined

29. Vomiting and diarrhea may be of special concern in children because:
    a. children can dehydrate rapidly
    b. these signs indicate an underlying serious abdominal problem
    c. these signs are linked to febrile seizures
    d. children must be given intravenous fluids when these signs occur

30. Blood loss is more significant in children because:
    a. there is less circulating volume to begin with
    b. they are difficult to type and cross-match
    c. the normal clotting factors are not yet present
    d. the pneumatic anti-shock garment (PASG) cannot be used on children

31. A sign of hypoperfusion in infants would be:
    a. copious amounts of tears when crying
    b. decreased urine output
    c. frequent urination
    d. flushed skin

32. Secondary drowning syndrome refers to:
    a. drowning after being injured in the water
    b. drowning after developing respiratory arrest
    c. a medical condition wherein the patient drowns from fluid in the lungs
    d. deterioration that occurs following a near-drowning event and after the patient has resumed normal breathing

33. The primary cause of sudden infant death syndrome (SIDS) is:
    a. external suffocation
    b. unknown
    c. choking
    d. parental neglect

34. When a SIDS situation is encountered:
    a. question the parents regarding what they may have done to contribute to the death
    b. never institute CPR, as this may compromise the police investigation of the death
    c. think of the parents as patients also
    d. try to forget about the situation and do not discuss it with other crew members

35. The most common type of trauma in children is:
    a. open injury
    b. crush injury
    c. deceleration injury
    d. blunt injury

36. Blood loss in a child is considered serious if the amount lost exceeds:
    a. 5% of total blood volume
    b. ½ unit
    c. 500 cc
    d. 1 cup

37. When assessing a child who was in a motor vehicle crash and was restrained with only a lap belt, suspect:
    a. abdominal and lower spine injuries
    b. head injuries
    c. chest and arm injuries
    d. leg injuries

38. An area that commonly needs to be padded when a child is affixed to a backboard is:
    a. under the shoulders
    b. under the head
    c. under the lower back
    d. under the occiput

39. A correct statement concerning PASG use on children is that it should be used:
    a. if the patient can be placed in a leg of the garment
    b. any time hypoperfusion is present
    c. only if the child fits properly in the garment
    d. any time the blood pressure is below 90 mm Hg systolic

40. When using the PASG on children, inflate the:
    a. legs and then the abdominal compartment
    b. abdominal compartment and then the legs
    c. abdominal compartment only
    d. legs only

41. Physical abuse may be defined as:
    a. giving insufficient attention to a child
    b. improper or excessive action that injures or causes harm
    c. striking a child as a form of discipline
    d. all of the above

42. Suspect child abuse if:
    a. an isolated bruise in the process of healing is noted
    b. an injury is inconsistent with its described mechanism
    c. an isolated scar from a burn is found while examining the patient
    d. the parents tell the same story about how the injury occurred

43. If child abuse is suspected:
    a. privately report suspicions to the emergency department staff
    b. attempt to get the parents to confess to child abuse
    c. advise the parents you are going to have them investigated for child abuse
    d. take the child to the hospital without parental consent

44. When a child on a home ventilator is encountered:
    a. refer to the instruction manual to determine how to operate the unit
    b. remove the patient from the ventilator and place him or her on a nonrebreather mask at 15 L/min
    c. have the parents assist in managing the patient
    d. start CPR and transport if the ventilator malfunctions

45. If bleeding is noted in the area where a central IV line enters the skin:
    a. soak up the blood with loose, bulky dressings
    b. apply ice to the area
    c. clamp off the IV tubing
    d. control the bleeding by applying pressure

46. A gastrostomy tube:
    a. hooks directly into a major blood vessel
    b. is placed directly into the brain to relieve intracranial pressure
    c. is placed directly into the trachea through a hole in the neck
    d. is placed directly into the stomach for feeding

47. Two positions in which an infant or child with a gastrostomy tube may be transported are:
    a. lying on the back, or lying on the left side with the head lower than the trunk
    b. sitting, or lying on the right side with the head elevated
    c. in a position of comfort, or prone with the head lower than the trunk
    d. supine, or prone with the head elevated

48. A shunt runs from:
    a. the brain to the abdomen to drain excess cerebrospinal fluid
    b. the heart to the lungs to reoxygenate blood
    c. the ears to the throat to relieve pressure behind the eardrum
    d. the kidneys to the bladder to drain excess urine

49. Infants or children with shunts are particularly prone to:
    a. high fevers
    b. rapid heart rates
    c. respiratory arrest
    d. hypoperfusion

❋ **ENRICHMENT QUESTIONS**

50. An important consideration when caring for newborns is that they:
    a. primarily breathe through their mouth
    b. primarily breathe through their nose
    c. breathe through both the mouth and nose
    d. breathe more slowly than adults

51. The single most important factor in
accurately obtaining a child's blood
pressure is the:
   a. child's emotional state
   b. limb used
   c. age of the patient
   d. size of the blood pressure cuff

52. The most accurate indicator of early shock
in an infant or child with trauma is:
   a. blood pressure
   b. pale, cool, and clammy skin
   c. a pulse rate greater than 120 beats
   per minute
   d. capillary refill time

53. Two common upper respiratory infections
in children that the EMT may encounter are:
   a. croup and epiglottitis
   b. asthma and bronchitis
   c. epiglottitis and asthma
   d. bronchiolitis and emphysema

54. A child who presents with a high
fever, very sore throat, pain when
swallowing, and drooling, should be
suspected of having:
   a. croup
   b. bronchitis
   c. epiglottitis
   d. asthma

55. A respiratory disease that gets worse
at night and is characterized by a loud
"seal bark" cough is:
   a. epiglottitis
   b. croup
   c. tonsillitis
   d. asthma

■ Additional Points for Discussion ■

1. What are your local and state laws
regarding reporting suspected child
abuse cases?

2. What are your local protocols regarding
the handling of a SIDS situation?

3. Is there a SIDS crisis group in your area?
If so, how can they be contacted?

4. What hospital(s) in your area are able to
handle a child with severe trauma?

5. Are there any children within your
response area with medical problems
who are receiving special medical
care at home?

   • If so, what type of medical problems do
   they have?

   • What special medical care is
   being provided?

   • Is there anything that would need to be
   done differently when responding to an
   EMS call on those patients?

ANSWERS TO CHAPTER 14 REVIEW QUESTIONS

1. **c.** Infants and children tend to be more fearful than adults and may have difficulty communicating. The ambulance may present a frightening environment for a child.

2. **a.** Unless a serious emergency exists, take a little more time when dealing with a child to explain and perform the examination. This will help put the child at ease. Alter the examination to fit the circumstances but do not skip the assessment. Infants and children should not be thought of as "little adults."

3. **c.** Tell a child in advance if a procedure will hurt. If a child is lied to or surprised, he or she may not trust the EMT for the remainder of the care period. Parents can be used to lend support provided they can handle the situation. Do not restrain a child unless absolutely necessary.

4. **d.** Make judicious use of the parents to assist in examining and caring for infants and children. Parents can be used to calm the child. If a parent is agitated, however, this will agitate the child.

5. **a.** When assessing a child, the first concern is the patient's breathing status. This is especially important with young children and infants, as cardiac arrest is normally secondary to respiratory arrest. Aggressive airway management can make a difference.

6. **a.** The EMT's general impression of the child's well-being is an important consideration. Physical signs may not always be as valuable as the EMT's impression of how serious the child's injuries are. Although it is best to have the permission of one parent to institute care, care can be rendered under implied consent if no parents are present.

7. **d.** When performing a detailed physical exam on a newborn or infant, examine the heart and lungs first and the head last. It is best to obtain heart and lung sounds before the child becomes agitated by the rest of the examination.

8. **b.** When performing a detailed physical exam on a toddler, use a trunk-to-head approach. This approach is used to build confidence and should be taken before the child becomes agitated. Airway, breathing, and circulation still take priority over vital signs.

9. **a.** Traumatic injury is the number-one cause of death among infants and children.

10. **d.** When opening the airway of an infant or child, do not hyperextend the neck. Hyperextending the neck can cause airway obstruction.

11. **a.** A child who is breathing rapidly and displaying signs of increased breathing effort is compensating. The child's condition may deteriorate rapidly due to rapid respiratory muscle fatigue or general fatigue.

12. **a.** Oral airways are inserted differently in children than in adults. Because of loose teeth and soft tissue, the airway should be inserted right-side-up rather than upside-down and rotated. A tongue blade should be used to assist in placement.

13. **d.** When suctioning an infant or young child, continually monitor the child's heart rate. Suctioning can stimulate nerves in the throat and cause the child's heart rate to slow.

14. **d.** Oxygen should be carefully administered to newborns with breathing problems. Local protocols should be followed regarding the exact means for administering oxygen to both newborns and infants. In most cases, oxygen can be carefully administered via a nonrebreather mask or through use of a blow-by method where appropriate. Avoid directing the oxygen at the infant's face, as this can irritate the trigeminal nerve and cause the baby to stop breathing. This situation can be minimized by using warm oxygen and directing the flow to one side of the baby's nose.

15. **b.** If a seriously ill or injured infant or child will not tolerate an oxygen mask, use a blow-by technique. This can be accomplished using a variety of methods. Oxygen tubing can be held about 2 inches from the patient's face, or it may be inserted into a paper cup held near the child's face. As an alternative, an oxygen mask may be held near the child's face. The objective is to increase the concentration of oxygen in the surrounding air. A good indication of the child's need for oxygen is whether he or she will accept it. Seriously ill or injured infants or children do not usually fight the oxygen mask.

16. **a.** The best way determine the breathing rate of a newborn or infant is to watch the chest rise from a distance. Touching the child can cause agitation that will affect the breathing rate.

17. **b.** Infants and children have relatively small respiratory reserves and may deteriorate quickly. Signs of respiratory distress include nasal flaring, use of accessory muscles, and "see-saw" breathing, that is, the abdomen and chest move in opposite directions with each respiration.

18. **a.** The best place to check for cyanosis in an infant or child is the oral mucosa, lips, or tongue. Use caution if checking the nail beds of an infant; they may not be an accurate indicator of central circulation status even when they appear cyanotic.

19. **b.** The pulse rate of infants and children is normally faster than that of adults because of their faster metabolic rate.

20. **c.** Blood pressure should be assessed only on children older than 3 years.

21. **a.** Stridor is heard on inspiration and is a sign of upper airway obstruction.

22. **b.** If the EMT notes wheezing on expiration, lower airway disease should be suspected.

23. **b.** An infant or child is considered to be in respiratory arrest when the breathing rate drops below 10 breaths per minute. The patient may also exhibit limp muscle tone, unconsciousness, slow or absent heart rate, and weak or absent distal pulses. Artificial ventilations should be started immediately.

24. **c.** Any time a breathing emergency is present, administer oxygen.

25. **d.** The occurrence of a febrile seizure is linked to a rapid rise in temperature and not the final degree of the fever. They usually occur in children 6 months to 5 years old and are generalized seizures. Approximately 5% of children with fevers experience febrile seizures, but most never have a repeat episode. The child should be evaluated at a hospital.

26. **a.** If a child with a history of seizures has just experienced a seizure, determine whether the seizure is similar to others the child has experienced or if anything is different. Also ask if the child is taking antiseizure medication.

27. **d.** When a child ingests poison, contact medical direction concerning whether to administer activated charcoal. The patient should be assessed at a hospital, since the effects of some poisons may not be seen for some time after the ingestion.

28. **b.** Fever accompanied by a rash may signify a serious situation.

29. **a.** Vomiting and diarrhea can cause rapid dehydration in infants and children. These signs do not always indicate serious illness (gastrointestinal upset may even accompany an ear infection). Administration of intravenous fluids is not always necessary.

30. **a.** Since children have less circulating blood volume, a loss of what seems to be even a small amount of blood may lead to shock.

31. **b.** Decreased urine output is a sign of hypoperfusion in infants. To determine if this sign is present, ask parents about diaper wetting. The patient will be pale, and tears will be absent even when the child is crying.

32. **d.** Secondary drowning syndrome refers to deterioration that occurs following a near-drowning event and after the patient resumes normal breathing. This syndrome may occur minutes to hours later.

33. **b.** The cause of sudden infant death syndrome (SIDS) is largely unknown.

34. **c.** Parents of SIDS babies should be viewed as patients also. Do not question them about what they may have done to contribute to the death; there are usually no external factors involved. They will already feel guilty, and questioning will add to the guilt. CPR may be initiated and the child transported if appropriate. The situation may be very stressful to the EMT as well, and it should be discussed if the crew wishes.

35. **d.** Blunt injury is the leading causes of traumatic death in children.

36. **c.** Blood loss exceeding 500 cc in a child is considered serious.

37. **a.** When a child who was restrained with only a lap belt is involved in a motor vehicle crash, suspect abdominal and lower spine injuries. With children, lap belts are often improperly positioned with the lap belt above the pelvis. In a crash, compression injuries to the soft abdominal organs can occur. If the child is not wearing a diagonal shoulder strap, the uncontrolled forward movement of the upper body can cause spinal injuries.

38. **a.** Because children have proportionally larger heads than adults, it is often necessary to pad under the shoulders and/or upper torso to keep the spine in a neutral, in-line position. Padding under the head or occiput (the posterior part of the skull) is inappropriate because it will tilt the head even further forward.

39. **c.** Use the PASG on children only if the child fits properly in the garment. Do not place the child in one leg of the garment. The device may be used in cases of trauma with signs of severe hypotension and pelvic instability. Follow local protocols on indications for use.

40. **d.** When using the PASG on children, inflate the legs only; do not inflate the abdominal compartment because children use their abdominal muscles for breathing. The younger the child, the more he or she uses these muscles to breathe. Inflation of the abdominal compartment can greatly interfere with the child's breathing. Consult local protocols for precise guidelines on inflating the PASG for children.

41. **b.** Physical abuse is improper or excessive action that injures or causes harm to a child. Giving insufficient attention to a child is considered neglect. Physical abuse and neglect are the two forms of child abuse the EMT-Basic is likely to suspect.

42. **b.** Suspect child abuse if the injury is inconsistent with its described mechanism or if parents cannot account for all of the child's injuries. If the child displays different injuries, such as burns or bruises in various stages of healing, this should also alert the EMT to the possibility of child abuse. Repeated calls to the same residence or for the same child to provide care for various injuries may also be a clue. An isolated injury or burn does not necessarily signal abuse.

43. **a.** If child abuse is suspected, report it privately to the emergency department staff. It should also be reported to the appropriate authorities as specified by state and local laws. Do not discuss it with the parents. Parental consent normally must still be obtained before the child can be transported.

44. **c.** When a child on a home ventilator is encountered, have the parents assist in managing the patient since they should be familiar with the operation of the ventilator. Do not remove the patient from the ventilator since it is breathing for the patient. If the ventilator malfunctions, manually ventilate the patient.

45. **d.** If bleeding is noted in the area where a central IV line enters the skin, control the bleeding by applying pressure. Do not apply ice to the area or clamp off the IV tubing.

46. **d.** A gastrostomy tube is placed directly into the stomach for feeding.

47. **b.** Two positions in which an infant or child with a gastrostomy tube may be transported are sitting, or lying on the right side with the head elevated.

48. **a.** A shunt runs from the brain to the abdomen to drain excess cerebrospinal fluid.

49. **c.** Infants and children with shunts are particularly prone to respiratory arrest.

✳ ENRICHMENT QUESTIONS

50. **b.** Newborns primarily breathe through the nose. In many cases, suctioning the secretions from an infant's nasopharynx can improve breathing problems.

51. **d.** The single most important factor in accurately obtaining a child's blood pressure is the size of the cuff.

52. **d.** Delayed capillary refill time is the most accurate indicator of shock in infants and children. Adequate blood pressure in children can often be maintained until the end, and tends to drop only immediately before death.

53. **a.** Croup and epiglottitis are two common upper respiratory tract infections the EMT may encounter when managing a child with respiratory difficulty. Bronchiolitis is a lower respiratory tract disease frequently caused by respiratory syncytial virus (RSV) infection. Although generally benign and self-limiting, severe bronchiolitis can be life-threatening. Respiratory syncytial virus is the leading cause of lower respiratory tract disease in infants and young children. Symptoms of RSV infection range from those of a bad cold to severe bronchiolitis or pneumonia.

54. **c.** Epiglottitis should be suspected in children who complain of a very sore throat and pain when swallowing that begins suddenly and may be accompanied by a fever and drooling. Epiglottitis is a bacterial illness and is a true emergency since the patient is in danger of developing a complete airway obstruction due to swelling of the epiglottis and supraglottic structures. The EMT should allow the child to remain in whatever position makes it easiest to breathe. No attempt should be made to visualize the airway if the child is still ventilating adequately. The receiving hospital should be notified prior to EMS arrival so they may prepare for what may be a very difficult patient management scenario.

55. **b.** Croup is a viral illness that results in inflammation of the larynx, trachea, and bronchi. The child will normally display mild symptoms including fever and respiratory difficulty during the day, but at night the child's condition will worsen. A loud "seal bark" cough is characteristic of the illness.

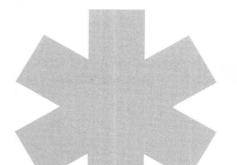

15

Miscellaneous

D.O.T. Curriculum Objectives
Covered in This Chapter:

Lesson 1-1
Lesson 1-2
Lesson 1-3
Lesson 1-6
Lesson 3-7
Lesson 3-8
Lesson 7-1
Lesson 7-2

CHAPTER 15 REVIEW QUESTIONS

■ LEGAL ASPECTS

1. A contractual or legal obligation that may exist that requires an EMT to provide emergency medical care is:
   a. Good Samaritan act
   b. medico-ethical act
   c. statute to act
   d. duty to act

2. Deviating from the accepted standard of care that a reasonable, prudent EMT would render is:
   a. abandonment
   b. breach of contract
   c. negligence
   d. breach of duty

3. Assistance may be rendered to an unconscious patient or to an ill child whose parents or guardians cannot be reached under the law of:
   a. actual consent
   b. informed consent
   c. implied consent
   d. minor's consent

4. Terminating care of a patient without ensuring continuation of care at the same or higher level, or without the patient's consent to stop rendering care is:
   a. breach of contract
   b. assault and battery
   c. breach of consen
   d. abandonment

5. The four elements necessary to prove negligence are:
   a. duty to act, breach of duty, injury, and proximate cause
   b. actual consent, breach of duty, damage, and breach of confidentiality
   c. duty to act, breach of contract, injury, and abandonment
   d. lack of informed consent, duty to act, breach of contract, and damage

6. An EMS report or record:
   a. should be thorough and accurate
   b. cannot be changed after the patient is transferred to the hospital
   c. is of little value if an EMT is sued
   d. cannot be used in court

7. Guidelines for the EMT that are established by local and state laws or protocols, professional organizations or societies, and acceptable case law precedents make up the:
   a. patient's right to emergency care
   b. standard of care
   c. local tort laws
   d. civil EMS code

8. Generally, if there are no written Do Not Resuscitate (DNR) orders present:
   a. attempt to contact the family doctor before starting CPR
   b. begin resuscitation efforts
   c. consult law enforcement officers on the legality of starting CPR
   d. accept the family's word that DNR orders exist

9. To refuse medical care, the patient must:
   a. refuse any and all care the EMT may provide
   b. be 15 years of age or older
   c. not have received any medical care prior to the point of refusing
   d. be mentally competent

10. An EMT may be required to report a suspected situation involving:
    a. child abuse
    b. commission of a crime
    c. abuse of the elderly
    d. all of the above

■ AMBULANCE OPERATIONS

11. Most accidents involving emergency vehicles occur:
    a. due to skids
    b. during U-turns
    c. while en route to the hospital
    d. at intersections

12. The recommended number of feet an ambulance should be parked from wreckage is:
    a. 50
    b. 100
    c. 150
    d. 200

13. Generally, ambulances should be escorted by police or other emergency vehicles:
    a. only if the crew is unfamiliar with the location of the patient or receiving facility
    b. whenever possible
    c. whenever responding to a potentially violent situation
    d. only when a operator with minimal experience is driving

14. A helicopter landing zone should ideally:
    a. be a maximum of 90 feet by 90 feet square
    b. be fenced off to keep onlookers away
    c. be at least 100 feet by 100 feet square
    d. have no more than a 15-degree slope

15. A medical helicopter should initially be approached:
    a. from the rear
    b. immediately after it lands
    c. from the front
    d. in a standing position

✳ ENRICHMENT QUESTIONS

16. The most important safety equipment in an ambulance:
    a. are goggles and hard hats
    b. are safety belts
    c. is a fire extinguisher
    d. are traffic flares

17. The "2-second rule" refers to:
    a. the amount of time the ambulance should remain stopped at a traffic light before proceeding
    b. the length of time a driver should look in the sideview mirror
    c. the maximum amount of time it should take an EMT to make a driving decision
    d. the safe distance that should be maintained between the ambulance and a vehicle it is following

18. Before crossing an intersection, the emergency vehicle driver should:
    a. look to the left, then to the right, and then again to the left
    b. turn off the siren and listen for other emergency vehicles
    c. look to the right, and then to the left
    d. turn on the vehicle's 4-way flashers

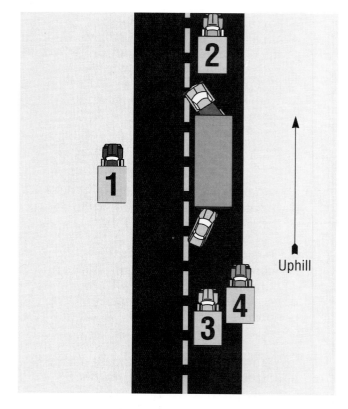

Figure 15-2

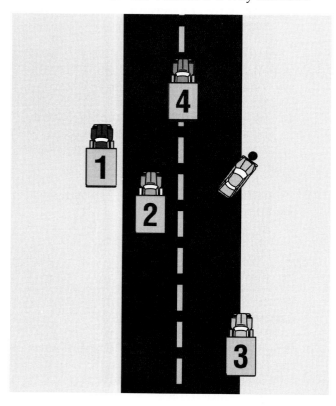

Figure 15-1

19. Your unit responds to the scene of a motor vehicle crash where a car has struck a tree. The road is a level 2-lane street with 2-way traffic. No police units are available to provide traffic control. Referring to Figure 15-1, the best place to position your emergency vehicle would be location:
    a. 1
    b. 2
    c. 3
    d. 4

20. While traveling uphill, a fast-moving car runs underneath the back end of a slower-moving tanker truck carrying diesel fuel. There is no fuel leakage present, although the integrity of the tank is questionable. Referring to Figure 15-2, the best place to position your emergency vehicle would be location:
    a. 1
    b. 2
    c. 3
    d. 4

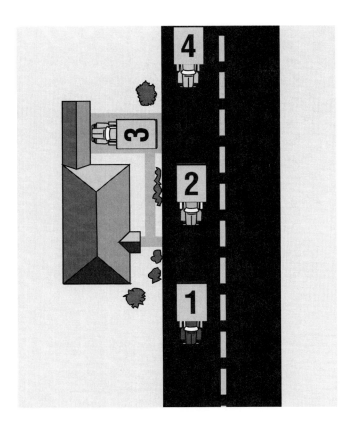

Figure 15-3

21. You are dispatched to the scene of a domestic squabble that resulted in a shooting. As you near the house in a quiet, suburban neighborhood, the communications center advises that police units are en route but will not arrive before your unit. Referring to Figure 15-3, the safest place to park your vehicle would be location:
    a. 1
    b. 2
    c. 3
    d. 4

■ PATIENT LIFTING AND MOVING

22. Lifting should be done using the:
    a. legs
    b. arms
    c. back
    d. waist

23. When lifting, keep the weight:
    a. as far from the body as possible
    b. a comfortable distance from the body
    c. as close to the body as possible
    d. to the side of the body

24. Prior to lifting, the feet should be:
    a. together
    b. shoulder-width apart
    c. one in front of the other
    d. as far apart as possible

25. When lifting a stretcher or backboard, keep the back:
    a. locked into normal curvature
    b. bent forward
    c. bent backward
    d. twisted to one side

26. When grasping a stretcher, place the hands:
    a. next to each other
    b. at least 6 inches apart
    c. at least 10 inches apart
    d. at least 18 inches apart

27. If possible, lifting partners should:
    a. be approximately the same age
    b. have different amounts of physical strength
    c. be approximately the same height
    d. be of the same sex

28. Unless there is a medical contraindication, the best way to move a patient up or down stairs is with:
    a. a backboard
    b. a scoop stretcher
    c. an ambulance cot
    d. a stair chair

29. When reaching:
    a. do not reach more than 15 to 20 inches
    b. do not reach for more than 30 seconds
    c. try to reach to the side
    d. all of the above

30. Whenever possible in situations involving pulling or pushing:
    a. keep the elbows locked
    b. it is preferable to push rather than pull
    c. keep the weight below waist level
    d. keep the line of pull to the side of the body

31. The primary danger of moving a patient too soon is:
    a. further injury or illness may occur if the patient is not properly packaged
    b. a thorough examination cannot be performed once a patient is on an ambulance cot
    c. the patient may need Advanced Life Support intervention from a paramedic unit prior to being moved
    d. there may not have been enough time to obtain consent to treat

32. An emergency move is used when:
    a. the patient's condition may deteriorate
    b. there are not enough EMTs to properly move the patient
    c. there is an immediate threat to the life of the patient
    d. maximum control of the spine is needed

33. If an emergency move must be made:
    a. roll the patient
    b. pull the patient in the direction of the long axis of the body
    c. pull the patient sideways in the direction of the shoulder
    d. lift the patient in any way possible and carry him or her away from danger

34. When performing an urgent move on a person injured in a vehicle crash:
    a. one EMT must continue to maintain cervical spine stabilization
    b. take extra time to properly immobilize the spine
    c. there is no time to perform spinal immobilization
    d. a backboard is not used

35. The two types of non-urgent moves that are commonly used to move a patient from the ground to the cot when no injuries to the spine or extremities are suspected are the:
    a. power lift and leg lift
    b. direct ground lift and extremity lift
    c. immediate lift and non-urgent lift
    d. stretcher lift and backboard lift

36. The two primary methods used to transfer a patient from a bed to a cot are the:
    a. push method and pull method
    b. slide method and roll method
    c. immediate method and urgent method
    d. direct carry method and draw-sheet method

37. When using a wheeled ambulance cot:
    a. three EMTs are needed
    b. the EMTs should stand at the sides
    c. the foot end should be pulled
    d. smooth terrain should be avoided

38. When moving a wheeled ambulance cot over rough terrain, use:
    a. two rescuers, with one rescuer placed at each end facing each other
    b. two rescuers, with one rescuer placed at each end facing the same direction
    c. four rescuers, with one rescuer at each end facing each other and one rescuer on each side facing each other
    d. four rescuers, with one rescuer placed at each corner of the cot

39. Using the following list of patient positions, fill in the position most likely to be used to transport a patient suffering from the various problems listed:
**legs elevated 8 to 12 inches
on left side
position of comfort
supine on backboard**

_____ conscious patient who is nauseated or vomiting

_____ hypotensive pregnant patient

_____ patient complaining of severe difficulty breathing

_____ semi-conscious seizure patient

_____ patient with chest pain

_____ patient with spinal injury

_____ patient with a medical or nontraumatic head injury

_____ patient displaying signs of shock without spinal injury

✳ **ENRICHMENT QUESTIONS**

40. When two patients on backboards are to be transported in the same ambulance, load the:
a. patient who is to be placed on the ambulance benchseat first
b. patient who will stay on the wheeled cot first
c. heaviest patient first
d. most critical patient first

41. A type of patient lifting device that can be separated lengthwise into halves and placed under a patient without log-rolling and with a minimum amount of movement is a:
a. basket stretcher
b. scoop stretcher
c. pole stretcher
d. SKED stretcher

■ **COMMUNICATION AND DOCUMENTATION**

42. The difference between protocols and standing orders is that:
a. protocols outline procedures an EMT may perform, and standing orders outline medications an EMT can administer or assist a patient in administering
b. protocols are overall steps in patient care treatment, and standing orders outline procedures an EMT may perform without contacting medical direction
c. protocols outline when to call medical direction, and standing orders outline how to perform procedures ordered by medical direction
d. protocols cover only medical procedures, whereas standing orders outline department policies

43. To correct an error made on an EMS report that is discovered when the report is being written:
a. obliterate the error and write the correct information next to it
b. add a note at the end of the report indicating what incorrect information was recorded earlier in the report
c. draw a single line through the error, initial it, and write the correct information next to it
d. after returning to the station, write an addendum that contains the correct information that should be in the report

44. When examining your patient, you notice a large laceration on his left thigh. Noting this on the patient report is an example of recording:
    a. objective information
    b. subjective information
    c. circumstantial information
    d. positive information

45. During your questioning of the patient, she tells you about some symptoms she is having. Her family tells you about some things they have observed as well. What you record on your report would be considered:
    a. objective information
    b. unreliable information
    c. unproved information
    d. subjective information

46. The absence of a sign or symptom that may be expected to be present when assessing a patient with a particular medical problem is known as:
    a. a pertinent positive
    b. a pertinent negative
    c. a nonspecific complaint
    d. extraneous information

47. You are called for a person with difficulty breathing. When listening to lung sounds, you note wheezing in both sides. Recording this finding on your report is an example of documenting:
    a. a pertinent negative
    b. a subjective observation
    c. a pertinent positive
    d. pertinent subjective information

48. When writing an EMS report, a proper observation to include would be that the patient:
    a. described the pain as sharp and stabbing
    b. is obviously intoxicated
    c. is having a heart attack
    d. suffered a stroke

49. To communicate with a patient with a hearing impairment, the EMT may try all of the following *except*:
    a. speaking clearly with his lips visible to the patient
    b. using basic sign language
    c. exchanging written notes
    d. speaking from the patient's side

50. Two important points to remember when communicating with elderly patients are that:
    a. their memory is usually clearer and their speech is more intelligible
    b. they may have difficulty hearing and poor vision
    c. they are often shy and emotionally overwhelmed
    d. they often have a fear of strangers and are intimidated by authority figures

51. Two important aspects to communicating with children are:
    a. tell the child he or she will feel better and treat children like little adults
    b. always be truthful and assume a position at eye level with the child
    c. try to avoid having parents present when questioning the child and be honest with the child
    d. do not explain what you are doing since the child will not understand and may become more afraid, and always assume a position higher than the child

52. When communicating with elderly patients:
    a. avoid eye contact, which could be considered disrespectful
    b. stand in front of the patient as a gesture of respect
    c. speak clearly, distinctly, and loud enough to be heard
    d. use exact medical terms to describe what is going on

53. When addressing a patient, it is best to:
    a. ask the patient how he or she would like to be addressed
    b. use terms such as "dear" or "hon" when addressing the elderly
    c. always call the patient by his or her first name
    d. always use the patient's last name

54. A radio that is located at a stationary site, such as in a hospital, is an example of a:
    a. repeater radio
    b. digital radio
    c. base station radio
    d. mobile radio

55. To speak with medical direction from an incident scene, an EMT uses a hand-held radio. This type of radio is an example of a:
    a. portable radio
    b. base station
    c. mobile radio
    d. high-power transmitter

56. Two major reasons it is good for the EMT to contact the receiving hospital are:
    a. to speed ambulance turnaround time and to allow medical records to be retrieved
    b. to receive instructions and allow admitting to start appropriate paperwork
    c. to receive advice and instructions and to allow the hospital to prepare to receive the patient
    d. to allow hospital personnel to prepare to receive the patient and to allow insurance information to be retrieved

57. After receiving an order from medical direction to administer a medication or perform a procedure, the first thing the EMT should do is:
    a. immediately carry out the order
    b. relay the order to the EMT who will carry out the order
    c. immediately document the order on the patient care report
    d. repeat the order back word for word

58. An important reason for relaying accurate information when giving a radio report to medical direction is:
    a. all communications are recorded and checked later for accuracy
    b. orders for medication and procedures will be based on the information the EMT presents
    c. patients may hear the report and wish to ask questions about what is being done
    d. a copy of the radio report will become part of the patient's hospital medical records

59. When speaking on the radio:
    a. show courtesy by using words such as "please," "thank you," and "you're welcome"
    b. use codes whenever possible to reduce transmission time
    c. speak clearly and slowly
    d. try to speak as fast as possible to reduce transmission time

■ GERIATRIC EMERGENCIES

60. The leading cause of death in elderly patients is:
    a. cardiovascular disease
    b. stroke
    c. cancer
    d. falls

61. The increased porosity of bone that occurs in elderly patients and that contributes to a high incidence of musculoskeletal injuries is known as:
    a. kyphosis
    b. osteoarthritis
    c. Alzheimer's disease
    d. osteoporosis

62. A contributing factor to the frequency of falls experienced by elderly patients is:
    a. a heightened sense of balance
    b. loss of muscle mass
    c. an increase in bone mass
    d. an increase in skin elasticity

63. Due to having diminished liver and kidney functions, geriatric patients tend to:
    a. have an enhanced ability to form blood clots
    b. need reduced doses of medication
    c. need higher doses of medication
    d. be less sensitive to the effects of alcohol

64. A major complication related to the decrease in the elasticity of the lungs of the geriatric patient is:
    a. the development of asthma
    b. an increased ability to clear foreign matter from the lungs
    c. the development of pneumonia
    d. the development of congestive heart failure

65. When assessing a geriatric patient with an acute illness, the EMT should:
    a. only consider information gathered from the family or bystanders as being reliable
    b. not involve the family when obtaining a history
    c. consider an altered mental status to be normal for the patient
    d. plan on taking more time than normal to gather information and gain a history

66. An important aspect of managing geriatric patients as opposed to younger patients is that elderly patients tend to experience a:
    a. higher incidence of motor vehicle crashes
    b. lower incidence of abuse and neglect
    c. higher incidence of mental health problems
    d. lower incidence of falls

■ GAINING ACCESS

67. When arriving at the scene of a vehicle crash, the first thing an EMT should do is:
    a. make sure the scene is safe
    b. assess the patient's airway
    c. gain access to the patient
    d. stabilize the vehicle

68. As a general rule, when dealing with downed wires at a crash scene:
    a. there is no danger if they are telephone wires
    b. manipulation is possible using heavy, insulated gloves
    c. there is no danger if they are cable television wires
    d. always consider wires energized

69. If a downed power line is in contact with a car at the scene of a crash, the best course of action is to:
    a. wait for the electric company
    b. remove the wire with a hotstick
    c. tell the occupants to jump clear of the car
    d. remove the wire with lineman's gloves

70. The best way to gain quick access to a patient who is still in a vehicle following a crash is to:
    a. pry the door closest to the patient with a crowbar or hydraulic tool
    b. break a side window farthest from the patient and crawl in
    c. have the patient reach over and unlock an undamaged door
    d. check all doors to see if one will open

71. During the extrication process, patient care is generally:
    a. discontinued until the patient is out of the vehicle
    b. limited to assessment and vital signs
    c. continued to the greatest extent possible
    d. performed by firefighters

72. As rescuers work to extricate a patient, the patient should be:
    a. protected by a heavy, fireproof covering, and a rescuer should remain in the vehicle
    b. protected by a heavy, fireproof covering and be left alone in the vehicle
    c. covered with a clear plastic sheet
    d. covered with wet blankets to reduce fire hazard

■ MULTIPLE-CASUALTY SITUATIONS

73. The responsibility of the first arriving EMS unit at a mass casualty incident is to:
    a. immediately transport the most critical patients to the nearest hospital
    b. assume command, assess the situation, and not perform any patient care
    c. start extricating patients
    d. start caring for the most critically injured victims

74. A yellow triage tag signifies:
    a. a second-priority patient
    b. a patient who has minor injuries
    c. an obviously dead patient
    d. lowest priority patient

75. The position of triage officer should be assigned to:
    a. the highest ranking EMS officer
    b. the EMT with the most seniority
    c. the most qualified EMT
    d. a nurse, if available

76. A green triage tag signifies a patient:
    a. with moderate-priority injuries
    b. with low-priority injuries
    c. who is suffering psychological problems due to the inciden
    d. who is ready to be transported

77. Match the following sectors/groups/units with their primary responsibilities.
    extrication
    transportation
    treatment
    triage
    staging
    supply

    _____ sorts patients based on medical priority

    _____ obtains and distributes resources such as medical equipment and personnel

    _____ ascertains capabilities of receiving hospitals and coordinates loading of ambulances

    _____ rescues patients who are trapped at the scene

    _____ organizes incoming ambulances and coordinates the movement of ambulances to the loading zone

    _____ coordinates medical care for injured patients after they have been sorted and moved

78. Using the following descriptions to prioritize patients at a mass casualty scene, categorize them as: **first, second, third,** or **fourth.** (If you normally use the color system, mark the patients as: red, yellow, green, or black.)

_____ severe head injury, no pulse or breathing

_____ severe burns

_____ multiple bone or joint injuries

_____ minor soft-tissue injuries

_____ unconscious, unknown cause

_____ back injury without spinal damage

_____ a severe medical problem

_____ shock

_____ swollen extremity accompanied by minor pain

_____ multiple traumatic injuries accompanied by full cardiac arrest

_____ burns without airway problems

_____ active labor with a breech presentation

79. A red triage tag signifies a patient who is:
    a. a highest priority patient
    b. bleeding
    c. a delayed transport patient
    d. burned

■ WELL-BEING OF THE EMT

80. The three ways communicable diseases are normally transmitted include all of the following *except*:
    a. direct contact
    b. casual contact
    c. inhalation
    d. indirect contact

81. Patients with communicable diseases:
    a. can be easily identified by experienced EMTs
    b. generally look ill
    c. do not have a certain appearance
    d. pose no threat to an EMT wearing personal protective equipment

82. As an advanced safety precaution, it is generally recommended that an EMT receive an immunization to guard against:
    a. HIV
    b. tuberculosis
    c. AIDS
    d. hepatitis B

83. Gloves worn to protect the EMT against exposure to body fluids are:
    a. nitrile or latex
    b. rubber and butyl
    c. butyl and vinyl
    d. latex and rubber

84. As a general rule concerning the use of gloves:
    a. there are some situations in which gloves may not be needed
    b. gloves must be worn whenever a patient is touched
    c. gloves are needed only if blood is present
    d. the decision to wear gloves can be made based on the type of dispatch

85. Handwashing should be performed:
    a. only if the EMT was not wearing gloves
    b. for at least 10 to 15 seconds
    c. at least twice during a shift
    d. using only a bactericidal cleaner

86. EMTs should wear protective eyewear:
    a. whenever a patient with an infectious disease is encountered
    b. only if they are susceptible to eye infections
    c. if they have recently been ill
    d. in situations where blood splatter may occur

87. When a patient suspected of having tuberculosis is encountered, wear:
    a. self-contained breathing apparatus (SCBA)
    b. a disposable surgical mask
    c. appropriate respiratory protection
    d. a full face shield

88. Gowns should be worn when the EMT:
    a. is working with any patient with a communicable disease
    b. expects to have direct contact with a patient
    c. expects to encounter large amounts of blood or body fluids
    d. does not have a commercially manufactured EMS uniform

89. HIV can be transmitted in all of the following ways *except*:
    a. sharing of intravenous drug needles and syringes
    b. sexual contact
    c. casual contact
    d. from an infected mother to her baby

90. A federal agency that develops and enforces many regulations regarding infection control guidelines that apply to EMTs is the:
    a. Department of Transportation (DOT)
    b. National Highway Traffic Safety Administration (NHTSA)
    c. National Fire Protection Association (NFPA)
    d. Occupational Safety and Health Administration (OSHA)

91. After transporting a patient with an infectious disease, clean the ambulance by:
    a. washing with a germicidal and viricidal agent
    b. airing it out
    c. wiping all surfaces with alcohol
    d. using a commercially available aerosol spray

92. If it is known in advance that a patient with an infectious disease is to be transported:
    a. remove unnecessary equipment from the ambulance prior to responding to the call
    b. request police backup
    c. attempt to convince the patient to be transported by a friend or family member
    d. remove all linens from the ambulance cot and cover it with plastic sheets

93. One of the best ways to protect against infectious diseases is to:
    a. wear a mask and gown on all runs
    b. wash the hands after every run
    c. screen patients and not transport those with infectious diseases
    d. ride in the cab when an infectious disease patient is transported

94. High-efficiency particulate air (HEPA) respirators would be most commonly worn by EMTs when managing a patient with active:
    a. meningitis
    b. pneumonia
    c. tuberculosis
    d. hepatitis

95. A piece of equipment used by EMTs that it is appropriate to clean and reuse is:
    a. a stethoscope
    b. a rigid suction catheter
    c. an oropharyngeal airway
    d. a nonrebreather oxygen mask

96. Sexually transmitted diseases that may present a risk of exposure to the EMT include all of the following *except*:
    a. syphilis
    b. genital herpes
    c. gonorrhea
    d. rubella

97. If called to a scene where the death of a patient is imminent:
    a. immediately transport the patient to a hospital
    b. have the family leave the room
    c. allow the family to be with the patient
    d. transfer care of the patient to law enforcement officials

98. To help the body deal with stress, increase intake of:
    a. carbohydrates
    b. caffeine
    c. sugar
    d. fatty foods

99. The purpose of Critical Incident Stress Management (CISM) is to:
    a. allow EMTs to talk to a psychiatrist
    b. identify EMTs who require remedial training
    c. identify things that were done wrong during an emergency
    d. help EMTs work through their emotional and physical responses to an emergency incident

100. Ideally, a formal Critical Incident Stress Debriefing should be conducted:
    a. no later than 24 hours after the incident
    b. within 24 to 72 hours after the incident
    c. 1 week from the incident
    d. within a month of the incident

101. Professional attributes that the EMT should strive to possess include all of the following *except*:
    a. maintaining a neat appearance
    b. having a positive attitude
    c. a willingness to take care of the patient regardless of the risk of personal harm
    d. maintaining up-to-date knowledge and skills

■ HAZARDOUS MATERIALS

102. The primary responsibility of an EMT at an incident involving hazardous materials is:
    a. identifying the hazardous material
    b. controlling any spills or leaks
    c. the safety of self, the public, and any patients
    d. removing patients in the immediate vicinity of the hazardous material

103. Hazardous material transported by motor vehicles may be identified by:
    a. calling Chemical Transportation Emergency Center (CHEMTREC)
    b. obtaining a sample and sending it to a laboratory
    c. referencing the number on the placard
    d. smelling or feeling the substance

104. Information about a hazardous material used at an industrial or commercial site is best obtained:
    a. from the NFPA 704 symbol on the building
    b. from a material safety data sheet
    c. by interviewing plant employees
    d. by reading the label on the container from which the substance came

105. Generally, an EMT should enter an area where hazardous materials are found:
    a. any time a patient's life is in danger
    b. if the EMT has completed a hazmat "Awareness" course
    c. whenever firefighting turnout gear is available
    d. only if the EMT has proper training in wearing hazmat equipment and SCBA

106. EMS vehicles and personnel at a scene involving hazardous materials should be positioned:
    a. close enough to quickly reach anyone who is sick or injured as a result of the incident
    b. upwind from the incident, and at safe distance
    c. downwind from the incident
    d. downhill from the incident

■ MEDICAL TERMINOLOGY MATCHING

107. Match the following definitions to their corresponding medical terms. Terms followed by (2) correspond to two different medical terms.

abdomen	eye
above/over	fast
after/behind	fever
against	front
against/opposite	gland
air/breath	head
an abnormal	heart
condition	joint
around	kidney (2)
around/	large
surrounding	larynx
artery	liver
back	located behind
before	lung
belly	much/many
below normal	muscle
between	neck
beyond normal/	nerve
excessive	one half
bile	paralysis
blood	rib
blood vessel	skin
bone	skull
both	slow
both sides	small intestine
brain	speech
breath/	stomach
breathing	surgical removal
cancer	surgical repair
cartilage	tongue
cell	tooth (2)
chest	throat
clot	trachea
colon	upper arm
condition	uterus
destruction	vein (2)
diaphragm	with
difficult/	within (2)
bad/abnormal	without
disease	woman
disease of a part	

Medical terms ending in "o" are combining forms. Terms preceded by a hyphen are suffixes, and terms followed by a hyphen are prefixes.

Medical Term	Definition
a, an	_____
abdomin o	_____
aden o	_____
ambi-	_____
angi o	_____
ant-, anti-	_____
antero-	_____
arteri o	_____
arthr o	_____
bi-	_____
brachi o	_____
brady-	_____
carcin o	_____
cardi o	_____
cephal o	_____
cervic o	_____
chol e	_____
chondr o	_____
circum-	_____
col o	_____
con-	_____
contra-	_____
cost o	_____
crani o	_____

cyt o   _____

dent o   _____

derm o/dermat o   _____

dors o   _____

dys-   _____

-ectomy   _____

encephal o   _____

end-, endo-   _____

enter o   _____

febr o   _____

gastr o   _____

gloss o   _____

gynec o   _____

hem o/hemat o   _____

hepat o   _____

hyper-   _____

hypo-   _____

hyster o   _____

-iasis   _____

inter-   _____

intra-   _____

laryng o   _____

-lysis   _____

mega-, megal o   _____

my o   _____

nephr o   _____

neur o   _____

ocul o/ophthalm o   _____

odont o   _____

-osis _____

oste o _____

path o _____

pathy _____

peri- _____

pharyng o _____

phas o _____

phleb o _____

phren o _____

-plasty _____

-plegia _____

-pnea _____

pneum o/pneumat o _____

poly- _____

post- _____

pre- _____

pulmon o _____

ren o _____

retro- _____

semi- _____

supra- _____

tachy _____

thorac o _____

thromb o _____

trache o _____

ven o _____

ventr o _____

■ Additional Points for Discussion ■

1. What office in your state certifies and governs EMTs?

   - What is the address and phone number?

2. Does your state recognize Do Not Resuscitate (DNR)/Do Not Attempt Resuscitation (DNAR) orders?

   - Is there a standard state form?

   - Does it have to be signed by the patient's doctor?

   - What are your local and departmental procedures for dealing with a DNR/DNAR order?

3. Review your department's guidelines for performing a mechanical check on your ambulances and for performing an inventory check of supplies.

4. What criteria does your department follow for deciding when to call for helicopter transport?

5. What are the guidelines of the local helicopter service for setting up a landing zone?

6. What are your state laws regarding the following?

   - Motorists yielding the right-of-way to emergency vehicles

   - Driving emergency vehicles

   - The use of red lights and sirens

   - Operating an ambulance through a school zone

   - Passing a school bus while on an emergency run

7. Answer the following questions regarding an ambulance involved in an accident.

   - Which police unit(s) would be responsible for investigating and filing a report?

   - Is there a specific form (departmental, county, or state) that must be completed?

8. What are some common situations (such as where there is a potential for violence directed at EMTs or potential situations involving hazardous materials) that may be encountered in your area that could be potentially dangerous for EMS personnel?

   - What might you be able to do to protect yourself or lessen the chances of becoming involved in such a situation?

9. What is the role of your EMS at the scene of a vehicle crash with entrapment?

10. What is the role of your EMS at an incident involving hazardous materials?

11. Is there a hazardous materials team available in your area? When would you summon this team and how?

12. What hazardous materials reference books are carried on your ambulances?

   • Where are they kept?

13. Review your department's guidelines for the following.

   • Dealing with patients with infectious diseases

   • Reporting exposure to an infectious disease

14. In your state or county, what types of incidents (such as child or elder abuse) must be reported to other agencies such as the police?

ANSWERS TO CHAPTER 15 REVIEW QUESTIONS

■ LEGAL ASPECTS

1. **d.** Duty to act refers to the responsibility of an EMT, either by statute or function, to provide patient care when the opportunity presents itself.

2. **c.** A deviation from the accepted standard of care that a reasonable, prudent EMT would render is considered negligence.

3. **c.** Implied consent allows the EMT to assist an unconscious patient or a minor child if a true emergency situation exists. The basis of implied consent is that a rational and reasonable person who is similarly ill or injured but able to communicate would want medical care.

4. **d.** Abandonment is terminating care of a patient without ensuring continuation of care at the same level or higher, or without the patient's consent to stop rendering care.

5. **a.** The four elements necessary to prove negligence are a duty to act, breach of duty, an injury, and proximate cause.

6. **a.** Because they are important safeguards in protecting EMTs, EMS reports and records must be thorough and accurate. No one has a memory good enough to remember everything about a call, and lawsuits may occur years later. The EMS report is a legal document that is admissible in court. The document, if sloppy and incomplete, can be detrimental as it implies that the EMT's abilities are also sloppy and incomplete. Testimony from memory may not be enough — the court will generally view a procedure or action not documented as not having been performed.

7. **b.** The standard of care is established by local and state laws or protocols, professional organizations and societies, and acceptable case law precedents.

8. **b.** Although EMTs should honor written DNR orders, it is generally recommended that resuscitation efforts be started if the DNR orders are not physically present.

9. **d.** To refuse medical care, the patient must be mentally competent. A patient is allowed to refuse a particular form of therapy or one aspect of care. The patient can refuse further care after the EMT has started treatment procedures. Although there are some exceptions, patients generally must be at least 18 years of age to refuse treatment.

10. **d.** In most areas, EMTs are required to report a situation that they suspect involves abuse of a child or an elderly person, or the commission of a crime.

■ AMBULANCE OPERATIONS

11. **d.** Approximately 50% of crashes involving emergency vehicles occur at intersections; 25% of emergency vehicle crashes occur while backing.

12. **b.** It is generally recommended that an ambulance be parked at least 100 feet from wreckage.

13. **a.** If the crew is unfamiliar with how to get to the location of the patient or how to get to the receiving facility, it is generally acceptable for the police or other emergency vehicles to escort an ambulance. Even in these cases, however, escorts should be avoided if possible because of the dangers involved in escort situations. In these cases, it is best if an experienced driver is operating the ambulance.

14. **c.** Ideally, a helicopter landing zone should be at least 100 feet by 100 feet square. For larger helicopters, 125 feet by 125 feet is desirable (consult local air medical services for recommended size). The ground should have no more than a 10° slope and should be clear of fences or other obstructions.

15. **c.** Most medical helicopters should initially be approached only from the front, and individuals should approach only after being directed to do so by the pilot or flight crew. Stay low when approaching the helicopter, as rotor blades can dip low to the ground and cause injury.

✱ ENRICHMENT QUESTIONS

16. **b.** Safety belts are the most important safety equipment in an ambulance and should be used by all personnel.

17. **d.** The "2-second rule" refers to the distance that should be maintained between an emergency vehicle and the vehicle in front of it. Using a fixed object as a reference point, it should take the emergency vehicle at least 2 seconds to reach the object after the vehicle ahead has passed the object. This following distance should be increased if driving conditions are hazardous or if the emergency vehicle is a large fire or rescue truck.

18. **a.** Before crossing an intersection, the emergency vehicle driver should look to the left, then the right, and then again to the left.

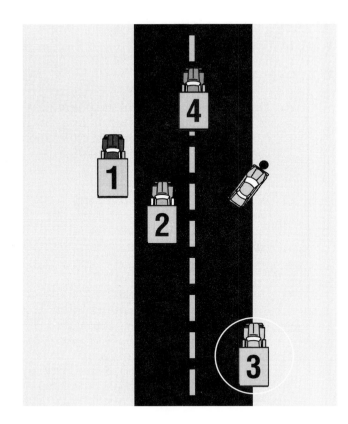

Figure 15-1

19. **c.** Because police units will not be available to provide traffic control, location 3 would be the best place to position the ambulance. This provides protection for the patient in the car as well as the EMTs while providing only minimal traffic obstruction. The ambulance should not be placed where it is a hazard to oncoming traffic (as in locations 2 and 4), nor should it be placed where the safety of personnel could be jeopardized by having to cross the road (location 1). If police units are available to block traffic, the ambulance can be pulled beyond the accident and to the right side of the road

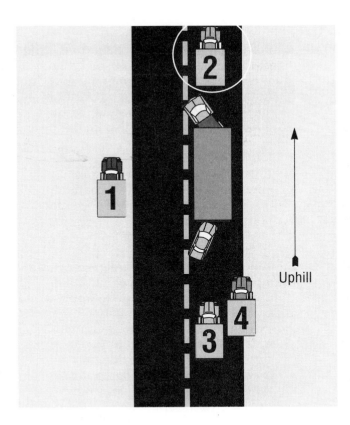

Figure 15-2

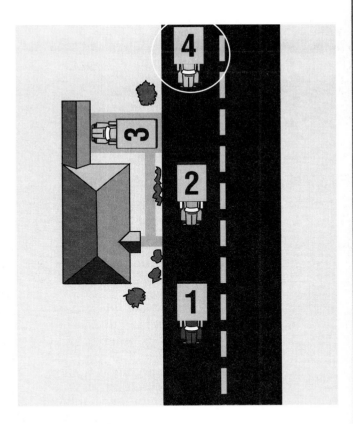

Figure 15-3

20. **b.** Due to the nature of the accident, location 2 would be the best location to position the ambulance. It is uphill and does not block traffic. Although a leak is not present, locations 3 and 4 are potentially dangerous if a leak develops because they are downhill. Additionally, if either accident vehicle is not stabilized, a danger of rolling is present. Location 1, although uphill, would place personnel in danger while trying to cross traffic.

21. **d.** Domestic violence situations can be hazardous to EMTs, and positioning the unit is important. Location 4 allows the EMTs to view the house for possible hazards while being in a position to back out of the scene quickly if the perpetrator appears with a weapon. Once the police arrive, the crew can quickly access the patient when the scene is made secure. Location 1 would require the unit to drive past the front of the house, thereby placing the crew in the line of fire. Locations 2 and 3 obviously place the crew in great danger, as there is a direct line of fire available to the gunman. Location 3 also necessitates backing up to escape the scene.

■ PATIENT LIFTING AND MOVING

22. **a.** Lifting should be done using the legs, not the back.

23. **c.** Keep the weight as close to the body as possible when lifting.

24. **b.** Keep the feet shoulder-width apart to provide firm footing when lifting.

25. **a.** Keep the back locked into normal curvature when lifting a stretcher or backboard.

26. **c.** Place the hands at least 10 inches apart when grasping a stretcher.

27. **c.** Ideally, lifting partners to be approximately the same height and strength. It is not necessary for them to be of the same sex or of similar ages.

28. **d.** Unless there is a medical contraindication, a stair chair is ideal for moving a patient up or down stairs.

29. **a.** When reaching, do not reach distances more than 15 to 20 inches. Avoid twisting when reaching and do not reach for periods longer than a minute.

30. **b.** Whenever possible, the EMT should push rather than pull.

31. **a.** The danger of moving a patient too soon is that further aggravation of injury or illness may occur if the patient is not properly stabilized. A full examination can be performed after a patient has been moved to the cot. Do not delay transport to wait for relatives or friends.

32. **c.** An emergency move is used when there is an immediate threat to the life of the patient. It is also used when lifesaving care cannot be rendered due to the patient's location or position, such as when a patient with cardiac arrest is found sitting in a chair.

33. **b.** If it is necessary to perform an emergency move, pull the patient in the direction of the long axis of the body, if possible.

34. **a.** When performing an urgent move on a person injured in a vehicle crash, there is not enough time to apply a short backboard or vest-style extrication device. However, one EMT must continue to manually maintain cervical spine stabilization and a cervical collar should be applied. When moving the patient to the backboard, the spine should be controlled as best as possible.

35. **b.** If there is no suspected injury to the spine or extremities, the direct ground lift and extremity lift are two types of non-urgent moves that can be used to move a patient from the ground to a cot.

36. **d.** The direct carry and draw-sheet method are two methods used to transfer a patient from a bed to a cot.

37. **c.** When using a wheeled cot, the foot end should be pulled. Two EMTs can use a wheeled cot and should be positioned at each end. This device works best over smooth terrain.

38. **d.** When a wheeled cot must be moved over rough terrain, use four rescuers with one placed at each corner of the cot.

39. Using the following list of patient positions, mark the position most likely to be used to transport a patient suffering from the various problems listed:
legs elevated 8 to 12 inches
on left side
position of comfort
supine on backboard

position of comfort	conscious patient who is nauseated or vomiting
on left side	hypotensive pregnant patient
position of comfort	patient complaining of severe difficulty breathing
on left side	semiconscious seizure patient
position of comfort	patient with chest pain
supine on backboard	spinal injury patient
on left side	patient with a medical or nontraumatic head injury
legs elevated 8 to 12 inches	patient displaying signs of shock without spinal injury

✳ **ENRICHMENT QUESTIONS**

40. **a.** When two patients on backboards are to be transported in one ambulance, the patient who is to be placed on the ambulance bench seat should be loaded first. Do not attempt to move a patient on a backboard over another patient on the ambulance cot.

41. **b.** The scoop stretcher can be separated lengthwise into two halves and slid under the patient with a minimal amount of movement. This type of stretcher is ideal for moving a patient up or down steps once the patient is secured with straps.

■ **COMMUNICATION AND DOCUMENTATION**

42. **b.** The difference between protocols and standing orders is that protocols are overall steps in patient care management and standing orders outline procedures an EMT may perform without contacting medical direction.

43. **c.** To correct an error made on an EMS report that is discovered when the report is being written, draw a single line through the error, initial it, and write the correct information next to it.

44. **a.** Objective information is information that is observable, verifiable, or measurable. Obvious injuries, such as lacerations, are examples of objective information.

45. **d.** Subjective information is information supplied by an individual from their point of view. For example, if a patient says he has a headache, this information cannot be verified by independent means.

46. **b.** The absence of a sign or symptom that may be expected to be present when assessing a patient is known as a pertinent negative. For example, a patient experiencing chest pain may have no radiation of the pain or no accompanying dyspnea. This is a pertinent negative. Although pertinent negatives do not warrant medical care, noting a pertinent negative is as important as noting a pertinent positive, that is, a positive finding. It also shows the thoroughness of the field assessment.

47. **c.** The presence of wheezing is considered a pertinent positive. It refers to the presence of a sign or symptom that helps to identify or substantiate something about a patient's condition.

48. **a.** When writing an EMS report, the EMT should avoid writing subjective statements that are merely his or her opinion. The EMT should also avoid writing what could be considered to be a diagnosis of a medical problem that the EMT cannot verify.

49. **d.** Since a patient with a hearing impairment may be able to read lips, speak clearly with your lips visible to the patient. Exchanging written notes may work but can be time-consuming. If the patient knows sign language, this may also be used to communicate if the EMT know some basic language. Avoid trying to speak from the patient's side where the patient cannot see you.

50. **b.** Elderly patients are more likely than other patient groups to have hearing and vision problems. This can present a communications problem. Although they are not likely to be as shy as children are, they may have memory problems, and if they have dentures but are not wearing them, their speech may be less intelligible.

51. **b.** When communicating with children, try to assume a position at eye level with the child. Also, always be honest since children can often sense lies. Although complex medical explanations can be confusing, try to explain what you are doing to the child in simple terms. Having parents present when assessing and questioning the child can be helpful and can alleviate fear.

52. **c.** Elderly patients may have difficulty hearing. Speaking clearly and distinctly, with sufficient volume to be heard will help the EMT achieve effective communication. Maintain eye contact and, when practical, position yourself at a level even with or lower than the patient. Patients may not understand exact medical terms, so explain what is wrong and what you are doing using words the patient can understand.

53. **a.** Ask the patient how he or she would like to be addressed. Some people prefer to be addressed by their first name or more formally using their last name. Avoid terms such as "dear," "hon," or "sweetie."

54. **c.** Radios located at a stationary site are referred to as base stations. These may or may not be digital. Mobile radios are vehicular mounted. Repeaters receive a transmission from another radio and then retransmit it.

55. **a.** A handheld radio is a portable radio. Portable radios are low power and have limited range.

56. **c.** Two major reasons it is good for the EMT to contact the receiving hospital are to receive advice and instructions and to allow the hospital to prepare to receive the patient.

57. **d.** The EMT should repeat the order back, preferably word for word, to ensure it was understood properly. Although it is a good idea to write down the order, it may not be practical to immediately document it on the report.

58. **b.** Since medical direction may give orders based on information received from the EMT, the radio report should be accurate. Depending on the hospital, radio report information may or may not be recorded on audiotape or on a written form for later review or inclusion with the patient's medical records.

59. **c.** When speaking on the radio, speak clearly and slowly. Avoid words such as "please," "thank you," and "you're welcome," and avoid the use of codes.

▪ GERIATRIC EMERGENCIES

60. **a.** Cardiovascular disease is the leading cause of death in elderly patients.

61. **d.** The increased porosity of bone that occurs in elderly patients and that contributes to a high incidence of injuries is known as osteoporosis. Kyphosis is curvature of the spine, osteoarthritis is a degeneration of the joints, and Alzheimer's disease a chronic organic disorder that affects the brain and results in dementia.

62. **b.** A contributing factor to the frequency of falls experienced by elderly patients is loss of muscle mass. Elderly patients also experience a loss of bone mass, a diminished sense of balance, and a decrease in skin elasticity

63. **b.** Due to having diminished liver and kidney functions, geriatric patients tend to need reduced doses of medication. They are therefore at risk of accidentally overdosing on medications even if the dose prescribed would be considered normal for most adults. Elderly patients are also more sensitive to the effects of alcohol and have a diminished ability to form blood clots.

64. **c.** Geriatric patients are at a higher risk of developing pneumonia and other respiratory infections due to the decreased elasticity of their lungs and the decreased activity of the cilia in the bronchial tree. The cilia protect the lower airway by sweeping mucus, bacteria, and other small particles toward the larynx, where they can then be expelled by coughing.

65. **d.** When assessing a geriatric patient with an acute illness, the EMT should plan on taking more time than normal to gather information and gain a history. The patient can be a reliable source of information, but family and bystanders may also be helpful. Unless someone who knows the patient confirms that an altered mental status is a chronic condition for the patient, suspect it to be the result of the present illness or injury.

66. **c.** Geriatric patients tend to experience a higher incidence of mental health problems. They also experience a higher incidence of falls, abuse, and neglect. Although motor vehicle crashes are still a concern, the incidence rate is not as high for the elderly as for younger motorists.

▪ GAINING ACCESS

67. **a.** The first thing the EMT should do when arriving at the scene of a vehicle crash is to make sure the scene is safe. This includes checking for downed wires, fire hazards, and other dangers. The safety of the EMTs and rescuers must come first. Dead EMTs don't save lives.

68. **d.** Always consider any downed wire energized and dangerous. Even a cable television or telephone wire may be energized if it has come in contact with electric wires down-line. Never attempt to manipulate the wire unless local protocols and proper training dictate otherwise.

69. **a.** The best course of action when energized wires have contacted a car is to wait for the electric company. Occupants should only be instructed to jump clear of the car if they are in immediate danger from fire or another life-threatening situation.

70. **d.** To gain access to a patient, check all the doors first. Although the EMT may be unable to open the door closest to the patient, other doors may be usable. Remember to "Try before you pry." If the doors will not open, it may be possible to roll down a window for access. Although the patient may be able to unlock a door, this may not be desirable if it will further aggravate an injury.

71. **c.** Generally, necessary care should be continued to the greatest extent possible during the extrication process.

72. **a.** During the extrication process, patients should be properly protected by a heavy, fireproof covering. A rescuer should also remain in the vehicle to monitor the patient and provide reassurance.

■ MULTIPLE-CASUALTY SITUATIONS

73. **b.** The first arriving EMS unit to arrive at a multiple casualty incident should assume medical command, assess the situation, start calling for additional aid, and direct incoming units. Patient care should not be started by this unit. Clear command must be established early if the incident is to be managed in an orderly fashion. If enough EMTs are present, triage may also be started.

74. **a.** A yellow triage tag signifies a second-priority or moderately injured patient.

75. **c.** The most qualified and competent EMT should assume the role of triage officer. Rank and seniority are unimportant at the scene of a multiple-casualty incident. Nurses, unless specially trained, lack the experience and expertise necessary to properly triage patients in the field.

76. **b.** A green triage tag signifies a patient with minor injuries. These are delayed-priority patients. Patients with green tags are sometimes referred to as the "walking wounded." This is not an accurate term since some walking patients may have severe injuries, and some patients with minor injuries may not be able to walk.

77. Match the following sectors/groups/units with their primary responsibilities.

extrication
transportation
treatment
triage
staging
supply

_____triage_____ sorts patients based on medical priority

_____supply_____ obtains and distributes resources such as medical equipment and personnel

___transportation___ ascertains capabilities of receiving hospitals and coordinates loading of ambulances

___extrication___ rescues patients who are trapped at the scene

___staging___ organizes incoming ambulances and coordinates the movement of ambulances to the loading zone

___treatment___ coordinates medical care for injured patients after they have been sorted and moved

78. Using the following descriptions to prioritize patients at a mass casualty scene, categorize them as: first, second, third, or fourth. (If you normally use the color system, mark the patients as: red, yellow, green, or black.)

___fourth (black)___ severe head injury, no pulse or breathing

___first (red)___ severe burns

___second (yellow)___ multiple bone or joint injuries

___third (green)___ minor soft-tissue injuries

___first (red)___ unconscious, unknown cause

___second (yellow)___ back injury without spinal damage

___first (red)___ a severe medical problem

___first (red)___ shock

___third (green)___ swollen extremity accompanied by minor pain

___fourth (black)___ multiple traumatic injuries accompanied by full cardiac arrest

___second (yellow)___ burns without airway problems

___first (red)___ active labor with a breech presentation

79. **a.** A red triage tag signifies a critical, first-priority patient.

■ WELL-BEING OF THE EMT

80. **b.** Communicable diseases are normally transmitted by direct contact, indirect contact, or inhalation. They are not normally transmitted by casual contact.

81. **c.** An EMT cannot recognize a patient with a communicable disease simply by his or her appearance.

82. **d.** Because EMS personnel are at greatest risk from hepatitis B, it is generally recommended that an EMT receive a hepatitis B immunization.

83. **a.** Gloves worn by EMTs are most commonly made from nitrile or latex.

84. **a.** Gloves protect from diseases transmitted by a variety of body fluids besides blood, and local protocols regarding their use should always be followed. There are some situations in which gloves may not be needed, however, such as when caring for a patient with a closed injury to the wrist or ankle.

85. **b.** When washing the hands, wash for at least 10 to 15 seconds. Hands should be washed after patient contact and after using the restroom. Hands should still be washed even if gloves were worn. Although antimicrobial or bactericidal cleaners are good, simple soap and water provides adequate protection against germs and bacteria.

86. **d.** In situations where blood may splatter, wear protective eyewear.

87. **c.** Wear appropriate respiratory protection, such as a high-efficiency particulate air (HEPA) respirator when working around a patient with suspected tuberculosis. Always follow local protocols.

88. **c.** When the EMT expects to encounter large amounts of blood or body fluid, it may be advisable to put on a gown if time permits.

89. **c.** HIV is primarily transmitted by the sharing of intravenous drug needles and syringes, by sexual contact, and from an infected mother to her baby. It is also transmitted by blood transfusions. Casual contact has not been linked to HIV transmission.

90. **d.** The Occupational Safety and Health Administration (OSHA) develops and enforces many regulations regarding infection-control guidelines for health care workers. EMS is subject to these regulations.

91. **a.** After transporting a patient with a communicable disease, the inside of the ambulance should be washed with a germicidal and viricidal agent. The use of aerosol sprays is not recommended as very little of the agent may reach the surface to be cleaned. Instead, use trigger-pump spray bottles to deliver the agent. Alcohol does not kill the germs and viruses. Research has shown airing out an ambulance is of no benefit.

92. **a.** If it is known in advance that a patient with an infectious disease is to be transported, unnecessary equipment may be removed from the ambulance to prevent contamination. A truly sick patient should be transported by ambulance. Linens may be exchanged or discarded at the hospital, but they should not be replaced with uncomfortable plastic sheets simply to avoid using linen.

93. **b.** Thoroughly wash the hands with a germicidal and viricidal solution following each run. Additional protection can be gained by having annual physical checkups and current vaccinations. It is not always necessary to wear a mask and gown, nor should the patient be left alone in the back of the ambulance.

94. **c.** High-efficiency particulate air (HEPA) respirators are most commonly worn by EMTs when managing a patient with active tuberculosis. This is because the tuberculosis bacilli are larger than the openings of the filter and therefore theoretically will not be able to pass through the filter.

95. **a.** Equipment such as stethoscopes and blood pressure cuffs are designed to be cleaned after each patient use and reused. Items such as suction catheters, airways, and oxygen masks and cannulas should be disposed of after a single use.

96. **d.** Syphilis, genital herpes, and gonorrhea are all sexually transmitted diseases that present a risk of exposure to EMTs. These communicable diseases may be transmitted in ways other than sexual contact, such as contact with drainage. Rubella is German measles, a common childhood disease.

97. **c.** If death is imminent, the family should be allowed to be with the patient whenever possible. It may not be appropriate to transport the patient to the hospital, for example, if there is a written DNR order on hand.

98. **a.** To help the body deal with stress, increase intake of carbohydrates. Decrease intake of caffeine, alcohol, sugar, and fat.

99. **d.** The purpose of a Critical Incident Stress Management (CISM) is to help EMTs work through their emotional responses to an incident and to accelerate the recovery process. It is not a disciplinary procedure designed to point out mistakes or areas that need improvement.

100. **b.** Ideally, a formal Critical Incident Stress Debriefing should be conducted within 24 to 72 hours of the critical incident.

101. **c.** There are a number of important professional attributes an EMT should strive to demonstrate, including a neat, presentable appearance. Initial training is just a start, and continuing education is necessary to keep knowledge and skills up to date. Remember, it's not whether you are paid or not that makes you a professional. Your attitude makes you a professional. Although EMTs try to make the patient's needs a top priority, they must not endanger their own lives.

■ HAZARDOUS MATERIALS

102. **c.** The primary responsibility of an EMT at a hazardous materials incident is the safety of the EMT, the public, and any patients. Access to patients should be accomplished only after personnel are properly protected with appropriate gear and breathing apparatus. Although early identification of the substance is important, it does not take priority over safety considerations. Identification is usually the responsibility of the fire department or hazardous materials team. Controlling the actual incident is not usually the job of EMS personnel.

103. **c.** Identification of hazardous materials transported by motor vehicles is best made by referencing the four-digit guide number found on placards and shipping information. The vehicle operator may not know what is being carried, and laboratory testing is a time-consuming process. Never smell or touch a potentially hazardous material. Identification should always be made while the EMT remains at a safe distance from the incident.

104. **b.** Information about a hazardous material used at an industrial or commercial site is best obtained by referencing a material safety data sheet. Plant employees may not be familiar with the material or may provide inaccurate information, and the container may be misleading.

105. **d.** Generally, only EMTs with proper training in wearing hazmat equipment and SCBA should enter an area where hazardous materials are found.

106. **b.** EMS vehicles and personnel at a scene involving hazardous material should be positioned upwind and uphill from the incident at a safe distance. Shouting distance is normally much too close, as fumes may quickly reach EMS personnel. In most instances, patients should be brought to the EMT, unless the EMT is properly trained and protected to enter the scene.

■ MEDICAL TERMINOLOGY MATCHING

Medical terms ending in "o" are combining forms. Terms preceded by a hyphen are suffixes, and terms followed by a hyphen are prefixes.

Medical Term	Definition
a, an	without
abdomin o	abdomen
aden o	gland
ambi-	both sides
angi o	blood vessel
ant-, anti-	against
antero-	front
arteri o	artery
arthr o	joint
bi-	both
brachi o	upper arm
brady-	slow
carcin o	cancer
cardi o	heart
cephal o	head
cervic o	neck
chol e	bile
chondr o	cartilage
circum-	around
col o	colon
con-	with
contra-	against, opposite
cost o	rib
crani o	skull

cyt o	cell
dent o	tooth
derm o/dermat o	skin
dors o	back
dys-	difficult, bad, abnormal
-ectomy	surgical removal
encephal o	brain
end-, endo-	within
enter o	small intestine
febr o	fever
gastr o	stomach
gloss o	tongue
gynec o	woman
hem o/hemat o	blood
hepat o	liver
hyper-	beyond normal, excessive
hypo-	below normal
hyster o	uterus
-iasis	condition
inter-	between
intra-	within
laryng o	larynx
-lysis	destruction
mega-, megal o	large
my o	muscle
nephr o	kidney
neur o	nerve
ocul o/ophthalm o	eye
odont o	tooth

-osis	an abnormal condition
oste o	bone
path o	disease
pathy	disease of a part
peri-	around, surrounding
pharyng o	throat
phas o	speech
phleb o	vein
phren o	diaphragm
-plasty	surgical repair
-plegia	paralysis
-pnea	breath, breathing
pneum o/pneumat o	air, breath
poly-	much, many
post-	after, behind
pre-	before
pulmon o	lung
ren o	kidney
retro-	located behind
semi-	one half
supra-	above, over
tachy	fast
thorac o	chest
thromb o	clot
trache o	trachea
ven o	vein
ventr o	belly

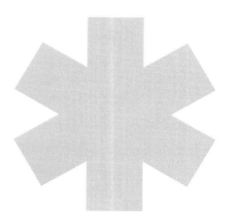

16

Cardiopulmonary Resuscitation, Basic Life Support, and Airway Obstruction

CHAPTER 16 REVIEW QUESTIONS

1. It is important for an EMT to have a good working knowledge of basic life support (BLS) because:
   a. most patients transported by ambulance require CPR
   b. most people having cardiac emergencies experience cardiac arrest before reaching the hospital
   c. most patients in cardiac arrest can be successfully resuscitated if high-quality CPR is performed
   d. a large percentage of cardiac arrests occur outside of the hospital

2. The percentage of oxygen present in standard room air is:
   a. 21%
   b. 35%
   c. 56%
   d. 78%

3. The percentage of oxygen in exhaled air is approximately:
   a. 5%
   b. 16%
   c. 21%
   d. 78%

4. Early opening of the airway and performance of artificial ventilations are important because brain damage can occur within:
   a. 2 to 4 minutes
   b. 4 to 6 minutes
   c. 8 to 10 minutes
   d. 10 to 12 minutes

5. In an unconscious patient, the most common cause of airway obstruction is:
   a. the tongue
   b. food
   c. blood
   d. small toys or marbles

6. After ensuring scene safety and taking body substance isolation precautions, the first thing a rescuer should do when a patient has collapsed due to illness or injury is:
   a. open the airway
   b. check for a medic alert tag
   c. call for help
   d. determine whether the patient is unresponsive

7. The preferred method of opening the airway of a patient without a suspected cervical spine injury is the:
   a. head-tilt/neck-lift
   b. modified jaw-thrust maneuver
   c. Heimlich maneuver
   d. head-tilt/chin-lift

8. The preferred method of opening the airway of a patient with a suspected neck injury is the:
   a. head-tilt/chin-lift
   b. head-tilt/neck-lift
   c. modified jaw-thrust maneuver
   d. Heimlich maneuver

9. After opening the airway, check for breathing for:
   a. 1 to 3 seconds
   b. 3 to 5 seconds
   c. 5 to 10 seconds
   d. at least 10 seconds

10. If an adult patient is not breathing, deliver:
    a. four quick breaths
    b. two slow breaths if alone, four quick breaths if a partner is present
    c. two full breaths of 2 seconds in duration
    d. one full breath of 1 to 1½ seconds in duration

11. Ventilate an adult patient who is not breathing but has a pulse at a rate of once every:
    a. 3 to 4 seconds
    b. 4 to 5 seconds
    c. 5 to 6 seconds
    d. 6 to 10 seconds

12. For a laryngectomy patient, ventilations should be delivered through the patient's:
    a. mouth and nose
    b. stoma
    c. mouth
    d. nose

13. To locate the carotid pulse:
    a. place the thumb on one side of the trachea and the forefinger on the opposite side at the level of the Adam's apple
    b. place two fingers in the notch directly below the Adam's apple
    c. place the thumb on the Adam's apple, then slide it into the groove between the neck muscles and trachea
    d. place two fingers on the Adam's apple, then slide them into the groove between the neck muscles and trachea

14. Initially assess the pulse for:
    a. 5 to 10 seconds
    b. 10 to 15 seconds
    c. 30 to 45 seconds
    d. 60 seconds

15. To properly receive CPR, the patient must be:
    a. in Trendelenburg position
    b. on a firm, flat surface
    c. at least 6 months of age
    d. in a prone position

16. To perform external chest compressions on an adult, use:
    a. two hands on a man, one hand on a woman
    b. the heel of one hand
    c. two hands, one placed on top of the other
    d. two hands, placed side by side

17. Chest compressions should be delivered to:
    a. the upper third of the sternum
    b. the xiphoid process
    c. the lower half of the sternum
    d. the manubrium

18. When adult CPR is being performed, the proper depth of chest compressions is:
    a. ¾ to 1½ inches
    b. 1½ to 2 inches
    c. 2 to 2½ inches
    d. as deep as necessary to produce a palpable pulse

19. Chest compressions should be:
    a. 25% compression, 75% relaxation
    b. 50% compression, 50% relaxation
    c. 75% compression, 25% relaxation
    d. varied to produce optimal cardiac output

20. The ratio of chest compressions to ventilations in one-rescuer adult CPR is:
    a. 5:1
    b. 15:1
    c. 5:2
    d. 15:2

21. In one-rescuer adult CPR, compressions should be delivered at a rate of:
    a. 60 to 70 per minute
    b. at least 80 per minute
    c. approximately 100 per minute
    d. at least 120 per minute

22. When performing two-rescuer adult CPR:
    a. pause after the fifth compression to allow the second rescuer to deliver a breath
    b. deliver a breath on the downstroke of the fifth compression
    c. pause after the fifth compression to allow the second rescuer to deliver two full breaths
    d. the second rescuer delivers a breath whenever possible

23. Patients in cardiac arrest should be reassessed:
    a. every 5 minutes
    b. after the first minute of CPR and every 10 minutes thereafter
    c. after the first minute of CPR and every few minutes thereafter
    d. only if the patient starts breathing on his or her own

24. When resuming one-rescuer adult CPR after reassessing the patient, give:
    a. no breaths and resume compressions
    b. one breath and resume compressions
    c. two breaths and resume compressions
    d. two breaths and recheck the pulse

25. For adults, activate the EMS system after:
    a. checking for a pulse
    b. the patient resumes a spontaneous pulse and breathing
    c. becoming too tired to continue CPR
    d. determining unresponsiveness

26. To find the proper hand position for adult external chest compressions:
    a. measure two fingers below the middle of the sternum
    b. measure one finger above the xiphoid process
    c. measure two fingers above the manubrium
    d. measure one finger below the nipple line

27. The ratio of chest compressions to ventilations for two-rescuer adult CPR is:
    a. 5:1
    b. 15:1
    c. 5:2
    d. 15:2

28. For two-rescuer adult CPR, the rate of compressions is:
    a. at least 60 per minute
    b. 40 to 60 per minute
    c. 60 to 80 per minute
    d. approximately 100 per minute

29. After reassessing the patient for return of breathing and circulation during two-rescuer adult CPR, the rescuer at the chest should:
    a. resume compressions after the rescuer at the head gives a breath
    b. pause after every four cycles of compressions to allow for a pulse check
    c. resume compressions without the rescuer at the head giving a breath
    d. intersperse an abdominal thrust after every cycle of five compressions

30. During two-rescuer CPR, a call for switching positions is made by the:
    a. rescuer performing ventilations
    b. rescuer performing compressions
    c. senior EMT
    d. rescuer who has been doing CPR the longest

31. After switching positions, the rescuer at the head:
    a. checks for a pulse and breathing
    b. immediately gives a breath
    c. waits for the rescuer at the chest to resume compressions
    d. gives two breaths and checks a pulse

32. Signs of effective CPR include all the following *except*:
    a. return of spontaneous pulses and breathing
    b. return of color to the patient (i.e., the patient "pinks" up)
    c. good pulses with compressions
    d. dilated pupils

33. When performing CPR, use supplemental oxygen:
    a. after the first pulse check
    b. when the rescuer starts to tire of rescue breathing
    c. as soon as it is available
    d. only if the patient has no history of respiratory problems

34. When managing a drowning patient in cardiac arrest:
    a. start chest compressions while the patient is still in the water
    b. wait until the patient is removed from the water to start CPR
    c. allow paramedics to assess the patient's electrocardiogram (ECG) before starting CPR
    d. start ventilations while the patient is still in the water

35. If air does not seem to enter the lungs during attempts to ventilate an unconscious patient:
    a. reposition the head and neck and reattempt ventilations
    b. perform abdominal thrusts
    c. perform a finger sweep
    d. perform chest thrusts

36. When a conscious adult patient has an obstructed airway:
    a. perform 6 to 10 abdominal thrusts
    b. administer four back blows followed by four abdominal thrusts
    c. perform abdominal thrusts until the obstruction is cleared or the patient becomes unconscious
    d. administer back blows only

37. A patient with a partial airway obstruction but good air exchange should be:
    a. managed in the same way as a patient with a full obstruction
    b. encouraged to cough and monitored closely
    c. given back blows only
    d. encouraged to drink a large glass of water to dislodge the obstruction

38. To relieve an airway obstruction in a pregnant or obese patient, use:
    a. abdominal thrusts
    b. chest thrusts
    c. back blows
    d. the Heimlich maneuver

39. To manage an airway obstruction in an unconscious adult patient, repeat cycles of:
    a. four abdominal thrusts followed by four chest thrusts, then reattempt to ventilate
    b. five abdominal thrusts followed by a finger sweep, then attempt to ventilate
    c. five back blows followed by five abdominal thrusts, then attempt to ventilate
    d. six to ten abdominal thrusts followed by one ventilation, then a finger sweep

40. After a foreign body is successfully dislodged, the patient should be:
    a. told to rest and not eat hard foods for a day or two
    b. advised to see their family physician the next day
    c. encouraged to go to a hospital and be examined by a physician
    d. observed for 5 minutes and not transported if no difficulties are noted

41. By American Heart Association (AHA) definition, a child is:
    a. 1 to 8 years old
    b. younger than 1 year old
    c. 2 to 10 years old
    d. 5 to 14 years old

42. To perform chest compressions on a child, use:
    a. the heel of one hand placed on the lower half of the sternum
    b. two hands placed on the middle of the sternum
    c. three fingers placed below the nipple line
    d. the heel of one hand placed on the upper third of the sternum

43. When performing chest compressions on a child, the hand closest to the patient's forehead should be:
    a. placed over the hand that is on the sternum
    b. kept on the patient's forehead to maintain head tilt
    c. placed under the patient's neck to maintain head tilt
    d. used to continually monitor a carotid pulse

44. The chest of a child should be compressed:
    a. ⅛ to ¼ the total depth of the chest
    b. ¼ to ⅓ the total depth of the chest
    c. ⅓ to ½ the total depth of the chest
    d. ½ to ⅔ the total depth of the chest

45. If a child is not breathing but has a pulse, the patient should be ventilated at a rate of:
    a. 10 times a minute, once every 6 seconds
    b. 12 times a minute, once every 5 seconds
    c. 15 times a minute, once every 4 seconds
    d. 20 times a minute, once every 3 seconds

46. By American Heart Association (AHA) definition, an infant is:
    a. <1 year old
    b. <18 months old
    c. 1 to 2 years old
    d. newborn to 3 years old

47. To assess the pulse of an infant, check the:
    a. brachial pulse
    b. apical pulse
    c. carotid pulse
    d. radial pulse

48. When opening the airway of an infant, avoid:
    a. using the jaw-thrust method
    b. hyperextending the neck
    c. suctioning
    d. using the head-tilt/chin-lift method

49. When ventilating an infant:
    a. give full breaths
    b. administer rapid breaths of ½ to 1 second duration
    c. perform mouth-to-mouth and nose breathing
    d. deliver four small puffs

50. To perform chest compressions on an infant when one rescuer is present, use:
    a. two fingers placed on the upper sternum
    b. two fingers placed one fingerwidth below the nipple line
    c. the heel of one hand placed on the middle of the sternum
    d. both thumbs placed on the upper sternum

51. The chest of an infant should be compressed:
    a. 1/16 to ⅛ the total depth of the chest
    b. ⅛ to ¼ the total depth of the chest
    c. ¼ to ⅓ the total depth of the chest
    d. ⅓ to ½ the total depth of the chest

52. For CPR on infants or children, the ratio of compressions to ventilations is:
   a. 15:2 regardless of the number of rescuers
   b. 5:1 for infants and 15:2 for children
   c. 15:2 for one rescuer CPR
   d. 5:1 regardless of the number of rescuers

53. If an infant is not breathing but has a pulse, the patient should be ventilated at a rate of:
   a. 10 times a minute, once every 6 seconds
   b. 12 times a minute, once every 5 seconds
   c. 15 times a minute, once every 4 seconds
   d. 20 times a minute, once every 3 seconds

54. If two healthcare providers are performing CPR on an infant, compressions should be performed:
   a. using the two thumb-encircling hand technique
   b. by placing the heel of the hand over the middle of the sternum
   c. using two fingers placed on the upper half of the sternum
   d. by placing the one thumb over the chest and one thumb over the abdomen

55. A conscious infant with a complete airway obstruction may be identified by:
   a. pink lips
   b. an absent pulse
   c. an inability to cry
   d. a persistent, forceful cough

56. One difference between managing an infant with an airway obstruction as opposed to an adult is that:
   a. back blows are not used
   b. abdominal thrusts are interspersed with chest thrusts
   c. ventilations are not attempted until the obstruction is relieved
   d. chest thrusts are used instead of abdominal thrusts

57. To relieve an airway obstruction in an infant, perform cycles of:
   a. six to ten abdominal thrusts
   b. five back blows followed by five chest thrusts
   c. six to ten chest thrusts, followed by a finger sweep
   d. five back blows followed by five abdominal thrusts

58. Manual removal of foreign bodies obstructing the airway in infants and children should be performed:
   a. only on patients older than 5 years of age
   b. only if the object can be visualized
   c. by using a blind finger sweep
   d. only on infants

59. When attempting to relieve an obstructed airway in an infant, position the infant:
   a. with the head and shoulders elevated
   b. with the head and trunk level
   c. upside down by the feet and ankles
   d. with the head lower than the trunk

60. If a rescuer is alone and finds a child or infant without a pulse and who is not breathing:
   a. perform CPR for 1 minute, then phone for help
   b. immediately phone for help
   c. perform CPR for 5 minutes, then phone for help
   d. open the airway, give two slow breaths, then phone for help

61. CPR should not be interrupted:
   a. when performing automated external defibrillation
   b. for more than a few seconds except in special situations
   c. for any reason
   d. for more than a few minutes unless performing endotracheal intubation

62. CPR may be discontinued for any of the following reasons *except*:
    a. the rescuer becomes too exhausted to continue
    b. spontaneous ventilations and circulation are restored
    c. the patient's pupils become fixed and dilated
    d. an authorized individual pronounces the patient dead

63. All of the following statements concerning complications from CPR are true *except*:
    a. they occur only when CPR is performed by poorly trained rescuers
    b. they include injuries to the lungs, heart, liver, and spleen
    c. they may occur even when compressions are properly performed
    d. they include fractures of the ribs and sternum

64. Generally, when ventilating a person wearing dentures:
    a. remove the dentures
    b. remove the dentures only if it is a partial plate
    c. leave the dentures in place
    d. leave the dentures in place only if it is a partial plate

65. If slight gastric distention is noted during CPR:
    a. relieve the distention by exerting moderate pressure with one hand over the upper abdomen
    b. discontinue CPR
    c. reposition the airway and ventilate less forcefully
    d. place the patient's head and neck in a neutral position

66. The chances of gastric distention and regurgitation can be reduced by:
    a. tilting the patient's head forward
    b. not using an adjunctive airway
    c. not pinching the patient's nose
    d. delivering ventilations with less force and speed

■ **Additional BLS Review** ■

After completing the statements below, fill in the answers in columns 2 and 3 of the charts.
Complete questions 1 through 5 regarding the steps an EMT takes after arriving on an accident scene.

1. Check for _____ .

2. Access the _____ system.

3. Open _____ and check for _____ .

4. Give _____ if breathing is absent:

   _____ seconds each breath for adults; _____ seconds each breath for infants and children.

5. Check for _____ and _____ .

Summary of Adult One- and Two-Rescuer CPR

	One Rescuer	Two Rescuer
Rate		
Ratio		
Hand placement		
Depth of compressions		
Location of pulse check		
Rescue breathing		

Summary of Infant and Child CPR

	Infant	Child
Age		
Rate		
Ratio		
Hand placement		
Depth of compressions		
Location of pulse check		
Rescue breathing		

■ Additional Points for Discussion ■

1. Identify specific buildings or locations in your area where it may be difficult to perform CPR while moving the patient.

2. If the patient must be moved, how will this be accomplished?

ANSWERS TO CHAPTER 16 REVIEW QUESTIONS

1. **d.** Because a large percentage of cardiac arrests occur outside of the hospital setting, it is imperative that EMTs have a good working knowledge of CPR and remain proficient in their skills. Not all patients experiencing cardiac emergencies will experience cardiac arrest, but the EMT must be ready if they do.

2. **a.** Oxygen makes up only 21% of room air.

3. **b.** Only 5% of the 21% of oxygen in room air is needed to sustain life. The air exhaled by a rescuer performing CPR contains 16% oxygen (21% minus 5%). This 16% oxygen exhaled by the rescuer is enough to sustain the life of the patient.

4. **b.** Without oxygen, brain damage occurs in 4 to 6 minutes.

5. **a.** The tongue is the most common cause of airway obstruction in an unconscious patient.

6. **d.** After ensuring scene safety and taking body substance isolation precautions, the first step in basic life support is to establish whether the patient is unresponsive. After establishing unresponsiveness, the rescuer should call for help and then open the airway.

7. **d.** The head-tilt/chin-lift maneuver is the preferred method of opening the airway of a patient without a suspected spinal injury. This method works better than the head-tilt/neck-lift because the chin lift moves the mandible forward, thereby lifting the tongue up out of the oropharynx.

8. **c.** The modified jaw thrust maneuver should be used to open the airway of a patient with a suspected cervical spine injury.

9. **c.** After opening the airway, check for breathing. This should take no more than 10 seconds. To check, look for chest movement, listen for breathing, and feel with your cheek for air movement.

10. **c.** Two slow breaths of 2 seconds in duration should be delivered to an adult patient who is not breathing. For infants and children, two slow breaths of 1 to 1½ seconds in duration should be delivered.

11. **b.** An adult patient who is not breathing but has a pulse should be ventilated once every 4 to 5 seconds.

12. **b.** To ventilate a laryngectomy patient, ventilations should be delivered through the patient's stoma. To accomplish this, a child- or infant-size ventilation mask can be placed over the stoma. Some patients may have only a partial or temporary tracheostomy. If this is the case, the rescuer may need to seal the patient's mouth and nose before ventilating to prevent air from leaking.

13. **d.** To locate the carotid pulse, the rescuer places two fingers on the Adam's apple and slides them toward the rescuer into the groove between the neck muscles and trachea. Do not attempt to palpate the pulse on the side of the trachea opposite the rescuer, and do not use the thumb to check a pulse.

14. **a.** The patient's pulse should initially be assessed for 5 to 10 seconds.

15. **b.** The CPR patient must be on a firm, flat surface to properly receive CPR. The patient should be in a supine position (on his or her back). There is no age limit for receiving CPR.

16. **c.** External chest compressions on an adult are performed using two hands on the sternum. The heel of the rescuer's hand closest to the patient's head should be placed on the sternum, and the rescuer's other hand should be placed on top of it.

17. **c.** Chest compressions should be delivered to the lower half of the sternum. The manubrium is the upper portion of the sternum.

18. **b.** The depth for chest compressions performed on an adult patient is 1½ to 2 inches.

19. **b.** Compressions should be delivered in a smooth manner, with 50% compression and 50% relaxation. The hands should not be removed from the patient's chest during the relaxation period.

20. **d.** The correct ratio of compressions to ventilations in one-rescuer adult CPR is 15:2.

21. **c.** Compressions should be delivered at a rate of approximately 100 per minute in one-rescuer adult CPR.

22. **a.** When performing two-rescuer adult CPR, if the airway is not controlled by an endotracheal tube, the rescuer performing compressions should pause after the fifth compression to allow the second rescuer to ventilate the patient.

23. **c.** After the first minute of CPR the patient's pulse and breathing should be reassessed. This equals four cycles of compressions and ventilations in one-rescuer or two-rescuer CPR. Thereafter, the patient should be reassessed every few minutes.

24. **a.** When resuming one-rescuer adult CPR after reassessing the patient, the rescuer begins with chest compressions. Give no breaths prior to resuming compressions.

25. **d.** When an adult is in cardiac arrest, the EMS system should usually be activated immediately after determining unresponsiveness. (Exceptions are cases of submersion or near-drowning, poisoning, drug overdose, and trauma.) If the rescuer is alone, he or she should call for additional help. If someone else is available, that person should call while the rescuer continues assessing the patient. Early delivery of defibrillation and Advanced Life Support is critical to survival of adult patients because ventricular fibrillation is the most common cause of arrest. If the rescuer is alone, rapid access to EMS may be more important than a short period of CPR, which will need to be interrupted anyway to summon help.

26. **b.** Measure one finger-width above the xiphoid process to find the proper hand position for adult chest compressions. Using the hand closest to the patient's feet, place the middle finger over the xiphoid process and the index finger next to it. Then place the heel of the hand closest to the patient's head next to the index finger, thereby positioning the hand one finger above the xiphoid.

27. **d.** The correct ratio of compressions to ventilations in two-rescuer adult CPR is 15:2.

28. **d.** In two-rescuer adult CPR, compressions should be delivered at a rate of approximately 100 per minute, the same rate as for one-rescuer adult CPR.

29. **c.** When resuming two-rescuer adult CPR after reassessing the patient, the rescuer at the chest begins performing chest compressions. The rescuer at the head does not give a breath prior to resuming compressions. The pulse should be checked every few minutes thereafter.

30. **b.** The rescuer performing compressions initiates a change in positions. The call usually is made when the rescuer becomes fatigued.

31. **a.** After changing positions, the rescuer at the head checks for a pulse and breathing. If neither are present, he or she calls for resumption of CPR.

32. **d.** Signs of effective CPR include a return of spontaneous pulses and breathing, return of color to the patient, and good pulses with compressions. Dilated pupils are not a sign of effective CPR.

33. **c.** Supplemental oxygen should be used as soon as it becomes available during CPR. All patients who are not breathing should be ventilated with 100% oxygen.

34. **d.** Ventilations should be started as soon as possible on drowning patients. If practical, this should be begun while the patient is still in the water. Because a hard surface is needed for chest compressions, patients will normally have to be removed from the water before compressions are initiated. Compressions should not be initiated while patients are still in the water unless the rescuer has special training in performing in-water CPR.

35. **a.** The rescuer should reposition the airway and attempt to ventilate a second time if air does not seem to enter the patient's lungs initially.

36. **c.** If a conscious adult has a complete airway obstruction, the rescuer should perform abdominal thrusts until the obstruction is relieved or the patient becomes unconscious. Back blows are not used on adults.

37. **b.** A patient with a partial airway obstruction and good air exchange should be encouraged to cough and monitored closely. A patient with a partial airway obstruction with poor air exchange should be managed in the same way as a patient with a complete obstruction.

38. **b.** Use chest thrusts instead of abdominal thrusts to relieve an airway obstruction in a pregnant or obese patient.

39. **b.** The rescuer should repeat cycles of up to five abdominal thrusts followed by a finger sweep and a ventilation attempt when managing an unconscious adult with an obstructed airway.

40. **c.** Patients who have experienced airway obstruction should be examined by a physician. Although the patient cannot be forced to go to a hospital, EMTs should strongly encourage the patient to do so. Trauma to the area of the larynx may not be readily recognized, and swelling may later compromise the airway.

41. **a.** By American Heart Association standards, a child is a patient 1 to 8 years old.

42. **a.** The heel of one hand is used when performing CPR on a child. It is placed over the lower half of the sternum.

43. **b.** When performing compressions on a child, the hand closest to the patient's head should be kept on the patient's forehead to maintain an open airway. After ventilating the patient, the rescuer replaces the hand performing compressions on the chest by sight.

44. **c.** The depth of compressions for child CPR is approximately one third to one half the depth of the chest, which is about 1 to 1½ inches on most children.

45. **d.** To perform rescue breathing on a child who has a pulse but is not breathing, ventilate the patient 20 times a minute, once every 3 seconds. This is the same rate as for an infant.

46. **a.** By American Heart Association standards, an infant is a patient younger than 1 year old.

47. **a.** The brachial pulse is used to assess the pulse of an infant. The carotid pulse is still used to assess the pulse of a child.

48. **b.** Avoid hyperextending the neck of an infant, which can be caused by excessive head tilt. The cartilaginous rings of the trachea are not fully formed; thus, hyperextension of the neck can kink the trachea (in the same way a garden hose may be kinked) and result in an airway obstruction.

49. **c.** When ventilating an infant, the rescuer should cover the infant's mouth and nose with his or her mouth, or a mask. The ventilations should be slow puffs (1 to 1½ seconds in duration), to avoid high pressure and gastric distention.

50. **b.** If only one rescuer is present, chest compressions should be performed by placing two fingers one finger-width below an imaginary line drawn between the infant's nipples.

51. **d.** The depth of compressions for infant CPR is approximately one third to one half the depth of the chest, which is about ½ to 1 inch on most infants.

52. **d.** The ratio of compressions to ventilations when performing CPR on infants or children is 5:1 regardless of the number of rescuers.

53. **d.** If an infant is not breathing but has a pulse, he or she should be ventilated 20 times per minute, once every 3 seconds. Newborns should be ventilated at 40 times a minute.

54. **a.** If two healthcare providers are performing CPR on an infant, compressions should be performed using the two thumb-encircling hand technique. To accomplish this, place both thumbs side by side over the lower half of the infant's sternum, approximately one finger-width below the intermammary line. Be sure the thumbs do not compress on or near the xiphoid process. The rescuer should also encircle the infant's chest and support the infant's back with the fingers of both hands.

55. **c.** Cyanosis and/or an inability to cry are signs that should alert a rescuer to a complete airway obstruction in a conscious infant.

56. **d.** Chest thrusts, rather than abdominal thrusts, should be performed on an infant with an airway obstruction.

57. **b.** Perform cycles of five back blows followed by five chest thrusts to relieve an airway obstruction in an infant. If the infant is unconscious, the rescuer should also attempt to ventilate following each set of five chest thrusts. Blind finger sweeps should not be performed on infants or children, as this can push the object back into the airway and cause further obstruction.

58. **b.** Manual removal of foreign bodies obstructing the airway in infants and children should be performed only if the object can be visualized.

59. **d.** The rescuer should keep the infant's head lower than the trunk while performing maneuvers to relieve an obstructed airway. The infant may be straddled over the rescuer's arm to accomplish this.

60. **a.** If a rescuer is alone and finds an unresponsive infant or child, the patient should be further assessed to see if rescue breathing or CPR is needed. If there no one else is available to call EMS, the rescuer should perform CPR for 1 minute, then activate the EMS system. CPR or rescue breathing should be resumed as quickly as possible after the phone call. Since the most common cause of arrest in infants and children is hypoxia, the minute of CPR or rescue breathing may make a critical difference in survival. If another person is present, he or she should immediately activate the EMS system while the rescuer provides medical support.

61. **b.** CPR should not be interrupted for more than a few seconds except in unusual situations. Such situations include moving a patient down stairs or placing an endotracheal tube. CPR must also be interrupted to perform automated external defibrillation.

62. **c.** Fixed and dilated pupils alone are not a reason to stop CPR. CPR may be discontinued if the rescuer is too exhausted to continue, if spontaneous pulses and breathing are restored, or if a patient is pronounced dead by an authorized individual, such as a doctor or coroner. The responsibility for performing CPR may also be turned over to a higher medical authority such as a physician or paramedic, but CPR should not be discontinued.

63. **a.** Complications may occur even if compressions are performed correctly by well-trained rescuers. Complications of CPR include fractures of the ribs and sternum, as well as laceration of the lungs, liver, spleen, and heart and damage to the pleura. Constant practice and skill maintenance can reduce the risk of such complications.

64. **c.** Dentures should normally be left in place when ventilating a patient. Creating a good seal may be difficult if dentures are removed, as they often provide underlying support to the soft tissue of the mouth and face.

65. **c.** If the rescuer notes slight gastric distention developing during CPR, the airway should be repositioned and ventilations delivered less forcefully.

66. **d.** The chance of gastric distention and regurgitation can be reduced by ventilating with less force and speed. On adults, ventilations should be delivered slowly over 1½ to 2 seconds. Do not continue to force air into the patient after the chest rises.

■ Additional BLS Review ■

After completing the statements below, fill in the answers in columns 2 and 3 of the charts. Complete questions 1 through 5 regarding the steps an EMT takes after arriving on an accident scene.

1. Check for <u>unresponsiveness (shake and shout)</u> .

2. Access the _____ <u>EMS</u> _____ system.

3. Open _____ <u>airway</u> _____ and check for _____ <u>breathing</u> _____ .

4. Give _____ <u>2 slow breaths</u> _____ if breathing is absent:

   _____ <u>2</u> _____ seconds each breath for adults; <u>1 to 1½</u> seconds each breath for infants and children.

5. Check for _____ <u>breathing</u> _____ and _____ <u>pulse</u> _____ .

Summary of Adult One- and Two-Rescuer CPR

	One Rescuer	**Two Rescuer**
Rate	Approximately 100 per minute	Approximately 100 per minute
Ratio	15 compressions/2 breaths	15 compressions/2 breaths
Hand placement	2 hands—heel of hand 1 or 2 fingers above xiphoid process	2 hands—heel of hand 1 or 2 fingers above xiphoid process
Depth of compressions	1½" to 2"	1½" to 2"
Location of pulse check	Carotid	Carotid
Rescue breathing	1 breath every 4 to 5 seconds	1 breath every 4 to 5 seconds

Summary of Infant and Child CPR

	Infant	**Child**
Age	0 to 1 year	1 to 8 years
Rate	>100 per minute	Approximately 100 per minute
Ratio	5 compressions/1 breath	5 compressions/1 breath
Hand placement	2 or 3 fingers—1 fingerwidth below line between nipples	Heel of 1 hand—lower half of sternum
Depth of compressions	⅓ to ½ depth of chest (approximately ½" to 1")	⅓ to ½ depth of chest (approximately 1" to 1½")
Location of pulse check	Brachial	Carotid
Rescue breathing	20 times per minute (1 breath every 3 seconds)	20 times per minute (1 breath every 3 seconds)

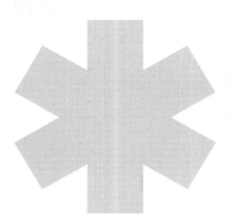

17

Evaluation and Situational Review

CHAPTER 17 REVIEW QUESTIONS

1. Your unit is summoned to a home for a child who has ingested an unknown quantity of children's aspirin. The patient is a 4-year-old boy. As you question him, you note that he is alert and oriented. You perform your assessment and find no immediately life-threatening problems. He admits to having taken the aspirin, but cannot tell you how many. After contacting medical direction by telephone, you are ordered to administer activated charcoal. The correct dose for this patient is:
   a. 1 milligram per kilogram of body weight
   b. 2 grams per kilogram of body weight
   c. 12.5 to 25 grams
   d. 25 to 50 milligrams

2. Prior to administering the charcoal:
   a. tell the child it is candy
   b. shake the container thoroughly
   c. mix the charcoal with water
   d. pour the fluid into a glass

3. Receiving an order for activated charcoal is an example of:
   a. up-line medical direction
   b. direct-line medical direction
   c. on-line medical direction
   d. straight-line medical direction

4. Your patient is a 28-year-old female in her eighth month of pregnancy. Her family called because she had been complaining of a severe, persistent headache and was vomiting. As you begin your evaluation, you notice that her face and hands appear swollen. She is somewhat confused and disoriented, and vital signs reveal a blood pressure of 162/100. Further questioning of the family reveals the patient experienced sudden weight gain prior to the onset of the other complaints. While caring for this patient, be alert for:
   a. a sudden drop in blood pressure
   b. sudden respiratory arrest
   c. uncontrolled vaginal bleeding
   d. seizures

5. While transporting your patient to the hospital, it is best to transport the patient:
   a. lying flat on her back
   b. with her shoulders and head elevated
   c. as quickly as possible using lights and sirens
   d. lying on her right side with her feet elevated

6. After arriving home from work, a man finds his wife unconscious in bed. Your patient is a 28-year-old woman. She is responsive only to painful stimuli. Her pulse is fast, and she is pale and sweating. The husband tells you she has a history of diabetes. Management of this patient would include:
   a. administering oral glucose
   b. placing the patient on her left side
   c. applying a cervical collar and backboard
   d. placing the patient on oxygen by cannula at 15 L/min

7. It is 2 AM. Parents called EMS to evaluate their sick child. Your patient is 3 years old. She had a cold but is only running a slight fever. Parents say the child usually is better during the day, but tonight the problem seems worse. As you enter the room, you hear a harsh, high-pitched sound with each of the child's inspirations. What you hear is:
   a. stridor
   b. crackles
   c. wheezing
   d. snoring

8. You also note that the child is hoarse and has an unusual cough that sounds like a "seal bark." Based on the child's signs and symptoms, you are most likely dealing with:
   a. croup
   b. epiglottitis
   c. asthma
   d. pneumonia

9. You attempt to place the child on oxygen, but she does not accept the mask. You try to calm her down, but each time you try to apply the mask she becomes very agitated. You should:
   a. leave the child off oxygen to avoid upsetting her
   b. restrain the child and administer the oxygen
   c. provide oxygen using a blow-by technique
   d. place a paper bag over the child's head and place oxygen tubing inside the bag

10. The patient is a 12-year-old boy who sustained a leg injury while playing soccer. Upon examination, you note the patient has a painful, swollen, deformed lower right leg. After applying a splint and moving the patient to the cot:
    a. lower the leg, and apply a heat pack to the injury site
    b. elevate the leg, and apply a heat pack to the injury site
    c. lower the leg, and apply a cold pack to the injury site
    d. elevate the leg, and apply a cold pack to the injury site

11. While transporting, the EMTs should:
    a. obtain a pulse and blood pressure every 10 minutes
    b. position the patient in the recovery position
    c. recheck pulses, motor function, and neurological function
    d. position the patient's leg so that it is lower than his body

12. You are dispatched for a sick child having a seizure. Upon arrival, you find a 2-year-old girl lying on the living room couch. Her mother tells you a 103° F temperature developed relatively quickly. The child has no history of seizures. This seizure was most likely:
    a. a febrile seizure
    b. due to a head injury
    c. a petit mal seizure
    d. due to low blood sugar

13. The EMTs should:
    a. perform an alcohol rub down
    b. have the parents monitor the child and call back if another seizure occurs
    c. transport the child to a hospital for evaluation
    d. place the child in a cool bath

14. You have been summoned to the local shopping mall to examine a pregnant female experiencing an "unknown problem." She is pale, her pulse is rapid, and she is complaining of severe, localized abdominal pain. She is in her eighth month of pregnancy. Physical examination reveals steady bleeding from the vagina. The bleeding most likely indicates:
    a. a meconium emergency
    b. premature labor
    c. postpartum hemorrhage
    d. a problem with the placenta

15. At this time, your major concern is that the patient:
    a. may have a breech delivery
    b. is experiencing hypovolemic shock
    c. is likely to have seizures during transport
    d. may have a miscarriage

16. You are summoned in the morning to check on a patient injured in a "previous" auto crash. After arriving at the scene, you find the crash occurred late last evening. Your patient is a 16-year-old male with no significant medical history who seems disoriented and at times does not respond to verbal stimuli. When he is able to answer your questions, his replies are inappropriate. Family members tell you the accident occurred just down the road and he walked home. They advise you that, at the time, he seemed to be more concerned that he could not afford car repairs than with any injuries he may have sustained. Your partner examines the car that is now in the driveway and notes a "spiderweb" pattern crack on the driver's side of the windshield. You suspect his altered mental status is most likely the result of:
    a. a head injury
    b. a diabetic emergency
    c. drinking alcohol
    d. seizure activity

17. The appropriate way to transport this patient is to:
    a. place him in a prone position on the ambulance cot
    b. apply a cervical collar and backboard prior to moving the patient
    c. place him in the recovery position on his left side in case he loses consciousness
    d. place him in the shock position

18. You are dispatched to a "sick person" at a local restaurant. Upon arrival, you find a female patient reclining in a booth. Friends say she was talking but suddenly became unresponsive. She is breathing and responds somewhat to verbal stimuli, but can only utter sounds. Upon examination you notice that she is unable to move her extremities on the left side, and her mouth tends to droop on the left side. She also appears to have difficulty swallowing. Her vital signs are within normal range. This patient should be transported:
    a. in a supine position
    b. in a prone position
    c. on her left side
    d. sitting upright

19. Based on the clinical presentation, you suspect the patient is likely experiencing:
    a. a myocardial infarction
    b. an allergic reaction to food
    c. seizure activity
    d. a stroke

20. A 54-year-old man is experiencing chest pain and difficulty breathing. The pain started after he had walked up three flights of stairs to his apartment, which was approximately 10 minutes prior to your being dispatched. The patient states the pain is mostly on the left side and feels like a tremendous pressure. The pain radiates down his left arm. You notice also that he is pale and diaphoretic. Part of your care may likely include:
   a. placing the patient on oxygen by cannula at 4 L/min
   b. assisting the patient to take nitroglycerin
   c. assisting the patient down the stairs to the cot
   d. transporting the patient on his back with his legs elevated

21. While reassessing the patient during transport, the patient advises you the pain is not getting any better. If anything, it is getting worse. On the way to the hospital, the EMT should be especially alert for:
   a. sudden cardiac arrest
   b. the development of hypoglycemia
   c. the sudden development of left-sided weakness
   d. an increase in difficulty breathing

22. It is a hot summer day and your unit is sent to a metal foundry for a "man down." Upon arrival you find a 22-year-old unresponsive male patient. His pulse is rapid, and he is flushed. His skin is hot and dry to the touch. Management of this patient would include:
   a. giving the patient cool water to drink
   b. covering the patient with a light blanket to prevent rapid heat loss
   c. applying cold packs to the armpits, neck, and groin
   d. washing the patient down with rubbing alcohol

23. The local high school has called your unit for a "sick" juvenile in the gymnasium. As you start your evaluation, you find your patient is conscious but is weak and somewhat confused. He is pale and is sweating, although his vital signs are normal. His friends tell you he skipped lunch to play basketball with them. Halfway into the game he became weak, sat down, and soon thereafter started to demonstrate signs of illness. The school nurse arrives with the patient's records and advises you that he does take insulin. You suspect:
   a. a drug overdose
   b. a head injury
   c. a diabetic emergency
   d. a heat emergency

24. An important aspect of care for this patient will most likely include:
   a. applying cold packs to cool the patient down
   b. administering oral glucose
   c. checking the patient's locker for illegal drugs
   d. placing the patient in the recovery position

25. The patient is a full-term pregnant female in labor. When you examine the vaginal area, you notice a section of the cord protruding from the vaginal opening. As part of your management, you may need to:
   a. tell the patient to push as hard as possible to assist with delivery
   b. use two gloved fingers to push the presenting part of the fetus away from the cord
   c. pull on the cord
   d. tell the patient to cross her legs and not to push

26. The patient should be transported:
   a. on her back with her buttocks elevated
   b. without using lights and siren
   c. on her left side with her head slightly elevated
   d. sitting upright

27. Proper care of the exposed umbilical cord includes:
    a. attempting to push the cord back into the birth canal
    b. wrapping the cord in a dry trauma dressing
    c. covering it with a moist, sterile dressing
    d. placing cord clamps on the exposed section

28. For the second time in the day, you are dispatched to a local retirement home. Your patient is 72 going on 32 and is very independent. She is not pleased that her neighbors summoned you, but she is obviously having a lot of difficulty breathing. She states she has been short of breath for about the past 4 hours, but did not want to bother anyone. She has no chest pain. Her pulse is 96 and irregular, her B/P is 144/82, and breathing rate is 26 and labored. When you listen to her chest, you note wheezing on both inspiration and expiration. Questioning about medical history reveals she has a history of emphysema. The correct way to administer oxygen to this patient is by:
    a. nonrebreather mask at 15 L/min
    b. nonrebreather mask at 3 L/min
    c. nasal cannula at 6 L/min
    d. nasal cannula at 3 L/min

29. It is a sunny fall day. The patient is a 9-year-old girl who was outside playing in the leaves with her friends when she experienced difficulty breathing. Her parents tell you that she has a history of asthma, but this attack seems much worse than others. When listening to breath sounds, you hear pronounced wheezing, primarily on expiration. Part of the management of this patient may include:
    a. administering epinephrine
    b. inserting a nasopharyngeal airway
    c. ventilating the patient with a bag-valve-mask
    d. assisting with a prescribed inhaler

30. This incident was likely precipitated by:
    a. an emotional stress
    b. an allergic reaction
    c. an infection
    d. a drop in the patient's blood sugar level

31. If this patient's parents were not available to give permission to aid and transport the patient, the EMTs:
    a. could transport but only if a police officer placed the child in protective custody
    b. could aid and transport under the law of implied consent
    c. would have to wait to transport until another blood relative could be contacted
    d. could transport but could not give oxygen or perform any other aid without parental consent

32. Upon reassessing the patient, you notice the wheezes have disappeared but the patient still appears to be in distress. At this point, you suspect:
    a. the patient is now not moving enough air to cause wheezing
    b. the patient's condition has improved
    c. the carbon dioxide level in the patient's bloodstream has become too high
    d. pulmonary edema is developing

33. Your unit is called to a feed store for a person injured in the storeroom. Your patient is a 15-year-old teenager who was moving inventory when a shelf containing unmarked bags of dry powder fell over. Many of the bags have burst, and your patient is covered with the unknown powder. He is complaining of nausea, abdominal cramps, and moderate difficulty breathing. While performing your examination, you notice that he is sweating and salivating profusely, and his eyes are watery. There is some uncontrolled muscle twitching present. You suspect his problems to be related to:
    a. shock
    b. head injury
    c. chemical poisoning
    d. seizures

34. Early management of the patient would include:
    a. brushing off as much powder as possible and washing off the rest
    b. placing the patient in shock position and conserving body heat
    c. wiping off the powder with a damp rag
    d. wrapping the patient in a plastic sheet

35. You are called to a bar and find a patient with multiple stab wounds to the chest. The knife is still in place. The EMT should:
    a. remove the knife since it may interfere with breathing
    b. apply pressure to the knife to help control bleeding
    c. leave the knife in place and stabilize it with a bulky dressing
    d. place cold packs around the knife blade

36. The other chest wounds should be:
    a. covered only if bleeding is severe
    b. covered with a loose, bulky dressing
    c. left uncovered to allow rapid evaluation by hospital personnel
    d. covered with an occlusive dressing

37. Your patient is a 39-year-old male who has been experiencing persistent abdominal pain for the previous 12 hours with no relief. He has a history of alcoholism but takes no medications. He states he has been vomiting and that it "looks funny." You notice the vomitus in a trash can, and it resembles coffee grounds His abdomen is generally tender. Vital signs reveal a slightly rapid pulse and breathing, but blood pressure is normal. You suspect this patient has:
    a. alcohol poisoning
    b. gastrointestinal bleeding
    c. appendicitis
    d. cardiac compromise

38. The patient states that he is extremely thirsty. You should:
    a. avoid giving the patient anything by mouth
    b. give the patient water, but less than one cup
    c. encourage the patient to drink as much as possible to replenish lost fluids
    d. allow the patient to take a drink, but only if the liquids are at room temperature

39. A patient is in active labor. Upon your arrival, you follow all the local protocols for handling imminent delivery. Everything seems to be going routinely, but immediately after moving your patient to the cot, her bag of waters breaks. You notice that the fluid is thick and resembles pea soup. You become concerned because you are now dealing with a:
    a. breech delivery
    b. meconium emergency
    c. preeclampsia emergency
    d. prepartum hemorrhage

40. If the baby is delivered before reaching the hospital, your primary action should be to:
    a. immediately cut the cord
    b. immediately calculate an APGAR score
    c. monitor the mother for seizures
    d. aggressively suction the baby's airway

41. You are called to a construction site for a person with a leg injury. You find a 19-year-old man who was struck in the leg by a steel beam. His mid-thigh is painful, swollen, and deformed. Co-workers state he immediately fell to the ground after being struck, but he denies hitting his head or having any neck or back pain. The splint of choice for managing this injury is a:
    a. pneumatic splint
    b. traction splint
    c. soft splint
    d. ladder splint

42. A major concern with this type of extremity injury is:
    a. there is a high incidence of infection
    b. it may become a closed injury
    c. serious blood loss
    d. amputation below the injury is often indicated

43. The patient is a 72-year-old male who complains of back pain that became increasingly worse since yesterday. He tells you that he was weeding his garden and thinks he "just pulled something." His friends called EMS in spite of his objections. He does not want to go to the hospital. You should:
    a. explain the possible consequences of his action and allow him to sign a refusal if he still does not want to go
    b. restrain the patient and take him to a hospital since he may cause further harm to himself
    c. tell him you are obligated by law to transport him since an ambulance was called
    d. request a police officer to arrest the patient, at which time you may transport without his consent

44. You arrive at the scene of a single-car crash and find the patient has already been removed from the car by bystanders. He is standing and complains of neck and back pain. A check of the car reveals a "spiderweb" crack pattern to the windshield. Your partners have already placed a cervical collar on the patient. The best way to place this patient onto your ambulance cot is to:
    a. place a backboard on the cot and have the patient sit down on the board
    b. place a short backboard on the patient then have him lie down on the stretcher
    c. perform an emergency move to place him on the cot as quickly as possible
    d. place a backboard on the patient while he is still standing, then move him

45. A 6-year-old boy was discovered at the bottom of the community swimming pool located next door to your station. The lifeguards have been doing CPR for approximately 3 minutes prior to your arrival. Your first actions would include:
    a. attaching the patient to an automated external defibrillator
    b. assessing the adequacy of the CPR being performed
    c. performing abdominal thrusts on the patient
    d. ventilating the patient with a flow-restricted, oxygen-powered ventilation device

46. A critical part of the management of this patient involves:
    a. administering oxygen via cannula
    b. administering glucose since the patient is unconscious
    c. placing the patient on a backboard
    d. leaving the automated external defibrillator on during transport

47. The fire department has removed a man from a burning garage. Upon discovering the fire, the man went through a side door and attempted to open the garage door to remove an antique car. The man is conscious and obviously upset at the firefighters for not allowing him to remove the car. As you examine the patient, you notice what appears to be soot or burns around his mouth or nose. The patient is coughing, and his sputum appears to have black particles mixed with it. As he answers some of your questions, he sounds hoarse. He does not want to go to the hospital. You feel he may have:
    a. a diabetic emergency
    b. a closed head injury
    c. an allergic reaction to the smoke
    d. respiratory tract burns

48. Your management of this patient would include:
    a. administering oxygen for 15 minutes and advising him to see his doctor as soon as possible
    b. having him sign a witnessed refusal form and returning to the station
    c. explaining the complications associated with his problem, and strongly recommending that he go the hospital to be examined
    d. forcibly restraining him and transporting him to the hospital

49. Your unit is sent to the scene of a person who has fallen down a flight of steps at a college dormitory. The patient is a 20-year-old male who fell approximately three-quarters of the way down a long flight of steps. The patient is unconscious and lying on his back at the bottom landing. The patient is assessed, and no external bleeding is noted. Your primary concern is that this patient may:
    a. have a spinal injury
    b. have a history of seizures
    c. be hyperglycemic
    d. be faking unconsciousness

50. Assessment of the patient reveals he has a blood pressure of 76/40 and a weak, regular pulse with a rate of 64. He is not cool or clammy to the touch. You suspect he is suffering from:
    a. psychogenic shock
    b. neurogenic shock
    c. anaphylactic shock
    d. septic shock

51. You are dispatched to the city park for a person with difficulty breathing. Upon arriving, you encounter a distraught 19-year-old girl who has been stung by a bee. She is complaining of diffuse itching and a tightness in her throat and chest. Physical examination reveals a generalized rash accompanied by hives and a weak, rapid pulse. Wheezing is noted when you listen to the chest. This patient is experiencing:
    a. cardiac compromise
    b. hyperventilation syndrome
    c. an allergic reaction
    d. a diabetic emergency

52. You note that the stinger is still imbedded in your patient's arm. You should:
    a. remove the stinger with a pair of tweezers
    b. leave the stinger in place
    c. cover the stinger with a cold pack
    d. scrape the stinger out using the edge of a card

53. Management of this patient may include assisting with administration of:
    a. oral glucose
    b. epinephrine
    c. activated charcoal
    d. nitroglycerin

54. Before assisting with this particular medication, it is important to check:
    a. the medication's date of manufacture
    b. to be sure that the patient is not allergic to the medication
    c. the expiration date of the medication
    d. the name of the doctor who prescribed the medication

55. Your patient is an 82-year-old woman with severe difficulty breathing. As you enter the house, you hear gurgling breathing from the back bedroom. She is sitting upright in bed and coughing up frothy sputum. When you listen to her chest, you hear wet breath sounds. She has difficulty speaking, but denies any pain. You notice her neck veins are distended, and examination of her ankles and feet reveal marked swelling. This patient should be transported:
    a. supine with high-flow oxygen
    b. sitting upright with high-flow oxygen
    c. laying flat with oxygen via cannula
    d. in a position of comfort with low-flow oxygen

56. You are called to the scene of a chainsaw accident. A 31-year-old man was working in a tree when the saw hit his thigh. His co-workers helped him out of the tree, but he is still bleeding profusely. The first attempts to control bleeding should be performed using:
    a. arterial pressure points
    b. a tourniquet
    c. venous pressure points
    d. direct pressure over the wound

57. If the initial attempts at controlling bleeding do not work, the EMT should next:
    a. apply pressure to venous pressure points
    b. place a cold pack over the wound
    c. apply a tourniquet to the leg
    d. apply pressure to arterial pressure points

58. It is the first cold day of winter. Along with the fire department, you respond to a call for a furnace explosion. The owner was asleep when he heard a loud bang in the basement and awoke to find smoke billowing from the heat registers. He was not burned or injured, but tells you he has a severe headache, nausea, and "feels real bad." He denies having felt that way before he went to bed. He was the sole occupant of the house. You suspect that the patient is suffering from:
    a. the flu
    b. a head bleed
    c. inhalation poisoning
    d. a nervous disorder

59. Initial management would include:
    a. administering high-flow oxygen
    b. applying a cervical collar
    c. placing the patient in Trendelenburg position
    d. cooling the patient

60. Your patient was recently released from the hospital after undergoing abdominal surgery. The patient had a coughing spell that caused his stitches to rupture. Upon your arrival you find part of the man's intestines protruding through the open incision. Management would include:
    a. replacing the organs in the abdominal cavity
    b. covering the organs with a moist, sterile dressing
    c. applying direct pressure on the organs to prevent internal bleeding
    d. covering the organs with a dry, sterile dressing

61. The patient should be transported:
    a. on his left side with his knees and hips flexed
    b. sitting up with his knees straight
    c. on his back with his knees and hips flexed
    d. on his right side with his knees and hips straight

62. It's another Friday night at the local high school football game. As usual, your team is losing. You and your partner are standing by at the game trying to make the best of the last 10 minutes before returning to the station when spectators nearby start yelling that someone has "passed out." It takes you only about a minute to reach a 58-year-old man who is in cardiac arrest. Your first action is to:
    a. attach the patient to an automated external defibrillator
    b. begin two-rescuer CPR
    c. administer oxygen
    d. insert an oral airway

63. Despite your efforts, the man remains in cardiac arrest. Removing this patient from the stands is best accomplished using a:
    a. stair chair
    b. backboard
    c. half backboard
    d. direct carry

64. You are dispatched to a possible behavioral emergency. When you enter the house, police are already on the scene arguing with a 43-year-old male. You notice the inside of the house has been demolished prior to your arrival. The patient tells you that foreign agents are trying to kill him by letting tarantulas loose in his house. From time to time the patient claims to see one going under a piece of overturned furniture. He also tells you that he is convinced that the agents operate out of the local hospital and that he is not going to be taken alive. Discussion with the patient's family reveals that he has a long history of behavioral problems and he has not been taking his prescribed medication. He also has a history of violence. You should:
    a. offer to help the patient kill all the tarantulas if he goes with you to the hospital
    b. tell him you are just taking him to see his family doctor
    c. join the police in arguing with him about going to the hospital
    d. consider restraining the patient

65. You arrive at the scene of a call for a female patient experiencing chest pain. Your patient is complaining of substernal chest pain radiating to the left arm. She was cleaning her house when the pain started. She is on an unknown medication for high blood pressure but takes no other prescribed drugs. Her vital signs are normal and she complains of only minimal shortness of breath. Her husband has a history of heart problems, and she advises you that she has access to his "little white pills" that he puts under his tongue when he gets chest pain. Your actions should include:
    a. contacting medical direction for permission to assist the patient with taking her husband's nitroglycerin
    b. administering high-flow oxygen by nonrebreather mask
    c. connecting the patient to an automated external defibrillator
    d. contacting the patient's family doctor for further instructions

66. While returning from the hospital, you and your partner notice a crowd gathered on a downtown street corner. A man is lying on the ground actively seizing. Bystanders say he was jogging down the street when he suddenly fell to the sidewalk and starting to jerk violently. You notice blood coming from the vicinity of the left side of his head. Your first action in assisting the patient is to:
    a. protect him from further injury
    b. insert an oral airway
    c. control the bleeding from his scalp
    d. restrain him

67. After the seizure stops, the best course of action before transporting the patient to the hospital is to:
    a. place the patient in a supine position and monitor his airway
    b. place the patient directly on the ambulance cot on his side
    c. secure the patient to a backboard
    d. sit the patient upright

68. A 52-year-old male has gone into cardiac arrest while at work in a fabricating plant. He is currently one level above the main floor lying on a metal grate deck. Co-workers are doing CPR. A high priority in this situation is to:
    a. defibrillate the patient with an automated external defibrillator
    b. move the patient off of the metal decking
    c. insert a nasopharyngeal airway
    d. check for a blood pressure

69. A 26-year-old woman went into active labor at home. Just prior to your arrival, police advise you the baby has been born. When you reach the scene, you find a newborn who is limp and has a heart rate of 88. Your first action is to:
    a. begin ventilating the infant with 100% oxygen
    b. begin chest compressions
    c. position the baby on its left side
    d. administer oxygen by nonrebreather mask

70. When you reassess the newborn, you find the infant's heart rate has now dropped to 62. At this point, you should:
    a. ventilate the infant but not perform chest compressions
    b. attempt to stimulate the baby by flicking the soles of its feet
    c. begin chest compressions
    d. suction the infant

71. There has been a serious motor vehicle crash on the expressway. You and your partner have just removed an injured patient who is 7 months pregnant. Your assessment reveals that she has a pulse rate of 132 and a blood pressure of 82/58. During transport, it is best to position your patient:
    a. on her right side with her head slightly elevated
    b. flat on her back
    c. in a position of comfort
    d. on her left side

72. A man has been injured in a boiler explosion at a local factory. He has partial-thickness burns over 50% of his body. Your examination reveals that he has a pulse of 116 and a blood pressure of 90/68. The likely cause of the hypoperfusion is that:
    a. the patient has a spinal injury with accompanying neurogenic shock
    b. the patient has another serious injury causing blood loss
    c. a large volume of fluid has been lost through seepage from the burns
    d. hypothermia has developed due to heat loss through the area of the burn

73. It is mid-December. You and your partner respond to a report of an unconscious man in the park. You find a male who appears to be in his mid-40s lying on a park bench partly covered with newspapers. An almost empty alcohol bottle is next to the bench. You notice the patient is semi-responsive, has a slow breathing rate, and his extremities look cyanotic. The most likely probability is that this patient is:
    a. postictal
    b. suffering from a stroke
    c. hypothermic
    d. intoxicated

74. Treatment of the patient on the park bench would include:
    a. gently handling the patient when moving him to the ambulance
    b. trying to get the patient to drink warm fluids
    c. gently massaging the patient's arms and legs
    d. applying heat packs to the arms and legs

75. At 3:00 AM a local resident awoke when she heard the sound of metal hitting a solid object. A car has struck a large tree head on and now you and your crew must take care of the severely injured 23-year-old driver. He is unresponsive and was obviously unrestrained. The steering wheel of the car is severely bent. Your patient is having trouble breathing; his breathing is shallow and slow. He is also cyanotic. Based on your observations, your major concern is that this patient may:
    a. have suffered a pelvic fracture
    b. be experiencing a diabetic emergency
    c. have a serious chest injury
    d. be experiencing a severe asthma attack

76. Treatment of this patient would likely include:
    a. administering oxygen by nonrebreather mask
    b. supporting ventilations with a bag-valve-mask
    c. administering oxygen by nasal cannula
    d. inserting a nasopharyngeal airway

77. There has been an explosion at a local industry with reports of a man burned. On arrival, you find a 31-year-old male patient with burns on the front of his body that are red and blistered. He is complaining of severe pain. Referring to Figure 17-1, you calculate the approximate percentage of burned area to be:
    a. 9% to 13%
    b. 16% to 18%
    c. 22% to 24%
    d. 30% to 32%

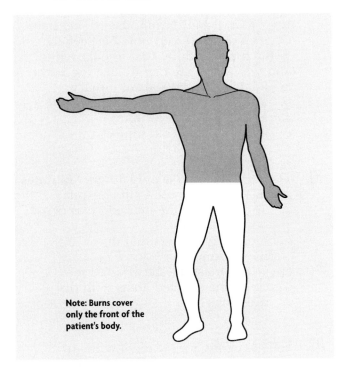

Note: Burns cover only the front of the patient's body.

Figure 17-1

78. Based on the description of the burns, you would classify them as:
    a. superficial
    b. partial thickness
    c. medium thickness
    d. full thickness

79. Based on the type, percentage, and location of the burns, this patient is considered to have a:
    a. minor burn
    b. superficial burn
    c. moderate burn
    d. critical burn

80. Your patient was stranded on a rural road when her car broke down in a freezing rainstorm. She was wearing only a pair of open-toed high-heel shoes and had to walk to a distant farmhouse to find help. On examination, you note her feet are cold to the touch and her toes appear white and waxy. You are mainly dealing with:
    a. a late or deep local cold injury
    b. a superficial local cold injury
    c. an early local cold injury
    d. a generalized cold injury

81. The local hospital is only about 9 minutes away. While en route to the hospital:
    a. apply heat to the injured areas of her feet and toes
    b. break any blisters that may have formed
    c. rub or massage the affected toes
    d. cover the affected areas with dry dressings

82. You are caring for a patient with an obvious head injury due to trauma. During your assessment, you note the patient has a blood pressure of 76/48 and pulse rate of 130 beats per minute. You should:
    a. position the patient on the right side with the head lower than the feet
    b. suspect other injuries or bleeding
    c. place the patient in a sitting position
    d. suspect a diabetic emergency

83. During your examination of a 4-year-old child experiencing breathing difficulty, you note wheezing on expiration. The wheezing is most likely caused by:
    a. throat inflammation
    b. upper airway obstruction
    c. constriction of the lower airways
    d. dilated bronchioles

84. Your patient is semi-conscious and having difficulty maintaining an airway but still has a gag reflex. The airway you would consider using is the:
    a. oropharyngeal airway
    b. nasopharyngeal airway
    c. Pharyngo-tracheal Lumen (PtL) airway
    d. endotracheal airway

85. Following delivery of a healthy infant, you prepare to cut the umbilical cord. The first clamp should be placed about:
    a. 4 inches from the mother
    b. 4 inches from the baby
    c. 10 inches from the mother
    d. 10 inches from the baby

86. Your patient has a history of violent behavioral problems and is extremely agitated. Your best course of management is to:
    a. approach the patient alone to gain his confidence
    b. surprise the patient and overpower him
    c. leave the patient for the police to deal with
    d. approach the patient only with backup assistance

87. You and your partner are dispatched to a middle-class residential neighborhood for a male patient with abdominal pain. The patient is reluctant to discuss his problem, but when questioning him about his recent medical history, he finally informs you that he has been vomiting what appears like coffee grounds. You suspect this patient has:
    a. appendicitis
    b. gastrointestinal bleeding
    c. diverticulitis
    d. gallbladder problems

88. A 38-year-old man got lost while out hunting. Upon examination, you find he has pale, cold, dry skin, and is shivering. He is alert and responding appropriately. Care for the patient would include:
    a. rewarming him by applying heat packs to the groin, armpits, and neck areas
    b. having him walk vigorously
    c. massaging his arms and legs to stimulate circulation
    d. giving him hot coffee or alcohol to drink

89. Your patient is a 16-year-old female who experienced a seizure while in bed. She is still unresponsive. Since your assessment reveals no reasons to suspect spinal injury, the position of choice when transporting this patient is:
    a. prone
    b. supine
    c. the recovery position
    d. the shock position

90. A young male patient is found in an alley. He is unresponsive, and his respirations are slow and shallow. Pulses are slow and weak. When assessing the patient, you note bruising around his eyes and behind his ears in the mastoid region. You suspect the patient has a:
    a. narcotics overdose
    b. history of diabetes
    c. skull injury
    d. seizure disorder

91. While transporting this patient, the EMT should be particularly alert for the development of:
    a. hypoglycemia
    b. seizures
    c. a myocardial infarction
    d. difficulty breathing

92. A high school student was accidentally hit in the head with a baseball bat during a practice game. He is bleeding from an area of what you suspect to be an open or depressed skull injury. The bleeding is best controlled by:
    a. applying firm pressure to the wound
    b. applying digital pressure to both carotid arteries
    c. packing the wound with gauze
    d. using a loose, bulky dressing

93. You have been ordered to assist a patient with the administration of nitroglycerin. Before administering the medication, the EMT should:
    a. verify the medication was prescribed by a local doctor
    b. check the patient's blood pressure
    c. assess capillary refill
    d. verify the pulse is greater than 100 beats per minute

94. Your patient has fallen from a roof. He has open fractures to both legs and an angulated fracture of the right forearm. His pulse is 132 beats per minute and his blood pressure is 76/58. Your best course of action is to:
    a. splint all injuries prior to moving the patient to prevent further blood loss
    b. perform full-body immobilization with a backboard and immediately transport
    c. splint only open musculoskeletal injuries prior to moving the patient
    d. quickly move the patient to the ambulance cot in whatever way necessary and rapidly transport

95. Your patient has a history of bronchitis and is complaining of shortness of breath and a productive cough that brings up thick, greenish mucus. While transporting, this patient should generally be placed:
    a. flat on his back
    b. on his left side
    c. in a position of comfort
    d. in Trendelenburg position

96. A 32-year-old female is found unconscious in a garage with a car still running. After ensuring personal safety, donning appropriate personal protective equipment, and reaching the patient, the first step in caring for her is to:
    a. apply a cervical collar and remove her on a backboard
    b. remove her from the hazardous environment
    c. determine the type of toxic gas involved
    d. open her airway and assess breathing

97. Your patient has a severe laceration to the forearm and direct pressure is not adequately controlling the bleeding. The pressure point of choice for controlling this patient's bleeding is over the:
    a. temporal artery
    b. popliteal artery
    c. brachial artery
    d. tibial artery

98. You encounter a 62-year-old male patient who is complaining of minor respiratory distress, a tight feeling in the throat, and itching. Your examination reveals some wheezing in the lungs and hives all over the patient's arms. You suspect this patient is experiencing:
    a. cardiac problems
    b. a drug overdose
    c. an allergic reaction
    d. a diabetic emergency

99. It may be appropriate to contact medical command for instructions regarding the management of this patient due to the fact that:
    a. the patient is over age 50
    b. the patient may need glucose
    c. toxic chemicals may be involved
    d. he may take nitroglycerin

100. While assessing a 65-year-old man who is complaining of shortness of breath, you hear wheezes. This means that the patient:
    a. must have asthma or COPD
    b. is hyperventilating
    c. may have fluid in his lungs from CHF or pneumonia causing the wheezing sound
    d. needs to cough

101. Your patient was working on his car when the battery blew up in his face. He has obvious chemical burns to his face and is complaining of burning in his eyes. The patient's eyes should be irrigated:
    a. with a neutralizing solution
    b. for not more than 15 minutes
    c. until the patient reaches the hospital
    d. only while on the scene of the incident

102. A 34-year-old male has had a finger amputated in an industrial accident. The proper way to package the finger for transportation to the hospital is to:
    a. pack it in ice
    b. wrap it in a sterile dressing and keep it cool
    c. immerse it in sterile water
    d. wrap it in a wet, sterile dressing and keep it warm

103. You are preparing to transport a child with a gastrostomy tube. The two positions in which the patient may be transported are:
    a. lying on the back, or lying on the left side with the head lower than the trunk
    b. in a position of comfort, or prone with the head lower than the trunk
    c. sitting, or lying on the right side with the head elevated
    d. supine, or prone with the head elevated

104. You and your partner are sent to evaluate a female patient experiencing a behavioral emergency. A sign that she may potentially become violent would be if she is:
    a. sitting on the edge of a seat
    b. lying on a bed or couch
    c. using monotone speech
    d. exhibiting open hands

105. While listening to the patient's chest, you hear the "wet" sounds of rales, which:
    a. are caused by fluid in the air sacs resulting from pneumonia
    b. are caused by the inability of the heart to handle the fluid being delivered to it, causing the fluid to "back up" into the lungs
    c. are due to swelling of the lower legs that is caused by the patient's drinking too much water
    d. indicates the patient needs to use his or her inhaler

106. A 24-year-old female patient admits to EMTs that she ingested approximately 50 aspirin tablets about 15 minutes ago. After consulting medical command, an order is given to a administer activated charcoal. The normal dose for this patient is:
    a. 12.5 to 25 grams
    b. 25 to 50 grams
    c. 50 to 75 grams
    d. 75 to 100 grams

107. Three 11-year-old boys were playing with a pile of tree limbs and brush, gasoline, and matches. One boy's t-shirt caught fire and burned completely off him before neighbors could come to his assistance and put the fire out. Referring to Figure 17-2, you calculate his percentage of burns to be:
    a. 14% to 16%
    b. 18% to 20%
    c. 24% to 26%
    d. 30% to 36%

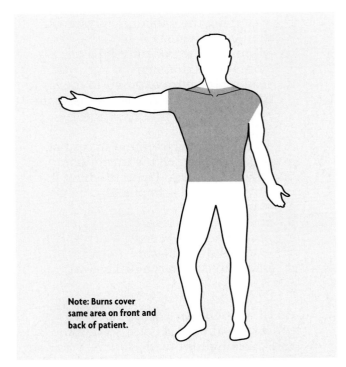

Note: Burns cover same area on front and back of patient.

Figure 17-2

108. When examining the burns, you notice that there are some burn areas that appear dry, white, and leathery. Based on this description, you would classify them as:
    a. superficial
    b. partial thickness
    c. moderate thickness
    d. full thickness

109. Based on the type, percentage, and location of the burns, this patient is considered to have a:
    a. minor burn
    b. superficial burn
    c. moderate burn
    d. critical burn

110. Management of these burns would include:
    a. covering the patient with clean, dry burn sheets
    b. wrapping the patient in moistened sterile bandages
    c. wrapping the patient with a non-porous dressing
    d. leaving the burn exposed to the air to allow heat in the tissues to dissipate

111. A 74-year-old male is found in cardiac arrest in his room on the third floor of an apartment building. Upon reaching the patient, your first action is to:
    a. start CPR
    b. check blood pressure
    c. attach the automated external defibrillator
    d. insert an oropharyngeal airway

112. As CPR continues, you opt to place an endotracheal tube. After inserting the tube and checking for breath sounds, you note that breath sounds are heard only on the right side. Your next action would be to:
    a. deflate the cuff, pull the airway out, and reattempt intubation
    b. deflate the cuff and pull the airway back slightly
    c. deflate the cuff and insert the airway slightly further into the lungs
    d. leave the airway in place and ventilate at a faster rate

113. The best way to move this patient is using a:
    a. stair chair
    b. bed sheet
    c. direct carry
    d. backboard

114. You are dispatched for a sick child with a high fever. Upon arrival, you find a 4-year-old female sitting on the edge of her bed. She is leaning slightly forward and drooling because she says it "hurts too much to swallow." Her mother tells you she started complaining of a sore throat just a short time earlier in the day and that she now has a 103° F temperature. You are concerned because you suspect the child may have:
    a. strep throat
    b. a foreign body airway obstruction
    c. epiglottitis
    d. meningitis

115. An important part of your management of this patient would be to:
    a. lay her flat on her back during transport
    b. avoid placing anything in her mouth or throat
    c. cool her off with towels soaked in tepid water
    d. examine her throat for signs of redness and swelling

ANSWERS TO CHAPTER 17 REVIEW QUESTIONS

1. **c.** The correct dose is 12.5 to 25 grams, or 1 gram per kilogram of body weight.

2. **b.** Prior to administering the charcoal, shake the container thoroughly. Do not lie to the child by saying it is candy. Also, do not put the charcoal in a glass because if the child sees the slurry, he may not be willing to drink it.

3. **c.** The order received over the telephone was an example of on-line medical direction.

4. **d.** The EMT should be alert for seizures.

5. **b.** This patient should be transported with her shoulders and head elevated.

6. **b.** The patient should be placed on her left side to facilitate drainage of secretions from her mouth. Because she is unresponsive, she should not be given oral glucose. Oxygen is indicated, but by nonrebreather mask at 15 L/min.

7. **a.** The sound is stridor, and it indicates an upper airway problem.

8. **a.** The child's signs and symptoms point toward the respiratory illness known as croup. Hoarseness, inspiratory stridor, "seal-bark" cough, and the fact that the child's condition gets worse at night are all clues that you are dealing with croup.

9. **c.** Because the child will not tolerate the oxygen mask, administer oxygen using a blow-by technique to enrich the air in the immediate vicinity of the child's mouth and nose.

10. **d.** After applying a splint, elevate the leg and apply cold packs to the area. This will help reduce swelling.

11. **c.** While transporting, the EMTs should regularly check pulses, motor function, and neurological function. Since the patient is stable, vital signs can be checked every 15 minutes. If possible, elevate the leg during transport.

12. **a.** The child has most likely suffered a febrile seizure.

13. **c.** The child should be taken to a hospital for evaluation. Although a febrile seizure is suspected, other causes should be ruled out by a doctor.

14. **d.** Vaginal bleeding that occurs during late pregnancy is usually associated with a problem with the placenta.

15. **b.** Looking at the clinical presentation of the patient, it is obvious she is developing hypovolemic shock. Although the life of the fetus is also a concern, if the mother dies, so might the fetus. Therefore, efforts should be focused on stabilizing the mother and transporting to an appropriate hospital.

16. **a.** The patient's altered mental status is most likely the result of a head injury that occurred in the auto crash. The "spiderweb" pattern on the windshield indicates that the patient's head struck the windshield.

17. **b.** The damage to the car, especially the "spider web" pattern cracks in the windshield, indicate a mechanism of injury consistent with cervical spine injury. Therefore, even though the patient has been up and walking around, it is appropriate to apply a cervical collar and transport the patient on a backboard.

18. **c.** Because the patient may be unable to protect her airway, she should be transported on her left side. This also allows her to move the unaffected extremities on her right side if her condition improves.

19. **d.** Although it must be confirmed at the hospital, this patient is displaying signs and symptoms consistent with those of a stroke. Recognizing this is important, since early treatment of stroke can make a significant difference in patient outcome. If possible, transport the patient to a hospital capable of providing cutting-edge evaluation and treatment of strokes.

20. **b.** If this patient has a prescription for nitroglycerin, you will probably be instructed to assist the patient in taking medication.

21. **a.** The EMT should be prepared to manage sudden cardiac arrest in this patient. It may be advisable to have an automated external defibrillator ready, as well as airway equipment.

22. **c.** This patient is experiencing a serious medical problem. Because rapid cooling is needed, cold packs should be applied to the armpits, neck, and groin area.

23. **c.** The patient is most likely experiencing a diabetic emergency.

24. **b.** Administration of oral glucose will probably be ordered.

25. **b.** Management of a prolapsed cord may include inserting two gloved fingers into the vagina to push the presenting part of the fetus away from the cord, thereby taking pressure of the cord.

26. **a.** Transport the patient on her back with the buttocks elevated, which will allow gravity to assist in taking some pressure off the cord. Because this is a true emergency situation, transport should be done using lights and sirens unless contraindicated by local protocols.

27. **c.** Proper care of the exposed umbilical cord includes covering it with a moist, sterile dressing.

28. **a.** This patient needs a lot of oxygen. Use a nonrebreather mask at 15 L/min.

29. **d.** Since this patient has a history of asthma, she may have a prescribed inhaler. If so, medical direction will probably order you to assist her in using it.

30. **b.** Since the patient was outside playing in leaves, it is most likely this incident was precipitated by an allergic reaction.

31. **b.** Even if the parents are not present, care and transport can proceed under the law of implied consent. A police officer need not be present.

32. **a.** When an asthma attack is severe, the patient may not be able to move enough air to cause wheezing. This is a bad sign because it indicates the patient may rapidly deteriorate and experience respiratory arrest.

33. **c.** This patient's problems are likely related to some sort of chemical poisoning.

34. **a.** Because the poison is entering the skin through absorption, it must be removed. Brush off as much of the chemical as possible, then wash off any remaining chemical with copious amounts of water. The patient's clothing should be removed. Wrapping the patient in a plastic sheet would keep the poison near the patient and allow continued absorption. Personnel treating the patient should also be careful not to become contaminated themselves.

35. **c.** The knife should be left in place and stabilized with a bulky dressing.

36. **d.** The other chest wounds should be covered with occlusive dressings.

37. **b.** This patient is presenting signs of gastrointestinal bleeding.

38. **a.** Although the patient is extremely thirsty, give no fluids by mouth because the patient may need to go into surgery. Even if he does not, the fluids may worsen the nausea.

39. **b.** Discharge of amniotic fluid that resembles thick, green pea soup indicates a meconium emergency.

40. **d.** Aggressive suctioning is a must. Pay particularly close attention to the baby's airway to keep the meconium from entering the lungs.

41. **b.** This type of musculoskeletal injury is best managed with a traction splint. A traction splint should not be used, however, if the injury is close to the knee or hip; if a partial amputation or avulsion with bone separation is present; or if the ankle, lower leg, knee, or pelvis is also injured.

42. **c.** A femur injury of this type can result in severe blood loss. The injury is already a closed injury, but mismanagement may turn it into an open injury.

43. **a.** Rational adult patients have the right to refuse any or all care. Thorough documentation is important whenever a patient refuses transport.

44. **d.** This patient should be backboarded while standing. Although he was moving around at the scene, a spinal injury may still be present.

45. **b.** Upon arrival, assess the adequacy of the CPR being performed. This patient is too young for the automated external defibrillator or flow-restricted, oxygen-powered ventilation device. Abdominal thrusts are not indicated in the initial management of all drowning patients.

46. **c.** Since it cannot be determined that the incident is not related to a diving accident, the EMTs must assume a neck injury may be present. Therefore, the patient must be transported on a backboard with a cervical collar in place.

47. **d.** The patient probably has respiratory tract burns. Signs include a history of being in an enclosed fire area, soot or burns around mouth and nose, coughing accompanied by black particles in the sputum, and hoarseness.

48. **c.** Explain the potential complications and strongly recommend that the patient go to the hospital. Also, administer high-flow oxygen for as long as possible.

49. **a.** The patient's presentation strongly suggests the possibility of spinal injury.

50. **b.** Neurogenic shock is associated with spinal injuries. Damage to the spinal cord produces dilation of the blood vessels, which causes the "container" to be too large for the normal amount of blood in the system. The patient will present with low blood pressure, but the pulse rate remains normal and the typical signs of cool, clammy skin are not present.

51. **c.** The patient is experiencing an allergic reaction. Clues include a bee sting, diffuse itching, tightness in the throat and chest, rash and hives, a rapid pulse, and wheezing.

52. **d.** Scrape the stinger out using the edge of a card or something similar. Using tweezers may force more poison into the wound. Do not leave the stinger in place, as muscles around the poison sac may continue to constrict, thereby forcing more poison into the patient.

53. **b.** Treatment of this patient may include administering epinephrine.

54. **c.** Check the expiration date of the epinephrine before administering it. There are no contraindications to using epinephrine in a life-threatening situation.

55. **b.** The patient has fluid in her lungs and should be transported sitting upright to allow gravity to keep the upper lungs as clear as possible. She also needs as much oxygen as possible.

56. **d.** Initial attempts at controlling bleeding should include applying direct pressure to the wound area.

57. **d.** If the bleeding cannot be controlled with direct pressure, pressure can be applied to an arterial pressure point. In this case, it would be the femoral artery.

58. **c.** This patient is most likely suffering from poisoning by inhalation.

59. **a.** This patient should immediately be given 15 L/min of oxygen by nonrebreather mask.

60. **b.** Management of an evisceration includes covering the organs with a moist, sterile dressing.

61. **c.** The patient should be transported on his back with the hips and knees flexed.

62. **a.** Early defibrillation is the key in managing this patient. If an automated external defibrillator is readily available, defibrillation takes priority over airway and CPR. If two EMTs are present, one can start one-rescuer CPR while the other connects the automated external defibrillator.

63. **b.** While moving the patient, CPR needs to be continued as much as possible. This is best accomplished by moving the patient using a long backboard.

64. **d.** Due to the violent nature of this patient's behavior, restraints will probably be needed to protect him and the rescuers. Do not argue with or lie to the patient, and do not go along with his hallucinations.

65. **b.** High-flow oxygen should be administered. Because she does not have her own prescription for nitroglycerin, she should not be assisted in taking the drug.

66. **a.** Your first action in assisting the patient is to protect him from injury. The violent, uncontrolled jerking associated with seizures can cause the patient to harm himself. It may be necessary to place padding between the patient and any hard objects while the seizure runs its course. It will be impossible to obtain an accurate blood pressure while the patient is seizing. Also, do not attempt to place anything in the patient's mouth while seizures are still actively occurring.

67. **c.** Since it is known that this patient fell to the ground, and since he has sustained a head laceration in the fall, the EMT must suspect a neck injury. Appropriate packaging of the patient includes applying a cervical collar and placing him on a backboard. If the patient remains unresponsive and secretions in the mouth cause potential for airway compromise, the backboard can be tilted to one side to allow secretions to drain. Suction should also be readily available.

68. **b.** A high priority in this case is to remove the patient from the metal decking in order to defibrillate the patient if appropriate. Defibrillating the patient while he is still on the metal decking can cause injury to the rescuers.

69. **a.** A heart rate of less than 100 beats per minute in a newborn is not adequate. Since slow heart rates are often associated with hypoxia, the baby should be ventilated with 100% oxygen. This will often help to improve the heart rate.

70. **c.** Any time a newborn infant's heart rate is below 60 beats per minute, or the heart rate remains between 60 and 80 beats per minute despite ventilations, the baby should be ventilated and chest compressions should be started.

71. **d.** This patient should be transported on her left side to relieve pressure on the vena cava and abdominal organs. The patient should still be secured on a backboard, but the board and patient can be tilted as a unit to avoid compromising spinal immobilization.

72. **b.** The most likely cause of hypoperfusion in this patient is hypovolemia due to other injuries. Burns, even those that cover a rather large area of the body, do not cause a rapid development of hypoperfusion and shock. Since burns look serious, they can often cause an EMT to overlook other less obvious but more severe injuries. A thorough patient examination and assessment will minimize the possibility of missing other injuries.

73. **c.** This patient is most likely hypothermic. Alcohol ingestion can especially predispose a patient to hypothermia, as can the use of drugs and various medical conditions.

74. **a.** Severely hypothermic patients should be handled gently. Rough handling can send cold, acidotic blood that has pooled in the extremities to the patient's core and cause ventricular fibrillation. Massaging the arms and legs or applying heat packs or hot water bottles to the extremities can do the same. Patients who are not responsive should not be given anything to drink.

75. **c.** Based on the mechanism of injury and the patient's signs and symptoms, your patient most likely has a serious chest injury. These patients are at high risk of experiencing cardiac arrest and need to be seen as quickly as possible at a trauma center.

76. **b.** Since this patient is cyanotic and has slow, shallow breathing, you must support ventilations using a bag-valve-mask.

77. **c.** Using the rule of nines for adults, the percentage of burns for this patient is approximately 22% to 24%. The fronts of the arms are approximately 4.5% each, the front of the chest is approximately 9%, and the front of the face is 4.5%.

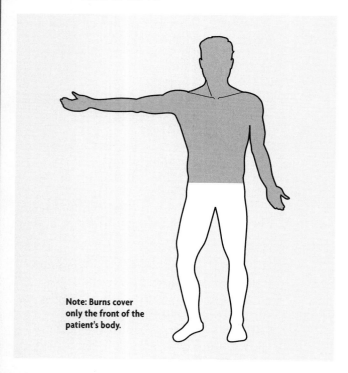

Note: Burns cover only the front of the patient's body.

Figure 17-1

78. **b.** A burn characterized by reddened skin, blister formation, and intense pain is classified as a partial-thickness burn.

79. **d.** Based on the percentage of burns and the fact that the patient's face and hands are involved, these burns would be considered critical.

80. **a.** This patient is suffering a late or deep local cold injury.

81. **d.** The patient's injured areas should be protected by covering them with dry dressings. Do not massage the areas and do not break any blisters that may have formed. In most cases, the injured parts should not be rewarmed. Always follow local protocols regarding management of late or deep local cold injuries including frostbite.

82. **b.** In any patient with a serious head injury who presents with low blood pressure and a rapid pulse, the EMT should suspect other injuries or bleeding. Such patients are of high priority and should be evaluated in a trauma center.

83. **c.** Wheezing is a result of constriction of the lower airways. In children, it is often associated with asthma or bronchiolitis.

84. **b.** Patients in need of an airway but who still have a gag reflex present are best managed using a nasopharyngeal airway.

85. **b.** The first clamp should be placed approximately 4 inches, or four finger-widths, from the infant. The second clamp is placed approximately 2 inches away from the first clamp on the side closer to the placenta.

86. **d.** When a violent patient is encountered, the best course is to approach the patient only with backup assistance, preferably from police. Since the patient may also be in need of medical care, EMS personnel should not leave the patient for police to deal with. This may be considered abandonment.

87. **b.** In a patient who is vomiting "coffee-ground" emesis, gastrointestinal bleeding should be suspected.

88. **a.** Since the patient is alert and responding appropriately, active rewarming may be accomplished using warm blankets, and/or by applying heat packs to the groin, armpits, and neck area. Always follow local protocols concerning the management of generalized cold exposure patients.

89. **c.** In the absence of spinal injuries, seizure patients may be transported in the recovery position, that is, lying on the left side.

90. **c.** Bruising around the eyes or behind the ears is indicative of a serious skull injury.

91. **b.** When transporting a patient with a severe head injury, the EMT should always be prepared to manage seizures should they develop.

92. **d.** Bleeding from an open or depressed skull injury is best controlled by using a loose, bulky dressing.

93. **b.** Prior to assisting a patient with taking nitroglycerin, it is important to check the blood pressure to ensure that it is greater than 100 mm Hg systolic.

94. **b.** Although this patient needs to get to a trauma center as quickly as possible, spinal immobilization still must be performed. Your best course of action is to perform full-body immobilization with a backboard and then rapidly transport to the closest appropriate facility.

95. **c.** Patients experiencing breathing difficulty are generally best transported in a position of comfort. This will normally be in a sitting position.

96. **b.** Although assessing the airway and breathing are important, the patient should be removed from the hazardous environment and placed in a safe area prior to starting an assessment.

97. **c.** Pressure should be applied to the brachial artery, which supplies blood to the arm.

98. **c.** Based on the patient's signs and symptoms, he is most likely experiencing an allergic reaction.

99. **a.** Although there is no age limit for using epinephrine in a severe allergic reaction, there are potential complications associated with its use in older patients. This includes the potential for causing a heart attack. Therefore, contacting medical control before giving epinephrine to patients over 50 years of age may be wise.

100. **c.** All that wheezes is not asthma. Any fluid collection in the airways may narrow them sufficiently to cause the sound of wheezing. Congestive heart failure may cause wheezing, which is often called "cardiac asthma." Coughing will not alleviate wheezing, and hyperventilation does not cause wheezing.

101. **c.** The patient's eyes should be irrigated until the patient reaches the hospital.

102. **b.** Generally, the proper way to package an amputated finger for transportation to the hospital is to wrap the finger in a sterile dressing and keep it cool. Do not immerse it in water, moisten it, or pack it in ice as this can cause tissue damage. Always follow local protocols regarding packaging of amputated body parts.

103. **c.** Children with gastrostomy tubes should normally be transported either sitting or lying on the right side with the head elevated.

104. **a.** Sitting on the edge of her seat may be a signal that the patient is posturing herself for action that may become violent. Potentially violent patients may also appear agitated; they may pace or be unable to sit still; speak loudly and quickly; and clinch their fists. Obtaining a thorough history may also reveal that the patient has displayed violent behavior in the past.

105. **b.** In congestive heart failure, the heart is unable to effectively pump the blood being supplied to it from the body and the lungs. The pressure of the blood backing up in the lungs forces the water (serum) it contains out of the vessels and into the alveoli. Pneumonia causes the pus in the bronchioles to make the sound of rhonchi, and inhalers are indicated for wheezing from bronchospasm.

106. **b.** The normal dose of activated charcoal for an adult patient is 25 to 50 grams, or 1 mg/kg.

107. **d.** Using the rule of nines for children, the front and back of the torso are 18% each. Considering the boy's t-shirt covered most of his torso, you calculate the patient's percentage of burns to be 30% to 36%.

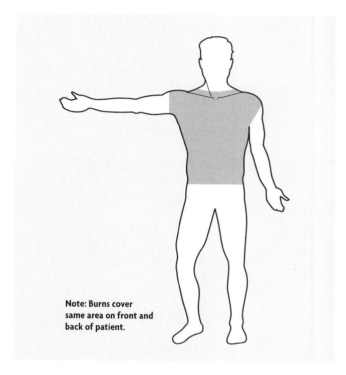

Note: Burns cover same area on front and back of patient.

Figure 17-2

108. **d.** Burns that appear as dry, white, leathery skin, or are charred black or brown, are classified as full-thickness burns.

109. **d.** Based on the percentage of burns and the fact that the burns are circumferential, that is, they encircle the torso, these burns would be considered critical.

110. **a.** The burns should be covered with a clean, dry burn sheet. Wet dressings should be avoided because the percentage of burn area is so large that covering them with wet dressings can cause hypothermia. Leaving the burn exposed to the air will increase the pain and chances for infection.

111. **c.** The first action upon reaching a patient experiencing cardiac arrest is to attach an automated external defibrillator if it is available.

112. **b.** If breath sounds are heard only on the right side, deflate the cuff and pull the airway back slightly until lung sounds are heard on both sides.

113. **d.** Since hallways and stairs or an elevator will have to be negotiated, and since CPR must continue if the patient does not regain a pulse, it is best to immobilize the patient on a backboard to move him to the ambulance.

114. **c.** This child probably has epiglottitis. With epiglottitis, the child's epiglottis swells and can totally obstruct the airway. Clues include a relatively rapid onset of a high fever, sore throat with reluctance to swallow, and that she is sitting forward and drooling.

115. **b.** Avoid placing anything in the child's mouth or throat, such as a tongue depressor to examine the throat, since this may cause complete obstruction of the airway by the swollen epiglottis.

18

100-Question Practice Test

1. You are caring for a patient with an obvious head injury due to trauma. During your assessment, you note the patient has a low blood pressure and rapid pulse. You should:
   a. position the patient on the right side with the head lower than the feet
   b. suspect other injuries or bleeds
   c. place the patient in a sitting position
   d. suspect a diabetic emergency

2. A patient with a minor injury, such as an ankle injury, should receive:
   a. an initial assessment followed by a focused history and physical exam
   b. an initial assessment only
   c. a detailed assessment only
   d. a focused history and physical exam followed by a detailed assessment

3. An EMT would perform an emergency move when:
   a. the patient's condition may deteriorate
   b. there are not enough EMTs present to properly move the patient
   c. there is an immediate threat to the life of the patient
   d. maximum control of the spine is needed

4. Bleeding that spurts with each heartbeat and is bright red in color is characteristic of:
   a. arterial bleeding
   b. primary bleeding
   c. venous bleeding
   d. consecutive bleeding

5. Your patient was stranded in freezing weather when her car broke down. To manage her late or deep cold injuries:
   a. apply heat to the injured areas
   b. break any blisters that may have formed
   c. rub or massage the affected areas
   d. cover the areas with dry dressings

6. During your examination of a 4-year-old child experiencing breathing difficulty, you note wheezing on expiration. You suspect this is linked to:
   a. throat inflammation
   b. upper airway obstruction
   c. lower airway disease
   d. dilated bronchioles

7. Your patient is semi-conscious and having difficulty maintaining an airway but still has a gag reflex. The airway you would consider using is the:
   a. oropharyngeal airway
   b. nasopharyngeal airway
   c. Pharyngeo-tracheal Lumen (PtL) airway
   d. endotracheal airway

8. Contraindication refers to:
   a. the way a medication affects the human body
   b. a side effect of a certain medication
   c. a medication that acts in an opposite way when administered with a different drug
   d. a situation in which a medication should not be administered because it may cause harm

9. Following delivery of a healthy infant, you prepare to cut the umbilical cord. The first clamp should be placed about:
   a. 4 inches from the mother
   b. 4 inches from the baby
   c. 10 inches from the mother
   d. 10 inches from the baby

10. After taking body substance isolation precautions, the first step in controlling bleeding is:
    a. placing the patient in shock position
    b. applying direct pressure
    c. applying digital pressure on an artery
    d. applying cold packs

11. The exchange of gases within the lungs takes place in the:
    a. bronchi
    b. pleural space
    c. alveoli
    d. trachea

12. Your patient has a history of violent behavioral problems and is extremely agitated. Your best course of management is to:
    a. approach the patient alone to gain his confidence
    b. surprise the patient and overpower him
    c. threaten the patient with physical harm if he becomes violent
    d. approach the patient only with backup assistance

13. A pedestrian has been struck by a car and is in shock. As part of the care rendered, the EMT should:
    a. control bleeding after ensuring an airway and breathing
    b. administer oxygen after splinting fractures
    c. apply heating pads or hot water bottles to warm the patient
    d. check vital signs every 15 minutes

14. The method used to determine which size oral airway to insert is to measure from the:
    a. Adam's apple to the corner of the mouth
    b. earlobe to the corner of the mouth
    c. angle of the jaw to the Adam's apple
    d. angle of the jaw to the clavicle

15. An EMT should insert fingers into a pregnant patient's vagina:
    a. to support the baby's head during delivery
    b. to assist the delivery of the shoulders
    c. only in the case of a breech delivery or prolapsed cord
    d. to check the baby's pulse in the case of a meconium emergency

16. An adult patient who is not breathing but has a pulse should be ventilated at a rate of once every:
    a. 3 to 4 seconds
    b. 4 to 5 seconds
    c. 5 to 6 seconds
    d. 6 to 10 seconds

17. A patient who is vomiting "coffee-ground" emesis should be suspected of having:
    a. appendicitis
    b. gastrointestinal bleeding
    c. diverticulitis
    d. gallbladder problems

18. Your male patient is hypothermic but is alert and responding appropriately. Care for the patient would include:
    a. having him walk vigorously
    b. massaging his arms and legs to stimulate circulation
    c. rewarming him by applying heat packs to the groin, armpits, and neck area
    d. giving him hot coffee or alcohol to drink

19. You and your partners have returned from a run involving a SIDS patient. If a Critical Incident Stress Debriefing is desired, it should take place:
    a. 1 to 2 weeks from the incident
    b. within a month of the incident
    c. no later than 24 hours after the incident
    d. within 24 to 72 hours after the incident

20. When a bone injury without distal pulses is encountered:
    a. realign the injury using gentle traction
    b. never straighten the injury
    c. realign the injury while pushing on the limb
    d. splint the injury with a traction splint

21. When using the mnemonic S-A-M-P-L-E, the letter *E* refers to:
    a. how long it took "EMS" to arrive
    b. whether the problem is a true "emergency"
    c. the "events" leading up to the injury or illness
    d. whether the patient was "extricated"

22. A nasal cannula may be used when:
    a. the patient complains of drying of the mouth
    b. the patient will not tolerate a nonrebreather mask
    c. pressure in the oxygen tank is low
    d. the patient is breathing primarily through the nose

23. Blood is pumped to the body by the:
    a. left atrium
    b. left ventricle
    c. right atrium
    d. right ventricle

24. When performing an assessment of a child, the most important thing is the:
    a. patient's pulse rate
    b. parent's general reactions
    c. patient's blood pressure
    d. EMT's general impression of the patient

25. Proper lifting should be performed using the:
    a. arms while keeping the feet as far apart as possible
    b. legs while keeping the feet shoulder-width apart
    c. waist while keeping the feet together
    d. back while keeping the feet shoulder-width apart

26. When using a nonrebreather mask, the proper oxygen flow rate is:
    a. 3 L/min if there is a history of breathing difficulty
    b. 6 L/min if the patient will not tolerate high flow
    c. 9 L/min if the patient complains of dry mouth and nose
    d. 15 L/min in all cases

27. A patient has just depressed her handheld inhaler and begins to inhale deeply. Immediately after the medication has been delivered, instruct the patient to:
    a. hold her breath
    b. exhale forcefully
    c. cough vigorously
    d. swallow

28. A wound characterized by irregular, jagged edges is:
    a. an avulsion
    b. a laceration
    c. an amputation
    d. an abrasion

29. EMTs should wear eye protection:
    a. whenever patients with infectious disease are encountered
    b. only if the EMT is susceptible to eye infections
    c. if the EMT has recently been ill
    d. in situations where blood splatter may occur

30. During your assessment, you decide you are dealing with a priority patient. Your action would be to:
    a. call an ALS unit for assistance and wait at the scene for its arrival
    b. immediately transport to a hospital of the patient's choosing
    c. call medical control and request further instructions for on-scene management
    d. expedite transport to an appropriate medical facility

31. An 18-year-old male has been involved in a fight and now has a knife protruding from his abdomen. Management of the impaled object would include:
    a. stabilizing the object with a bulky dressing
    b. applying pressure to the object for bleeding control
    c. removing the object immediately
    d. packing ice around the object

32. Your patient is a 16-year-old female who experienced a seizure while sitting on the couch. She is still unresponsive. Since your assessment reveals no reasons to suspect spinal injury, the position of choice for this patient is:
    a. prone
    b. supine
    c. in the recovery position
    d. in shock position

33. Restlessness and anxiety, a rapid pulse, cool clammy skin, and a drop in blood pressure are signs of:
    a. hyperglycemia
    b. a brain injury
    c. impending seizure
    d. hypoperfusion

34. Most accidents involving emergency vehicles occur:
    a. due to skids
    b. at intersections
    c. during "U" turns
    d. while en route to the hospital

35. The ratio of compressions to ventilations when performing CPR on infants or children is:
    a. 5:1 for infants and 15:2 for children
    b. 15:2 regardless of the number of rescuers
    c. 5:1 regardless of the number of rescuers
    d. 15:2 for one-rescuer CPR

36. Generally, joint injuries should be:
    a. realigned prior to splinting
    b. splinted with a traction splint
    c. splinted in the position found
    d. transported without splinting to reduce aggravation

37. Assistance may be rendered to an unconscious patient under the law of:
    a. implied consent
    b. actual consent
    c. informed consent
    d. minor's consent

38. A 25-year-old construction worker has been struck mid-femur by a steel beam. He is complaining of severe pain in the thigh area. The splint of choice for this injury is:
    a. a soft splint
    b. a pneumatic splint
    c. a traction splint
    d. an air splint

39. When using a tourniquet, an important point to remember is that it should be:
    a. placed below a knee or elbow to control severe bleeding from a foot or hand
    b. used whenever direct pressure alone will not control bleeding
    c. used whenever an amputation is encountered
    d. used only as a last resort

40. The first thing that should be done when a burn patient is encountered is to:
    a. stop the burning process
    b. apply sterile burn sheets
    c. estimate the percentage of burns
    d. assess breathing and circulation

41. Nitroglycerin should be:
    a. swallowed
    b. administered intramuscularly
    c. inhaled
    d. administered under the tongue

42. When a patient is encountered with bruising around the eyes or behind the ears, the EMT should suspect:
    a. a skull injury
    b. high blood pressure
    c. a history of violence
    d. a seizure disorder

43. The systolic pressure corresponds to:
    a. the difference between the resting pressure and pumping pressure
    b. the pressure exerted against the walls of the arteries during ventricular contraction
    c. the pressure exerted against the walls of the arteries when the left ventricle is at rest
    d. double the diastolic pressure

44. Your patient was the victim of an assault and has been struck multiple times in the head with a baseball bat. He is bleeding from the nose and ears. During your examination, you should be alert for the presence of:
    a. synovial fluid
    b. saline fluid
    c. cerebrospinal fluid
    d. aqueous fluid

45. To place a patient in the recovery position, you would:
    a. position the patient lying on his left or right side
    b. position the patient lying on his back and elevate his head about 6 inches
    c. elevate the foot end of the cot and position the patient lying face down
    d. elevate the foot end of the cot and position the patient lying face up

46. Bleeding from an open or depressed skull injury is best controlled by:
    a. applying firm pressure to the wound
    b. applying digital pressure to both carotid arteries
    c. packing the wound with gauze
    d. using a loose, bulky dressing

47. You have been ordered to assist a patient with the administration of a medication. Before administering the medication, the EMT should:
    a. be sure it was prescribed by a local doctor
    b. check the medication's expiration date
    c. note what pharmacy the prescription came from
    d. be sure the prescription belongs to someone in the patient's family

48. The assessment of a responsive medical patient:
    a. can usually wait until the patient is moved to the ambulance
    b. emphasizes the patient's vital signs
    c. is normally based on the patient's chief complaint
    d. is not as critical if there is no history of medical problems

49. Patients experiencing cardiac problems most commonly complain of pain described as:
    a. a pressure or crushing feeling
    b. worse when deeply inhaling
    c. sharp and stabbing like a knife
    d. cramping and intermittent

50. The primary purpose of a detailed assessment is to:
    a. check for signs of abuse or drug use
    b. help the EMT diagnose the patient's problem
    c. confirm that a medical problem exists
    d. find less-serious hidden injuries or medical problems

51. A patient is encountered with an altered mental status. After ensuring scene safety, the first priority in managing this patient is:
    a. administering sugar
    b. ensuring a patent airway
    c. performing a focused exam
    d. assessing baseline vital signs

52. You are readying a male patient with an evisceration with no accompanying spinal or leg injuries for transport. The preferred position for this patient is on his:
    a. stomach with the hips and knees straight
    b. back with the hips and knees flexed
    c. left side
    d. right side

53. Your patient is experiencing chest pain and has his own nitroglycerin with him. Before taking nitroglycerin, the patient's blood pressure should be:
    a. no more than 70 mm Hg diastolic
    b. at least 90 mm Hg diastolic
    c. greater than 100 mm Hg systolic
    d. no more than 130 mm Hg systolic

54. The airway of a patient with a suspected neck injury should be opened using the:
    a. modified jaw-thrust maneuver
    b. head-tilt/chin-lift maneuver
    c. head-tilt/neck-lift maneuver
    d. Heimlich maneuver

55. A 3-year-old child is having obvious difficulty breathing and is noted to be cyanotic but will not tolerate an oxygen mask. Your best option is to:
    a. restrain the child and force him or her to wear the mask
    b. wait for the child to become unconscious, then administer oxygen
    c. administer oxygen using a blow-by technique
    d. ventilate the patient with a flow-restricted, oxygen-powered ventilation device

56. EMTs are caring for a conscious patient with a history of diabetes and an altered mental status. Management of this patient would likely include:
    a. application of a cervical collar
    b. assisting with use of a prescribed inhaler
    c. oxygen by nonrebreather mask at 6 L/min
    d. administration of oral glucose

57. Your patient has fallen from a roof and presents with multiple musculoskeletal injuries and hypoperfusion. You would:
    a. splint all injuries prior to moving the patient to prevent further blood loss
    b. perform full-body immobilization with a backboard and immediately transport
    c. splint only open musculoskeletal injuries prior to moving the patient
    d. move the patient to the ambulance cot in whatever way necessary and rapidly transport

58. During transport, patients experiencing cardiac compromise should be placed:
    a. flat on their back
    b. on their left side
    c. in a position of comfort
    d. in a prone position

59. In any injured and unconscious patient, the EMT should suspect:
    a. a spinal injury
    b. high blood sugar
    c. heart problems
    d. an overdose

60. The proper method to perform chest compressions on a child is to use:
    a. the heel of one hand placed on the upper half of the sternum
    b. two hands placed on the middle of the sternum
    c. three finger-widths below the nipple line
    d. the heel of one hand placed on the lower half of the sternum

61. Early management of an open chest injury includes:
    a. covering the wound with a loose, bulky dressing
    b. sealing the wound with an occlusive dressing
    c. supporting the injured area with sandbags
    d. placing the patient on a backboard

62. A patient is found unconscious in a garage with a car still running. After ensuring personal safety and reaching the patient, the first step in caring for a victim of poison gas inhalation is to:
    a. place a cervical collar on the patient
    b. remove the patient from the toxic environment
    c. determine the type of gas involved
    d. open the airway and assess breathing

63. While being transported, a restrained patient starts spitting at the EMTs. This can be managed by:
    a. using surgical tape to tape the patient's mouth closed
    b. placing a pillow over the patient's face
    c. covering the patient's face with a surgical mask
    d. using a cravat to tie the patient's jaw shut

64. Upon reaching a cardiac arrest victim, if an automated external defibrillator is available, automated external defibrillation should be performed:
    a. after doing CPR for 1 minute
    b. unless bystander CPR is being performed
    c. after inserting an oral airway
    d. immediately after reaching the patient

65. Your patient has a severe laceration to the forearm, and direct pressure is not adequately controlling the bleeding. The pressure point of choice for this patient is the:
    a. temporal artery
    b. popliteal artery
    c. brachial artery
    d. tibial artery

66. Any suspicions of child abuse an EMT may have should be:
    a. reported to the child's parents
    b. privately reported to the appropriate authorities
    c. reported to the dispatcher
    d. anonymously reported by letter to the child-welfare authorities

67. The proper technique to insert an oral airway in an adult is to insert the airway:
    a. upside down then rotate it 180 degrees
    b. by pushing the tip along the tongue
    c. until the flange lies just behind the teeth
    d. so the flange lies 1 inch beyond the lips

68. When an unresponsive medical patient is encountered, after doing an initial assessment, perform:
    a. an assessment starting with the chest to evaluate the lungs and heart
    b. a thorough detailed physical exam
    c. a rapid head-to-toe assessment similar to the rapid trauma assessment
    d. an abbreviated focused history

69. When suctioning a newborn, the EMT should:
    a. wait until delivery is complete to perform suctioning
    b. squeeze the bulb syringe before inserting it
    c. insert the tip 2 to 3 inches into the mouth and each nostril
    d. lubricate the bulb syringe with petroleum jelly

70. When using O-P-Q-R-S-T to assess a patient, "Provocation" refers to:
    a. what time the pain started
    b. what makes the pain feel better or worse
    c. whether the patient has a violent history or easily loses his temper
    d. whether the patient has a previous injury or medical condition

71. An important early step in caring for a patient with skin that is hot to the touch is to:
    a. conserve body heat so as not to cause rebound hypothermia
    b. wipe down the patient with rubbing alcohol
    c. keep the skin dry
    d. apply cold packs to the neck, groin, and armpits

72. You encounter a patient who is complaining of respiratory distress, a tight feeling in the throat, and itching. Your examination reveals wheezing in the lungs and hives all over the patient's arms. You suspect this patient is experiencing:
    a. cardiac problems
    b. a drug overdose
    c. an allergic reaction
    d. a diabetic emergency

73. You are preparing to transport a pregnant female with a spinal injury who is on a backboard. When positioning the backboard, it should:
    a. be tilted to the right side
    b. be tilted to the left side
    c. have the head elevated
    d. have the head elevated

74. The EMT should evaluate motor, sensory, and circulatory status of an injured extremity:
    a. before and after splinting
    b. only if there is numbness or loss of sensation below the injury site
    c. only if a deformity is present
    d. only before splinting

75. CPR is being performed on a non-breathing child. Concerning the use of oral airways in children, the EMT should remember:
    a. to insert the airway upside down and rotate it once it is in the proper position
    b. medical control must order its use
    c. insert the airway right-side up without using a rotating maneuver like in an adult
    d. that oral airways should not be used on infants or children

76. Reddening, blister formation, and intense pain are characteristic of a:
    a. superficial burn
    b. partial-thickness burn
    c. medium-thickness burn
    d. full-thickness burn

77. Your patient has been exposed to toxic gases. One of your major concerns in dealing with this patient is that when a poison has been inhaled:
    a. it may be exhaled by the patient and contaminate the EMT
    b. it takes longer to enter the bloodstream
    c. oxygen should not be administered to the patient
    d. it may also damage the lining of the patient's airway

78. When performing one-rescuer adult CPR, the ratio of chest compressions to ventilations is:
    a. 5:2
    b. 15:2
    c. 5:1
    d. 15:1

79. A 22-year-old male patient has been involved in a knife fight and presents with an evisceration. Management would include:
    a. applying a moist sterile dressing to the area and covering it with an occlusive dressing
    b. replacing the organs in the abdominal cavity
    c. applying direct pressure to the organs and wound to control bleeding
    d. applying the PASG and inflating all three compartments

80. When a patient is encountered with chemical burns to the eyes, the patient's eyes should be irrigated:
    a. with a neutralizing solution
    b. for not more than 15 minutes
    c. until the patient reaches the hospital
    d. only while on the scene of the incident

81. To make breathing easier, patients experiencing breathing problems should be placed:
    a. flat on their back
    b. on their left side
    c. in Trendelenburg position
    d. in a position of comfort

82. Your patient has been poisoned by contact with a powdered chemical. Part of your management would include:
    a. leaving the chemical in place so the hospital can identify it
    b. brushing off any chemical
    c. removing the chemical with a wet towel
    d. wrapping the patient in a blanket to prevent spread of the chemical

83. You and your partner have just assisted with the delivery of a baby girl. The umbilical cord should be clamped and cut:
    a. after pulsations in the cord cease
    b. before the infant starts breathing
    c. after delivery of the placenta
    d. 10 to 15 minutes after delivery

84. A 32-year-old male has had a finger cut off in an industrial accident. The proper way to package the finger for transportation to the hospital is to:
    a. pack the finger in ice
    b. immerse the finger in sterile water
    c. wrap the finger in a sterile dressing and keep it cool
    d. wrap the finger in a wet, sterile dressing and keep it warm

85. The ongoing assessment repeats all of the components of the:
    a. detailed physical exam
    b. rapid trauma assessment
    c. SAMPLE history
    d. initial assessment

86. A dire emergency exists if a patient is encountered with:
    a. moist, pale, normal-temperature skin
    b. dry or moist, hot skin
    c. moist, pale, cool skin
    d. moist, pink, normal-temperature skin

87. The normal breathing rate for an adult is:
    a. 5 to 10 times per minute
    b. 8 to 16 times per minute
    c. 12 to 20 times per minute
    d. 16 to 28 times per minute

88. Consider delivery imminent when:
    a. contractions are less than
        2 minutes apart
    b. it is the mother's first pregnancy and
        contractions are 5 minutes apart
    c. contractions last longer than
        20 seconds
    d. the patient is experiencing lower
        abdominal pain with no back pain

89. You are preparing to transport a child with
    a gastrostomy tube. The two positions in
    which the patient may be transported are:
    a. lying on the back, or lying on the left
        side with the head lower than
        the trunk
    b. in a position of comfort, or prone with
        the head lower than the trunk
    c. sitting, or lying on the right side with
        the head elevated
    d. supine, or prone with the
        head elevated

90. A condition in which the body is unable to
    utilize glucose normally is:
    a. asthma
    b. diabetes mellitus
    c. epistaxis
    d. appendicitis

91. Ideally, the detailed physical examination
    should be performed:
    a. prior to leaving for the hospital
    b. after ALS personnel arrive
    c. before moving the patient
    d. while en route to the hospital

92. You and your partner are sent to evaluate
    a female patient experiencing a behavioral
    emergency. A potential sign of violence on
    the part of your patient is if she is:
    a. sitting on the edge of a seat
    b. lying on a bed or couch
    c. using monotone speech
    d. exhibiting open hands

93. Medical command advises you to
    administer activated charcoal to an adult
    patient. The usual dose is:
    a. 12.5 to 25 grams
    b. 25 to 50 grams
    c. 50 to 75 grams
    d. 75 to 100 grams

94. Management of an infant with an airway
    obstruction includes performing cycles of:
    a. 6 to 10 abdominal thrusts
    b. 5 backblows followed by
        5 abdominal thrusts
    c. 6 to 10 chest thrusts, followed by a
        finger sweep
    d. five backblows followed by
        five chest thrusts

95. A burn to the entire leg of an adult would
    comprise:
    a. 6% of body surface area
    b. 12% of body surface area
    c. 18% of body surface area
    d. 24% of body surface area

96. An indication for the use of the PASG
    would be:
    a. an unstable pelvic injury
    b. an open chest wound
    c. abdominal pain
    d. arterial bleeding

97. When caring for a sick or injured child, the EMT should:
    a. never allow parents to be present
    b. allow parents to be present only if absolutely necessary
    c. make judicious use of the parents to assist
    d. allow only one parent to be present at any time

98. Cardiac muscle differs from other muscle in that it:
    a. is a voluntary type of muscle
    b. can tolerate interruption of blood supply for long periods
    c. is found only in the heart and lungs
    d. has the ability to contract on its own

99. You and your partner are the first to arrive at the scene of an overturned truck carrying a hazardous material. Identification of the material can best be made by:
    a. calling the EPA
    b. referencing the number on the placard
    c. smelling or feeling the substance
    d. obtaining a sample and sending it to a laboratory

100. The operation of log rolling a patient is usually directed by:
    a. the EMT at the patient's waist
    b. the EMT at the patient's shoulders
    c. the EMT controlling the patient's head and neck
    d. the senior EMT on the crew

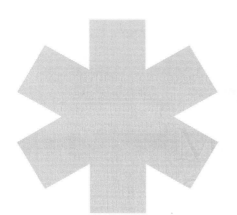

18
ANSWERS TO 100-QUESTION PRACTICE TEST

NOTE: More information on specific questions may be found by referencing the corresponding chapter and question number.

Test Question	Answer	Source Chapter	Source Question	Test Question	Answer	Source Chapter	Source Question
1.	b.	13	21	11.	c.	1	51
2.	a.	4	47	12.	d.	8	16
3.	c.	15	32	13.	a.	10	8
4.	a.	10	14	14.	b.	3	23
5.	d.	7	49	15.	c.	9	33
6.	c.	14	22	16.	b.	16	11
7.	b.	3	21	17.	b.	10	29
8.	d.	5	5	18.	c.	7	42
9.	b.	9	23	19.	d.	15	100
10.	b.	10	16	20.	a.	12	11

Test Question	Answer	Source Chapter	Source Question	Test Question	Answer	Source Chapter	Source Question
21.	c.	2	34	37.	a.	15	3
22.	b.	3	13	38.	c.	12	19
23.	b.	1	59	39.	d.	10	21
24.	d.	2	2	40.	a.	11	48
25.	b.	15	22	41.	d.	5	66
26.	d.	3	11	42.	a.	13	20
27.	a.	5	27	43.	b.	2	28
28.	b.	11	4	44.	c.	13	23
29.	d.	15	86	45.	a.	1	90
30.	d.	4	15	46.	d.	13	24
31.	a.	11	13	47.	b.	5	2
32.	c.	6	28	48.	c.	4	37
33.	d.	10	6	49.	a.	5	56
34.	b.	15	11	50.	d.	4	46
35.	c.	16	52	51.	b.	6	2
36.	c.	12	13	52.	b.	11	19

Test Question	Answer	Source Chapter	Source Question
53.	c.	5	67
54.	a.	16	8
55.	c.	3	20
56.	d.	6	10
57.	b.	12	5
58.	c.	5	61
59.	a.	13	1
60.	d.	16	42
61.	b.	11	15
62.	b.	7	9
63.	c.	8	21
64.	d.	5	70
65.	c.	10	19
66.	b.	14	43
67.	a.	3	24
68.	c.	4	36

Test Question	Answer	Source Chapter	Source Question
69.	b.	9	17
70.	b.	4	39
71.	d.	7	59
72.	c.	6	36
73.	b.	9	39
74.	a.	12	6
75.	c.	14	12
76.	b.	11	31
77.	d.	7	27
78.	b.	16	20
79.	a.	11	18
80.	c.	11	55
81.	d.	5	21
82.	b.	7	14
83.	a.	9	22
84.	c.	11	21

Test Question	Answer	Source Chapter	Source Question
85.	**d.**	4	55
86.	**b.**	7	57
87.	**c.**	2	5
88.	**a.**	9	12
89.	**c.**	14	47
90.	**b.**	6	4
91.	**d.**	4	52
92.	**a.**	8	12
93.	**b.**	7	20
94.	**d.**	16	57
95.	**c.**	11	32
96.	**a.**	10	33
97.	**c.**	14	4
98.	**d.**	1	21
99.	**b.**	15	103
100.	**c.**	13	9

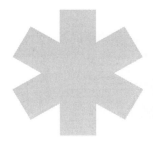

Appendix A

National Registry Skill Sheets

Patient Assessment/Management - Trauma

Start Time: _____

Stop Time: _____   Date: _____

Candidate's Name: _____

Evaluator's Name: _____

		Points Possible	Points Awarded
Takes, or verbalizes, body substance isolation precautions		1	
SCENE SIZE-UP			
Determines the scene is safe		1	
Determines the mechanism of injury		1	
Determines the number of patients		1	
Requests additional help if necessary		1	
Considers stabilization of spine		1	
INITIAL ASSESSMENT			
Verbalizes general impression of the patient		1	
Determines responsiveness/level of consciousness		1	
Determines chief complaint/apparent life threats		1	
Assesses airway and breathing	Assessment	1	
	Initiates appropriate oxygen therapy	1	
	Assures adequate ventilation	1	
	Injury management	1	
Assesses circulation	Assesses/controls major bleeding	1	
	Assesses pulse	1	
	Assesses skin (color, temperature and condition)	1	
Identifies priority patients/makes transport decision		1	
FOCUSED HISTORY AND PHYSICAL EXAMINATION/RAPID TRAUMA ASSESSMENT			
Selects appropriate assessment *(focused or rapid assessment)*		1	
Obtains, or directs assistance to obtain, baseline vital signs		1	
Obtains S.A.M.P.L.E. history		1	
DETAILED PHYSICAL EXAMINATION			
Assesses the head	Inspects and palpates the scalp and ears	1	
	Assesses the eyes	1	
	Assesses the facial areas including oral and nasal areas	1	
Assesses the neck	Inspects and palpates the neck	1	
	Assesses for JVD	1	
	Assesses for trachael deviation	1	
Assesses the chest	Inspects	1	
	Palpates	1	
	Auscultates	1	
Assesses the abdomen/pelvis	Assesses the abdomen	1	
	Assesses the pelvis	1	
	Verbalizes assessment of genitalia/perineum as needed	1	
Assesses the extremities	1 point for each extremity includes inspection, palpation, and assessment of motor, sensory and circulatory function	4	
Assesses the posterior	Assesses thorax	1	
	Assesses lumbar	1	
Manages secondary injuries and wounds appropriately 1 point for **appropriate management of the secondary injury/wound**		1	
Verbalizes re-assessment of the vital signs		1	

Critical Criteria   **Total:** 40

_____ Did not take, or verbalize, body substance isolation precautions
_____ Did not determine scene safety
_____ Did not assess for spinal protection
_____ Did not provide for spinal protection when indicated
_____ Did not provide high concentration of oxygen
_____ Did not find, or manage, problems associated with airway, breathing, hemorrhage or shock (hypoperfusion)
_____ Did not differentiate patient's need for transportation versus continued assessment at the scene
_____ Did other detailed physical examination before assessing the airway, breathing and circulation
_____ Did not transport patient within (10) minute time limit

Patient Assessment/Management - Medical

Start Time: _____

Stop Time: _____

Date: _____

Candidate's Name: _____

Evaluator's Name: _____

	Points Possible	Points Awarded
Takes, or verbalizes, body substance isolation precautions	1	
SCENE SIZE-UP		
Determines the scene is safe	1	
Determines the mechanism of injury/nature of illness	1	
Determines the number of patients	1	
Requests additional help if necessary	1	
Considers stabilization of spine	1	
INITIAL ASSESSMENT		
Verbalizes general impression of the patient	1	
Determines responsiveness/level of consciousness	1	
Determines chief complaint/apparent life threats	1	
Assesses airway and breathing — Assessment	1	
Assesses airway and breathing — Initiates appropriate oxygen therapy	1	
Assesses airway and breathing — Assures adequate ventilation	1	
Assesses circulation — Assesses/controls major bleeding	1	
Assesses circulation — Assesses pulse	1	
Assesses circulation — Assesses skin (color, temperature and condition)	1	
Identifies priority patients/makes transport decision	1	
FOCUSED HISTORY AND PHYSICAL EXAMINATION/RAPID ASSESSMENT		
Signs and symptoms (*Assess history of present illness*)	1	

Respiratory	Cardiac	Altered Mental Status	Allergic Reaction	Poisoning/ Overdose	Environmental Emergency	Obstetrics	Behavioral
*Onset? *Provokes? *Quality? *Radiates? *Severity? *Time? *Interventions?	*Onset? *Provokes? *Quality? *Radiates? *Severity? *Time? *Interventions?	*Description of the episode. *Onset? *Duration? *Associated Symptoms? *Evidence of Trauma? *Interventions? *Seizures? *Fever	*History of allergies? *What were you exposed to? *How were you exposed? *Effects? *Progression? *Interventions?	*Substance? *When did you ingest/become exposed? *How much did you ingest? *Over what time period? *Interventions? *Estimated weight?	*Source? *Environment? *Duration? *Loss of consciousness? *Effects - general or local?	*Are you pregnant? *How long have you been pregnant? *Pain or contractions? *Bleeding or discharge? *Do you feel the need to push? *Last menstrual period?	*How do you feel? *Determine suicidal tendencies. *Is the patient a threat to self or others? *Is there a medical problem? *Interventions?

	Points Possible	Points Awarded
Allergies	1	
Medications	1	
Past pertinent history	1	
Last oral intake	1	
Event leading to present illness (rule out trauma)	1	
Performs focused physical examination (*assesses affected body part/system or, if indicated, completes rapid assessment*)	1	
Vitals (*obtains baseline vital signs*)	1	
Interventions (*obtains medical direction or verbalizes standing order for medication interventions and verbalizes proper additional intervention/treatment*)	1	
Transport (re-evaluates the transport decision)	1	
Verbalizes the consideration for completing a detailed physical examination	1	
ONGOING ASSESSMENT (verbalized)		
Repeats initial assessment	1	
Repeats vital signs	1	
Repeats focused assessment regarding patient complaint or injuries	1	

Critical Criteria   Total: **30**

_____ Did not take, or verbalize, body substance isolation precautions when necessary
_____ Did not determine scene safety
_____ Did not obtain medical direction or verbalize standing orders for medical interventions
_____ Did not provide high concentration of oxygen
_____ Did not find or manage problems associated with airway, breathing, hemorrhage or shock (hypoperfusion)
_____ Did not differentiate patient's need for transportation versus continued assessment at the scene
_____ Did detailed or focused history/physical examination before assessing the airway, breathing and circulation
_____ Did not ask questions about the present illness
_____ Administered a dangerous or inappropriate intervention

Cardiac Arrest Management/AED

Start Time: _____

Stop Time: _____   Date: _____

Candidate's Name: _____

Evaluator's Name: _____

	Points Possible	Points Awarded
ASSESSMENT		
Takes, or verbalizes, body substance isolation precautions	1	
Briefly questions the rescuer about arrest events	1	
Directs rescuer to stop CPR	1	
Verifies absence of spontaneous pulse **(skill station examiner states "no pulse")**	1	
Directs resumption of CPR	1	
Turns on defibrillator power	1	
Attaches automated defibrillator to the patient	1	
Directs rescuer to stop CPR and ensures all individuals are clear of the patient	1	
Initiates analysis of the rhythm	1	
Delivers shock (up to three successive shocks)	1	
Verifies absence of spontaneous pulse **(skill station examiner states "no pulse")**	1	
TRANSITION		
Directs resumption of CPR	1	
Gathers additional information about arrest event	1	
Confirms effectiveness of CPR (ventilation and compressions)	1	
INTEGRATION		
Verbalizes or directs insertion of a simple airway adjunct (oral/nasal airway)	1	
Ventilates, or directs ventilation of, the patient	1	
Assures high concentration of oxygen is delivered to the patient	1	
Assures CPR continues without unnecessary/prolonged interruption	1	
Re-evaluates patient/CPR in approximately one minute	1	
Repeats defibrillator sequence	1	
TRANSPORTATION		
Verbalizes transportation of patient	1	
Total:	21	

Critical Criteria

_____ Did not take, or verbalize, body substance isolation precautions

_____ Did not evaluate the need for immediate use of the AED

_____ Did not direct initiation/resumption of ventilation/compressions at appropriate times.

_____ Did not assure all individuals were clear of patient before delivering each shock

_____ Did not operate the AED properly (inability to deliver shock)

_____ Prevented the defibrillator from delivering indicated stacked shocks

BAG-VALVE-MASK
APNEIC PATIENT

Start Time: _____

Stop Time: _____   **Date:** _____

Candidate's Name: _____

Evaluator's Name: _____	Points Possible	Points Awarded
Takes, or verbalizes, body substance isolation precautions	1	
Voices opening the airway	1	
Voices inserting an airway adjunct	1	
Selects appropriately sized mask	1	
Creates a proper mask-to-face seal	1	
Ventilates patient at no less than 800 ml volume *(The examiner must witness for at least 30 seconds)*	1	
Connects reservoir and oxygen	1	
Adjusts liter flow to 15 liters/minute or greater	1	
The examiner indicates arrival of a second EMT. The second EMT is instructed to ventilate the patient while the candidate controls the mask and the airway		
Voices re-opening the airway	1	
Creates a proper mask-to-face seal	1	
Instructs assistant to resume ventilation at proper volume per breath *(The examiner must witness for at least 30 seconds)*	1	
Total:	**11**	

Critical Criteria

_____ Did not take, or verbalize, body substance isolation precautions

_____ Did not immediately ventilate the patient

_____ Interrupted ventilations for more than 20 seconds

_____ Did not provide high concentration of oxygen

_____ Did not provide, or direct assistant to provide, proper volume/breath
(more than two (2) ventilations per minute are below 800 ml)

_____ Did not allow adequate exhalation

SPINAL IMMOBILIZATION
SEATED PATIENT

Start Time: _____

Stop Time: _____　　**Date:** _____

Candidate's Name: _____

Evaluator's Name: _____

	Points Possible	Points Awarded
Takes, or verbalizes, body substance isolation precautions	1	
Directs assistant to place/maintain head in the neutral in-line position	1	
Directs assistant to maintain manual immobilization of the head	1	
Reassesses motor, sensory and circulatory function in each extremity	1	
Applies appropriately sized extrication collar	1	
Positions the immobilization device behind the patient	1	
Secures the device to the patient's torso	1	
Evaluates torso fixation and adjusts as necessary	1	
Evaluates and pads behind the patient's head as necessary	1	
Secures the patient's head to the device	1	
Verbalizes moving the patient to a long board	1	
Reassesses motor, sensory and circulatory function in each extremity	1	
Total:	**12**	

Critical Criteria

_____ Did not immediately direct, or take, manual immobilization of the head

_____ Released, or ordered release of, manual immobilization before it was maintained mechanically

_____ Patient manipulated, or moved excessively, causing potential spinal compromise

_____ Device moved excessively up, down, left or right on the patient's torso

_____ Head immobilization allows for excessive movement

_____ Torso fixation inhibits chest rise, resulting in respiratory compromise

_____ Upon completion of immobilization, head is not in the neutral position

_____ Did not assess motor, sensory and circulatory function in each extremity after voicing immobilization to the long board

_____ Immobilized head to the board before securing the torso

SPINAL IMMOBILIZATION
SUPINE PATIENT

Start Time: _____

Stop Time: _____   Date: _____

Candidate's Name: _____

Evaluator's Name: _____

	Points Possible	Points Awarded
Takes, or verbalizes, body substance isolation precautions	1	
Directs assistant to place/maintain head in the neutral in-line position	1	
Directs assistant to maintain manual immobilization of the head	1	
Reassesses motor, sensory and circulatory function in each extremity	1	
Applies appropriately sized extrication collar	1	
Positions the immobilization device appropriately	1	
Directs movement of the patient onto the device without compromising the integrity of the spine	1	
Applies padding to voids between the torso and the board as necessary	1	
Immobilizes the patient's torso to the device	1	
Evaluates and pads behind the patient's head as necessary	1	
Immobilizes the patient's head to the device	1	
Secures the patient's legs to the device	1	
Secures the patient's arms to the device	1	
Reassesses motor, sensory and circulatory function in each extremity	1	
Total:	**14**	

Critical Criteria

_____ Did not immediately direct, or take, manual immobilization of the head

_____ Released, or ordered release of, manual immobilization before it was maintained mechanically

_____ Patient manipulated, or moved excessively, causing potential spinal compromise

_____ Patient moves excessively up, down, left or right on the patient's torso

_____ Head immobilization allows for excessive movement

_____ Upon completion of immobilization, head is not in the neutral position

_____ Did not assess motor, sensory and circulatory function in each extremity after immobilization to the device

_____ Immobilized head to the board before securing the torso

IMMOBILIZATION SKILLS
LONG BONE INJURY

Start Time: _____

Stop Time: _____   Date: _____

Candidate's Name: _____

Evaluator's Name: _____	Points Possible	Points Awarded
Takes, or verbalizes, body substance isolation precautions	1	
Directs application of manual stabilization of the injury	1	
Assesses motor, sensory and circulatory function in the injured extremity	1	
Note: The examiner acknowledges "motor, sensory and circulatory function are present and normal"		
Measures the splint	1	
Applies the splint	1	
Immobilizes the joint above the injury site	1	
Immobilizes the joint below the injury site	1	
Secures the entire injured extremity	1	
Immobilizes the hand/foot in the position of function	1	
Reassesses motor, sensory and circulatory function in the injured extremity	1	
Note: The examiner acknowledges "motor, sensory and circulatory function are present and normal"		
Total:	**10**	

Critical Criteria

_____ Grossly moves the injured extremity

_____ Did not immobilize the joint above and the joint below the injury site

_____ Did not reassess motor, sensory and circulatory function in the injured extremity before and after splinting

IMMOBILIZATION SKILLS
JOINT INJURY

Start Time: _____

Stop Time: _____   Date: _____

Candidate's Name: _____

Evaluator's Name: _____	Points Possible	Points Awarded
Takes, or verbalizes, body substance isolation precautions	1	
Directs application of manual stabilization of the shoulder injury	1	
Assesses motor, sensory and circulatory function in the injured extremity	1	
Note: The examiner acknowledges "motor, sensory and circulatory function are present and normal."		
Selects the proper splinting material	1	
Immobilizes the site of the injury	1	
Immobilizes the bone above the injured joint	1	
Immobilizes the bone below the injured joint	1	
Reassesses motor, sensory and circulatory function in the injured extremity	1	
Note: The examiner acknowledges "motor, sensory and circulatory function are present and normal."		
Total:	8	

Critical Criteria

_____ Did not support the joint so that the joint did not bear distal weight

_____ Did not immobilize the bone above and below the injured site

_____ Did not reassess motor, sensory and circulatory function in the injured extremity before and after splinting

IMMOBILIZATION SKILLS
TRACTION SPLINTING

Start Time: _____

Stop Time: _____   **Date:** _____

Candidate's Name: _____

Evaluator's Name: _____

	Points Possible	Points Awarded
Takes, or verbalizes, body substance isolation precautions	1	
Directs application of manual stabilization of the injured leg	1	
Directs the application of manual traction	1	
Assesses motor, sensory and circulatory function in the injured extremity	1	
Note: The examiner acknowledges "motor, sensory and circulatory function are present and normal"		
Prepares/adjusts splint to the proper length	1	
Positions the splint next to the injured leg	1	
Applies the proximal securing device (e.g... ischial strap)	1	
Applies the distal securing device (e.g...ankle hitch)	1	
Applies mechanical traction	1	
Positions/secures the support straps	1	
Re-evaluates the proximal/distal securing devices	1	
Reassesses motor, sensory and circulatory function in the injured extremity	1	
Note: The examiner acknowledges "motor, sensory and circulatory function are present and normal"		
Note: The examiner must ask the candidate how he/she would prepare the patient for transportation		
Verbalizes securing the torso to the long board to immobilize the hip	1	
Verbalizes securing the splint to the long board to prevent movement of the splint	1	
Total:	**14**	

Critical Criteria

_____ Loss of traction at any point after it was applied

_____ Did not reassess motor, sensory and circulatory function in the injured extremity before and after splinting

_____ The foot was excessively rotated or extended after splint was applied

_____ Did not secure the ischial strap before taking traction

_____ Final Immobilization failed to support the femur or prevent rotation of the injured leg

_____ Secured the leg to the splint before applying mechanical traction

Note: If the Sagar splint or the Kendricks Traction Device is used without elevating the patient's leg, application of manual traction is not necessary. The candidate should be awarded one (1) point as if manual traction were applied.

Note: If the leg is elevated at all, manual traction must be applied before elevating the leg. The ankle hitch may be applied before elevating the leg and used to provide manual traction.

BLEEDING CONTROL/SHOCK MANAGEMENT

Start Time: _____

Stop Time: _____ **Date:** _____

Candidate's Name: _____

Evaluator's Name: _____	Points Possible	Points Awarded
Takes, or verbalizes, body substance isolation precautions	1	
Applies direct pressure to the wound	1	
Elevates the extremity	1	
Note: The examiner must now inform the candidate that the wound continues to bleed.		
Applies an additional dressing to the wound	1	
Note: The examiner must now inform the candidate that the wound still continues to bleed. The second dressing does not control the bleeding.		
Locates and applies pressure to appropriate arterial pressure point	1	
Note: The examiner must now inform the candidate that the bleeding is controlled		
Bandages the wound	1	
Note: The examiner must now inform the candidate the patient is now showing signs and symptoms indicative of hypoperfusion		
Properly positions the patient	1	
Applies high concentration oxygen	1	
Initiates steps to prevent heat loss from the patient	1	
Indicates the need for immediate transportation	1	
Total:	**10**	

Critical Criteria

_____ Did not take, or verbalize, body substance isolation precautions

_____ Did not apply high concentration of oxygen

_____ Applied a tourniquet before attempting other methods of bleeding control

_____ Did not control hemorrhage in a timely manner

_____ Did not indicate a need for immediate transportation

AIRWAY, OXYGEN AND VENTILATION SKILLS
UPPER AIRWAY ADJUNCTS AND SUCTION

Start Time: _____

Stop Time: _____   Date: _____

Candidate's Name: _____

Evaluator's Name: _____

OROPHARYNGEAL AIRWAY

	Points Possible	Points Awarded
Takes, or verbalizes, body substance isolation precautions	1	
Selects appropriately sized airway	1	
Measures airway	1	
Inserts airway without pushing the tongue posteriorly	1	
Note: The examiner must advise the candidate that the patient is gagging and becoming conscious		
Removes the oropharyngeal airway	1	

SUCTION

	Points Possible	Points Awarded
Note: The examiner must advise the candidate to suction the patient's airway		
Turns on/prepares suction device	1	
Assures presence of mechanical suction	1	
Inserts the suction tip without suction	1	
Applies suction to the oropharynx/nasopharynx	1	

NASOPHARYNGEAL AIRWAY

	Points Possible	Points Awarded
Note: The examiner must advise the candidate to insert a nasopharyngeal airway		
Selects appropriately sized airway	1	
Measures airway	1	
Verbalizes lubrication of the nasal airway	1	
Fully inserts the airway with the bevel facing toward the septum	1	
Total:	13	

Critical Criteria

_____ Did not take, or verbalize, body substance isolation precautions

_____ Did not obtain a patent airway with the oropharyngeal airway

_____ Did not obtain a patent airway with the nasopharyngeal airway

_____ Did not demonstrate an acceptable suction technique

_____ Inserted any adjunct in a manner dangerous to the patient

MOUTH TO MASK WITH SUPPLEMENTAL OXYGEN

Start Time: _____

Stop Time: _____   Date: _____

Candidate's Name: _____

Evaluator's Name: _____

	Points Possible	Points Awarded
Takes, or verbalizes, body substance isolation precautions	1	
Connects one-way valve to mask	1	
Opens patient's airway or confirms patient's airway is open (manually or with adjunct)	1	
Establishes and maintains a proper mask to face seal	1	
Ventilates the patient at the proper volume and rate (800-1200 ml per breath/10-20 breaths per minute)	1	
Connects the mask to high concentration of oxygen	1	
Adjusts flow rate to at least 15 liters per minute	1	
Continues ventilation of the patient at the proper volume and rate (800-1200 ml per breath/10-20 breaths per minute)	1	
Note: The examiner must witness ventilations for at least 30 seconds		
Total:	8	

Critical Criteria

_____ Did not take, or verbalize, body substance isolation precautions

_____ Did not adjust liter flow to at least 15 liters per minute

_____ Did not provide proper volume per breath
(more than 2 ventilations per minute were below 800 ml)

_____ Did not ventilate the patient at a rate à 10-20 breaths per minute

_____ Did not allow for complete exhalation

OXYGEN ADMINISTRATION

Start Time: _____

Stop Time: _____   Date: _____

Candidate's Name: _____

Evaluator's Name: _____	Points Possible	Points Awarded
Takes, or verbalizes, body substance isolation precautions	1	
Assembles the regulator to the tank	1	
Opens the tank	1	
Checks for leaks	1	
Checks tank pressure	1	
Attaches non-rebreather mask to oxygen	1	
Prefills reservoir	1	
Adjusts liter flow to 12 liters per minute or greater	1	
Applies and adjusts the mask to the patient's face	1	
Note: The examiner must advise the candidate that the patient is not tolerating the non-rebreather mask. The medical director has ordered you to apply a nasal cannula to the patient.		
Attaches nasal cannula to oxygen	1	
Adjusts liter flow to six (6) liters per minute or less	1	
Applies nasal cannula to the patient	1	
Note: The examiner must advise the candidate to discontinue oxygen therapy		
Removes the nasal cannula from the patient	1	
Shuts off the regulator	1	
Relieves the pressure within the regulator	1	
Total:	**15**	

Critical Criteria

_____ Did not take, or verbalize, body substance isolation precautions

_____ Did not assemble the tank and regulator without leaks

_____ Did not prefill the reservoir bag

_____ Did not adjust the device to the correct liter flow for the non-rebreather mask
    (12 liters per minute or greater)

_____ Did not adjust the device to the correct liter flow for the nasal cannula
    (6 liters per minute or less)

Start Time: _____

Stop Time: _____

VENTILATORY MANAGEMENT
ENDOTRACHEAL INTUBATION

Candidate's Name: _____   Date: _____

Evaluator's Name: _____

Note: *If a candidate elects to initially ventilate the patient with a BVM attached to a reservoir and oxygen, full credit must be awarded for steps denoted by " ** " provided the first ventilation is delivered within the initial 30 seconds*

	Points Possible	Points Awarded
Takes of verbalizes body substance isolation precautions	1	
Opens the airway manually	1	
Elevates the patient's tongue and inserts a simple airway adjunct (oropharyngeal/nasopharyngeal airway)	1	
Note: The examiner must now inform the candidate "no gag reflex is present and the patient accepts the airway adjunct."		
** Ventilates the patient immediately using a BVM device unattached to oxygen	1	
** Hyperventilates the patient with room air	1	
Note: The examiner must now inform the candidate that ventilation is being properly performed without difficulty		
Attaches the oxygen reservoir to the BVM	1	
Attaches the BVM to high flow oxygen (15 liter per minute)	1	
Ventilates the patient at the proper volume and rate *(800-1200 ml/breath and 10-20 breaths/minute)*	1	
Note: After 30 seconds, the examiner must auscultate the patient's chest and inform the candidate that breath sounds are present and equal bilaterally and medical direction has ordered endotracheal intubation. The examiner must now take over ventilation of the patient.		
Directs assistant to hyper-oxygenate the patient	1	
Identifies/selects the proper equipment for endotracheal intubation	1	
Checks equipment — Checks for cuff leaks	1	
Checks laryngoscope operation and bulb tightness	1	
Note: The examiner must remove the OPA and move out of the way when the candidate is prepared to intubate the patient.		
Positions the patient's head properly	1	
Inserts the laryngoscope blade into the patient's mouth while displacing the patient's tongue laterally	1	
Elevates the patient's mandible with the laryngoscope	1	
Introduces the endotracheal tube and advances the tube to the proper depth	1	
Inflates the cuff to the proper pressure	1	
Disconnects the syringe from the cuff inlet port	1	
Directs assistant to ventilate the patient	1	
Confirms proper placement of the endotracheal tube by auscultation bilaterally and over the epigastrium	1	
Note: The examiner must ask, "If you had proper placement, what would you expect to hear?"		
Secures the endotracheal tube *(may be verbalized)*	1	
Total:	21	

Critical Criteria

_____ Did not take or verbalize body substance isolation precautions when necessary
_____ Did not initiate ventilation within 30 seconds after applying gloves or interrupts ventilations for greater than 30 seconds at any time
_____ Did not voice or provide high oxygen concentrations (15 liter/minute or greater)
_____ Did not ventilate the patient at a rate of at least 10 breaths per minute
_____ Did not provide adequate volume per breath (maximum of 2 errors per minute permissible)
_____ Did not hyper-oxygenate the patient prior to intubation
_____ Did not successfully intubate the patient within 3 attempts
_____ Used the patient's teeth as a fulcrum
_____ Did not assure proper tube placement by auscultation bilaterally over each lung **and** over the epigastrium
_____ The stylette (if used) extended beyond the end of the endotracheal tube
_____ Inserted any adjunct in a manner that was dangerous to the patient
_____ Did not immediately disconnect the syringe from the inlet port after inflating the cuff

**VENTILATORY MANAGEMENT
DUAL LUMEN DEVICE INSERTION FOLLOWING
AN UNSUCCESSFUL ENDOTRACHEAL INTUBATION ATTEMPT**

Start Time: _____

Stop Time: _____

Candidate's Name: _____   Date: _____

Evaluator's Name: _____	Points Possible	Points Awarded
Continues body substance isolation precautions	1	
Confirms the patient is being properly ventilated with high percentage oxygen	1	
Directs the assistant to hyper-oxygenate the patient	1	
Checks/prepares the airway device	1	
Lubricates the distal tip of the device (*may be verbalized*)	1	
Note: The examiner should remove the OPA and move out of the way when the candidate is prepared to insert the device		
Positions the patient's head properly	1	
Performs a tongue-jaw lift	1	

☐ USES COMBITUBE	☐ USES THE PTL		
Inserts device in the mid-line and to the depth so that the printed ring is at the level of the teeth	Inserts the device in the mid-line until the bite block flange is at the level of the teeth	1	
Inflates the pharyngeal cuff with the proper volume and removes the syringe	Secures the strap	1	
Inflates the distal cuff with the proper volume and removes the syringe	Blows into tube #1 to adequately inflate both cuffs	1	
Attaches/directs attachment of BVM to the first (esophageal placement)lumen and ventilates		1	
Confirms placement and ventilation through the correct lumen by observing chest rise, auscultation over the epigastrium and bilaterally over each lung		1	
Note: The examiner states, "You do not see rise and fall of the chest and hear sounds only over the epigastrium."			
Attaches/directs attachment of BVM to the second (endotracheal placement) lumen and ventilates		1	
Confirms placement and ventilation through the correct lumen by observing chest rise, auscultation over the epigastrium and bilaterally over each lung		1	
Note: The examiner states, "You see rise and fall of the chest, there are no sounds over the epigastrium and breath sounds are equal over each lung."			
Secures device or confirms that the device remains properly secured		1	
Total:		**15**	

Critical Criteria
_____ Did not take or verbalize body substance isolation precautions
_____ Did not initiate ventilations within 30 seconds
_____ Interrupted ventilations for more than 30 seconds at any time
_____ Did not hyper-oxygenate the patient prior to placement of the dual lumen airway device
_____ Did not provide adequate volume per breath (maximum 2 errors/minute permissible)
_____ Did not ventilate the patient at a rate of at least 10 breaths per minute
_____ Did not insert the dual lumen airway device at a proper depth or at the proper place within 3 attempts
_____ Did not inflate both cuffs properly
_____ **Combitube** - Did not remove the syringe immediately following the inflation of each cuff
_____ **PTL** - Did not secure the strap prior to cuff inflation
_____ Did not confirm, by observing chest rise and auscultation over the epigastrium and bilaterally over each lung, that the proper lumen of the device was being used to ventilate the patient
_____ Inserted any adjunct in a manner that was dangerous to the patient

VENTILATORY MANAGEMENT
ESOPHAGEAL OBTURATOR AIRWAY INSERTION FOLLOWING
AN UNSUCCESSFUL ENDOTRACHEAL INTUBATION ATTEMPT

Start Time: _____

Stop Time: _____   Date: _____

Candidate's Name: _____

Evaluator's Name: _____	Points Possible	Points Awarded
Continues body substance isolation precautions	1	
Confirms the patient is being ventilated high percentage oxygen	1	
Directs the assistant to hyper-oxygenate the patient	1	
Identifies/selects the proper equipment for insertion of EOA	1	
Assembles the EOA	1	
Tests the cuff for leaks	1	
Inflates the mask	1	
Lubricates the tube (*may be verbalized*)	1	
Note: The examiner should remove the OPA and move out of the way when the candidate is prepared to insert the device		
Positions the head properly with the neck in the neutral or slightly flexed position	1	
Grasps and elevates the patient's tongue and mandible	1	
Inserts the tube in the same direction as the curvature of the pharynx	1	
Advances the tube until the mask is sealed against the patient's face	1	
Ventilates the patient while maintaining a tight mask-to-face seal	1	
Directs confirmation of placement of EOA by observing for chest rise and auscultation over the epigastrium and bilaterally over each lung	1	
Note: The examiner must acknowledge adequate chest rise, bilateral breath sounds and absent sounds over the epigastrium		
Inflates the cuff to the proper pressure	1	
Disconnects the syringe from the inlet port	1	
Continues ventilation of the patient	1	
Total:	**17**	

Critical Criteria

_____ Did not take or verbalize body substance isolation precautions
_____ Did not initiate ventilations within 30 seconds
_____ Interrupted ventilations for more than 30 seconds at any time
_____ Did not direct hyper-oxygenation of the patient prior to placement of the EOA
_____ Did not successfully place the EOA within 3 attempts
_____ Did not ventilate at a rate of at least 10 breaths per minute
_____ Did not provide adequate volume per breath (maximum 2 errors/minute permissible)
_____ Did not assure proper tube placement by auscultation bilaterally and over the epigastrium
_____ Did not remove the syringe after inflating the cuff
_____ Did not successfully ventilate the patient
_____ Did not provide high flow oxygen (15 liters per minute or greater)
_____ Inserted any adjunct in a manner that was dangerous to the patient